D1031052

Normal Childbirth

Dedication

In memory of Tricia Anderson: her transformative
influence on the lives of childbearing women will
live on through generations to come.

All names used with participants' quotes are
pseudonyms.

Cover photograph reproduced with permission of
Martin Brown, Fairsnape Ltd

For Elsevier:
Commissioning Editor: Mairi McCubbin
Development Editor: Sheila Black
Project Manager: Gail Wright
Design: Charlotte Murray
Illustration Manager: Merlyn Harvey
Illustrator: Cactus

Bonnie Strickland

Normal Childbirth

Evidence and Debate

Second edition

Edited by

Soo Downe BA(Hons) MSc PhD RM

Professor of Midwifery Studies, University of Central Lancashire, Preston, UK

Foreword by

Robbie E. Davis-Floyd PhD

Senior Research Fellow, Department of Anthropology, University of Texas, Austin, Texas, USA

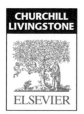

CHURCHILL LIVINGSTONE

ELSEVIER

Edinburgh London New York Oxford Philadelphia St Louis Sydney Toronto 2008

CHURCHILL LIVINGSTONE
ELSEVIER

An imprint of Elsevier Limited

© Elsevier Limited 2004
© 2008, Elsevier Limited. All rights reserved.

The right of Soo Downe to be identified as author of this work has been asserted by her in accordance with the Copyright, Designs and Patents Act 1988.

No part of this publication may be reproduced or transmitted in any form or by any means, electronic or mechanical, including photocopying, recording, or any information storage and retrieval system, without permission in writing from the publishers. Permissions may be sought directly from Elsevier's Rights Department: phone: (+1) 215 239 3804 (USA) or (+44) 1865 843830 (UK); fax: (+44) 1865 853333; e-mail: *healthpermissions@elsevier.com*. You may also complete your request on-line via the Elsevier website at http://www.elsevier.com/permissions.

First edition 2004
Second edition 2008

ISBN 978-0-443-06943-7

British Library Cataloguing in Publication Data
A catalogue record for this book is available from the British Library

Library of Congress Cataloging in Publication Data
A catalog record for this book is available from the Library of Congress

Notice
Neither the Publisher nor the Editor assumes any responsibility for any loss or injury and/or damage to persons or property arising out of or related to any use of the material contained in this book. It is the responsibility of the treating practitioner, relying on independent expertise and knowledge of the patient, to determine the best treatment and method of application for the patient.

The Publisher

ELSEVIER your source for books, journals and multimedia in the health sciences
www.elsevierhealth.com

Working together to grow
libraries in developing countries
www.elsevier.com | www.bookaid.org | www.sabre.org

ELSEVIER   BOOK AID International   Sabre Foundation

The publisher's policy is to use **paper manufactured from sustainable forests**

Printed in China

Contents

Contributors

The late Tricia Anderson (1957–2007) **BA(Hons) MSc PhD**
Formerly Research Midwife, Bournemouth University, UK, and Independent Midwife

Beverley A. Lawrence Beech
Chair, Association for Improvements in the Maternity Services

Sue Crabtree BM MA RM
Self-employed/Independent Midwife, Palmerston North, New Zealand

Soo Downe BA(Hons) MSc PhD RM
Professor of Midwifery Studies, University of Central Lancashire, Preston, UK

Amina M.R. El-Nemer BSc MSc PhD
Lecturer of Obstetric and Gynaecology Nursing, Faculty of Nursing, Mansoura University, Mansoura, Egypt

Debra Erickson-Owens PhD(c) CNM
Certified Nurse-Midwife; Doctoral Student, University of Rhode Island College of Nursing, Kingston, Rhode Island, USA

Jennifer Hall MSc PGDip(HE) ADM RN RM
Senior Lecturer in Midwifery, Faculty of Health and Social Care, University of West England, Bristol, UK

Victoria Hall Moran BSC MMedSci PhD
Senior Lecturer, Maternal and Infant Nutrition and Nurture Unit (MAINN), University of Central Lancashire, Preston, UK

Nicky Leap MSc DMid RM
Professor of Midwifery Practice Development and Research, University of Technology, Sydney and SE Sydney and Illawarra Area Health Service, Sydney, Australia

Christine McCourt BA PhD
Faculty of Health and Human Sciences, Centre for Research in Midwifery and Childbirth, London, UK

Marianne Mead BA(OU) MTD PhD RGN RM ADM
Reader in Midwifery, School of Nursing and Midwifery, University of Hertfordshire, Hatfield, UK

Judith Mercer PhD CNM FACNM
Certified Nurse-Midwife; Clinical Professor, University of Rhode Island College of Nursing, Kingston, Rhode Island, USA; Adjunct Professor of Pediatrics, Brown University, Providence, Rhode Island, USA

Belinda Phipps BSc(Hons) MBA
Chief Executive, National Childbirth Trust, London, UK

Rebecca Skovgaard CNM MS
Certified Nurse-Midwife, Strong Health Midwifery Group; Assistant Professor of Clinical Obstetrics and Gynecology, University of Rochester School of Medicine and Dentistry, Rochester, New York, USA

Denis Walsh MA DipEd DPSM RM
Reader in Normal Birth, Midwifery Research Department, University of Central Lancashire, Preston, UK

Carol Young BMedSci(Hons) DPMS RGM RM
Formerly Community Midwife, Derby City General Hospital, Derby, UK

Instead of approaching labour from a perspective of a catastrophe waiting to happen, it is time that professionals regain their trust in the physiology which enables healthy women to labour and deliver, mostly without interference. Pregnancy and labour should be seen as normal until proven otherwise.

– Marianne Mead, Chapter 5, 'Midwives' practices in 11 UK maternity units'

Let me be very clear. As the chapters in this book illustrate, the Western technocratic approach to birth, which has become the global technocratic approach to birth, is wrong. Simply and fundamentally wrong. It has nothing at all to do with the normal physiology of birth, and everything to do with the imposition of technocratic values and practices on birth.

For example, the rarity of normal birth in my country, the United States, is indicated in a profound scene in *The Business of Being Born*, a 2007 documentary film produced by actress Ricki Lake. In this scene, Ricki asks a group of white-coated obstetrical residents, 'Do you ever see normal birth?' Uneasily shaking their heads and glancing down and sideways at each other, they collectively respond, 'Um no, not really – *normal* birth? Um, no, we don't.' It is no wonder that, as Beech and Phipps point out in Chapter 4, 'much of the research that purports to be about normal birth is in fact about highly managed obstetric deliveries' – of course, because this research is conducted in hospitals where birth could theoretically be called 'normal' only because it is normal to give birth in hospital.

This book is not an indictment of obstetricians, only of the technocratic, pathology-oriented approach towards birth in which they are trained, and which puts a great deal of pressure on midwives and nurses as well, often impeding the efforts they make to foster normal birth. In Chapter 5, Marianne Mead notes that 'The situation we are experiencing today is primarily the result of good intentions, mainly the desire to reduce maternal and perinatal mortality and morbidity. However, in the absence of sound programmes of research, these good intentions have resulted in increased maternal morbidity... without a corresponding improvement in neonatal outcome.' And it's not just increased maternal morbidity that results from these good intentions. A recent study by a group of WHO researchers and affiliates found that while below 15% higher caesarean rates were unambiguously correlated with lower maternal and neonatal mortality, *above this range*, higher caesarean rates were predominantly correlated with higher maternal and neonatal *mortality* from complications of caesarean for mothers and increased prematurity and other factors for babies.[1]

What is normal birth? We find the following definitions in Chapter 4, 'Normal birth: women's stories' by Beverly Beech and Belinda Phipps:

The designation normal to describe labour and childbirth has been in use for centuries. The current UK Midwives Rules and Standards talk about a 'deviation from the norm' when referring to areas outside the midwives' competence. It is commonly taken to mean a physiological labour and a vaginal birth with little or no external intervention...

When parents talk about 'normal birth' or 'normal delivery' they mean a physiological birth where the baby is delivered vaginally following a labour which has not been altered by technological interventions...

There are indications that normal birth, in the widest sense of a spontaneous physiological, straightforward birth that occurs in the context of supportive, caring, respectful professional care, may enhance the woman's self-esteem, and her physical and mental health. It may also impact upon her relationship with her child and offer a good foundation for future family well-being.

Chapter 6 on midwifery in New Zealand illustrates the fragility of this concept of normal – a concept so easily co-optable that New Zealand midwives often find themselves saying that most of the births they attend are 'normal', then realizing upon reflection that these 'normal births' include huge percentages of labour induction and augmentation, epidurals and other interventions, leading the midwives to question to what extent they can in fact be the guides and guardians of normal birth. Author Sue Crabtree concludes, 'If we, as midwives, now support the view that "normal" includes a wide range of medical intervention, then we have little hope of educating women and the community that normal does not include those things. As a profession, I believe we need to increase our vigilance and challenge ourselves, asking: "from what basis am I making this decision or taking this action?"'

I am going to further address the issues raised in this book, and the value of its chapters, through four stories. The first goes as follows. Once upon a time (in 2002), I was being given a tour of the maternity ward of one of the premier hospitals in the United States. My tour guide was the Chief of Obstetric and Gynecological Anesthesia. He stopped me in front of the nursing station and said, 'What do you hear?' I listened carefully, and answered, 'Absolute silence.' He beamed, and said, 'There are thirty women in labour in this ward at this moment, and all you can hear is silence.' I said, 'But Bill, I would rather be hearing, "uuuuhhhhhhhhhhhhh, ooooohhhhhhhhhhhh, aaaaaaaaaahhhhhhhhhhh."' And he said, '*You* would, but *we* wouldn't. We like it this way!' Later, he ended an email to me saying, 'Gotta go, I'm off to administer more epidurals to more happy, smiling, grateful women. Love, Bill.'

He is as open-minded as any physician I know, so I am sure that he will read this book. While I doubt that it will change his practice, at least it will enhance his understanding of why I would personally rather have heard low guttural moans and why some women would want an atmosphere for birth in which they could make those kinds of noises. What is the problem, if you are healthy, your baby is healthy, you were treated with respect, and you had no pain? It is so very hard to explain to women and to healthcare practitioners exactly what is lost in the 'normal' American birth, and so very hard to get people to

think that technocratic birth is really not 'normal' – it is *typical*, but very far from normal. The chapters in this courageous book will help all of us in our efforts to explain exactly what is lost in 'typical birth', what 'normal birth' really is, and why it matters.

The chapter I most would like my friend to read for starters is the one telling women's stories (Chapter 4). The women quoted are eloquent in their explanations of what normal birth means to them and what importance it carries in their lives. Beverley Beech and Belinda Phipps have done a great service in offering us these women's words. Next I want him to read Chapter 2, in which Tricia Anderson and Nicky Leap finally break through the barriers that prevent us from talking about pain in childbirth and help us drop the euphemisms, like 'discomfort'. Such euphemisms allow women to be shocked when they experience real agony, and lack of advance discussion of labour pain means that women in their shock perceive it as negative instead of valuable. Anderson and Leap offer a new and clear identification of the differences between the 'pain relief paradigm' and the 'working with pain paradigm'. I deeply appreciate their clear identification of no fewer than ten aspects of the value of pain, of which, I am sure, few women are aware. Their discussion allows us to understand pain not as the curse of Eve but as a productive and positive phenomenon. Japanese anthropologist Etsuko Matsuoka[2] calls this phenomenon 'the metamorphic value of labour pain' – 'metamorphic' because, as the Japanese independent midwives Matsuoka interviewed describe, the pain of labour itself plays a major role in transforming a woman into a mother.

I think my anaesthesiologist friend will find it hard to relate to the chapter by Hall and Taylor on spirituality (Chapter 3). But for me spirituality is one of the most important subjects of this book, following through from Downe and McCourt's brilliant analysis in Chapter 1 of systems and chaos theory in relation to birth. So here comes another story.

In 1999 I was having lunch with a paediatrician who had sought me out because he wanted to know what American midwives did at home births when the baby came out and wasn't breathing. Amazed by the question, I told him that they all were trained in neonatal resuscitation, so they would do the same things he would do, but that there was one thing they would that he probably would not. Eagerly he asked me, 'What?' and I answered, 'They would call the baby.' 'Call the baby? What do you mean?' I explained that home birth midwives tend to believe that the baby plays a role in its own birth, that babies are born conscious and with their spirits present, and that the spirit has to make a decision whether to stay or go. A baby not breathing could mean that the spirit is hesitating. So as the midwives prepare to resuscitate, they ask the parents to start calling the baby, welcoming its spirit and asking it to come in. Often that works and there is no need for the actual resuscitation, or it can be a supplement to the process. At the very least, I said, it gives the parents a role to play in saving their baby; at the very most, the spirit hears and responds.

He didn't quite believe me, so he started asking every midwife he met, whether hospital or home-based, if she called the baby. Most of them said, 'Of course,' and many told him stories that so impressed him, he himself began to invite the parents to call the baby. He wrote me months later to tell me about all the times he had not needed the equipment by the time he got it ready to apply. (For more such stories from home birth midwives, see Davis-Floyd and Davis 1997[3] and Roncalli 1997.[4])

Few Western-trained practitioners have the courage to address the role of spirit in birth, or in healing in general. Yet for millennia the role of the shaman and often the midwife in birth has been to address the spirit of the mother and the spirit of the baby, perhaps in battle with other spirits, to facilitate a difficult birth. Modern science supposedly took us past all that 'superstitious nonsense', giving doctors 'real' ways to help. Is spirit 'real'? In *From Doctor to Healer: The Transformative Journey*, my co-author and I describe in detail the stories of 40 physicians who made a paradigm shift from the technocratic, through the humanistic, 'all the way' to the holistic model of medicine. They say 'all the way' because it is a long journey:

- from a paradigm (the technocratic model) that sees the body as a machine and treats the patient as an object
- through a paradigm (the humanistic model) that stresses mind–body connection and the importance of relationship but does not deal with spirit
- to a paradigm (the holistic model) that sees mind, body, and spirit as one. The holistic model not only sees mind/body/spirit as one, but also stresses the spiritual unity of patient and practitioner, that intangible energy that binds them in the healing dance and allows the energy of one to affect the energy and health of the other. (For full descriptions of these three paradigms, see Davis-Floyd and St. John 1998.[5])

Spirit does exist, these holistic physicians say, and if it exists, then it is always present, and to ignore it in the healing process is to leave out the most important element in illness and facilitator of wellness. In Chapter 1, Downe and McCourt critique the 'certainty' and 'linearity' that characterize authoritative obstetrical knowledge systems. These holistic MDs would fully agree that uncertainty and complexity characterize birth and that linear thinking cannot deal adequately with these complexities. They would also applaud Downe and McCourt's term 'salutogenesis', by which they mean the generation of well-being: a primary tenet of holistic healing is that creating wellness is far more important than curing illness. Understanding the non-linearity of many forms of illness and health, the holistic MDs I studied reject the routine, linear standardization of care in favour of individualization. Like the midwives Elizabeth Davis and I wrote about in *Intuition as Authoritative Knowledge in Midwifery and Home Birth* (available at www.davis-floyd.com), these physicians believe in normalizing uniqueness, or 'unique normality', as Downe and McCourt have so aptly transformed our phrase.

As an American reader, I am struck by the essential role that midwives play in birth in the UK. In my country midwives attend only around 10% of births and are still fighting for the existence and continued growth of their profession. Because of their small numbers, even nurse-midwives are still 'alternative' to some degree, and thus they tend to regard themselves as the alternative solution to the hegemonic obstetrical problem. But in the UK, it seems, midwives are so entrenched in the system that they themselves can become the problem. In this regard, readers will appreciate the variations in midwifery practice described by Marianne Mead in Chapter 5, 'Midwives' practices in 11 UK maternity units'. I was surprised by some of these variations and the ways in which they reflect midwives' self-perceptions as 'liberal' in relation to other midwives.

I was also surprised by the similarities between the problems midwives encounter as they try to practise 'the midwifery model' in the UK and in New Zealand, which I have tended to think of recently as a midwifery mecca. After all, the New Zealand midwives recreated themselves and their profession under a very holistic and woman-centred ideology some 15 years ago, and now attend about the same percentage of births as British midwives. But New Zealand midwife Sue Crabtree's description of midwives' efforts to construct birth as normal, to normalize uniqueness, clearly shows how they daily undergo the same struggles with the authoritative knowledge and power system of technocratic obstetrics. While New Zealand midwives believe in and strive to apply the kind of 'fluid definitions' of labour and birth stressed in Chapter 1 by Downe and McCourt, as elsewhere they succeed best in the home setting and experience extreme challenges to their desire to normalize uniqueness in the hospital.

Chapter 7 brings examples from Egypt to Walsh, El-Nemer and Downe's discussion of risk and safety. Sadly, their description of the treatment of Egyptian women in hospital resonates fully with many other ethnographic descriptions of what happens to women when the Western technocratic model is transported to the developing world (see Davis-Floyd 2000;[6] Davis-Floyd, Cosminsky and Pigg 2001[7] for summaries of this literature). Yet we cannot have too many such accounts – the growth of what the authors of this chapter term the 'risk culture in maternity care' is working to eliminate indigenous midwives and replace them with inadequate hospitals and clinics all over the Third World. Only awareness of the harm caused by this process can ever make it pause to create the systems of 'mutual accommodation' between biomedical and indigenous health care that Brigitte Jordan has been calling for since 1978. Such systems of mutual accommodation, where they currently exist, are almost always created by alliances – or at least mutual respect and cooperation – between indigenous and professional midwives (see Davis-Floyd 2000).[6] Thus this chapter is especially important for a book that will be read by the kind of professional midwives who can make this difference.

The construction of true systems of mutual accommodation will require the construction of new and comprehensive systems of authoritative midwifery knowledge that include the best of what traditional and professional midwives and obstetricians know. Walsh, El-Nemer and Downe describe how obstetrical knowledge has been constructed and accepted in an environment and with an ideology of birth as characterized by pathology and risk, in the 'linear thinking' mode. Chapter 8, by Downe et al., explores contestations of this kind of knowledge through 'the case of the early pushing urge'. Here she critiques the ironclad rule that women can't go from a few cm dilation to full in just a few minutes, citing many examples when they do just that, horrifying the midwife who just pronounced that 'it will be hours yet' even as the woman is insisting that she has to push. This chapter brings up questions about how exactly midwifery knowledge is constructed, which brings me to the third of my four stories.

In the summer of 2000, I was driving a carload of direct-entry American home birth midwives from Texas to Mexico. Part of the purpose of our trip was to visit the CASA School for Professional Midwives in San Miguel de Allende – a new experiment in midwifery education (see Davis-Floyd 2001).[8] One of these midwives was a preceptor at this school and the other, Patricia Kay, had played a key role in its founding. Sandi and Patricia got into a conversation about a problem that had recently arisen with the students, who seemed to be telling women to push too soon, resulting in swollen cervixes and difficult pushing. Trying to understand the source of the problem, Sandi did a repeat check after one of the students had checked a woman and pronounced her ready to push. But Sandi knew the mother wasn't ready at all. She gently conveyed this to the student, who, looking very confused, went off into a corner, surreptitiously got out a tape measure, and measured her fingers as she held them apart. Sandi suddenly realized that the problem was not the student but the teaching she had received, from Sandi herself. 'It's not about ten centimetres!' she exclaimed. 'When I checked the mother her cervix *was* ten centimetres dilated, but I could still feel the cervical lip. It's not about ten centimetres!'

In addition to that, the woman did not *feel* to Sandi like she was ready to push – she didn't have that certain look in her eyes, that certain grimace on her face, that certain something that Sandi could interpret when it happened but couldn't explain. And Sandi said to Patricia, 'We all are taught, and we all teach, ten centimetres. But it's not ten centimetres, it's where the cervix is – can you feel it or not? – and it's how the woman *is*.' Patricia heartily agreed, and I was struck once again by the embodied nature and verbal ineffability of what midwives know and how they know it.

Judith Mercer, Rebecca Skovgaard and Debra Erickson-Owens' chapter on fetal to neonatal transition, entitled 'First, do no harm', speaks directly to this midwifery construction of knowledge as well as to the issue of normalizing uniqueness. In this chapter they challenge accepted obstetrical authoritative knowledge about cord clamping, presenting the many good reasons for waiting until the baby receives all the blood and oxygen the cord has to give. Here is a practice I *do* wish we could standardize – so simple, so commonsensical, yet so antithetical to the technocratic paradigm's insistence on separation and the superiority of technological intervention.

And thus we come to my last story, which is about how an American obstetrician, Bethany Hays, figured out that she should stop early clamping of the cord. She was attending a hospital birth and decided the baby needed resuscitation. She cut the cord and started to run across the room to the resuscitation table when she slipped on a pool of amniotic fluid on the floor and fell. As she went down, she managed to twist around so that she landed on her back and the baby was safe on her stomach. Perhaps it was the stimulus of the fall, but the baby was suddenly breathing fine and screaming lustily. Later Bethany reflected on how 'stupid' the whole thing was. She said, 'I could have killed the baby trying to save him! If I hadn't cut the cord so fast, the baby probably would have not had so much trouble breathing in the first place. He was probably perfectly normal, and just needed more time to be connected.' (The evidence behind Bethany's realization can be found in Chapter 9 on the fetal to neonatal transition, which also, and very pertinently, explodes the myth that newborn suctioning should be routine.)

And that, primarily, is what this book is about. The editors and chapter authors are very aware that any deviation from what is medically defined as normal can easily derail what could have been a truly normal birth into a highly technocratic process. They point out that Friedman's curve tells us nothing about normal birth, as it was created using only women experiencing medicalized births in hospitals. Nor do studies of whether women prefer pethidine *versus* epidurals. This book and its title are important because, even in the early 21st century, we do not know what normal birth is, since we lost the experience of it when birth moved into hospitals, where almost all of the studies have been done. Chapter 10 by Walsh summarizes much of the evidence that supports the kind of normal birth this book is about, most especially the unequivocal evidence showing the benefits of social and emotional labour support.

I have long believed, and stated many times in my oral presentations, that the most important determinants of the outcome of a woman's birth are the attitudes and ideology of her primary caregiver(s). Recently a systematic review by Ellen Hodnett (2002)[9] of 137 studies reporting on factors influencing women's evaluations of their childbirth experiences confirmed my belief, which prior to this study was based primarily on my interviews and observations. The objective of Hodnett's review was to summarize what is known about satisfaction with childbirth, with particular attention to the roles of pain and pain relief. The reports included descriptive studies, randomized controlled trials, and reviews of intrapartum interventions. The results were as follows:

four factors – personal expectations, the amount of support from caregivers, the quality of the caregiver–patient relationship, and involvement in decision making – appear to be so important that they override the influences of age, socioeconomic status, ethnicity, childbirth preparation, the physical birth environment, pain, immobility, medical interventions, and continuity of care, when women evaluate their childbirth experiences.

The review's conclusion is that 'The influences of pain, pain relief, and intrapartum medical interventions on subsequent satisfaction are neither as obvious, as direct, nor as powerful as the influences of the attitudes and behaviors of the caregivers.'

Because what is defined as a deviation from normal is always in relation to the standardized rules and procedures for hospital birth, it has become absolutely essential for any practitioner interested in helping women achieve normal birth to gain the knowledge, the courage, and enough trust in their intuition to normalize uniqueness – to acknowledge that what is right or wrong for this woman at this moment in this birth may have little or nothing to do with standardized rules or randomized controlled trials. It might be about a knot in the cord, or a placenta previa, or it might be about spirit, and fear, and emotion, and love. Maybe a woman's labour stalls because she is terrified that she won't be able to mother this baby, or because there is anger and tension in the room. Maybe she needs to push for three hours because that's how long it takes her to find that deep place in herself from within which she can give birth, not only to her baby but also to herself. Maybe it's intuition that tells a midwife whether or not the baby and the mother are fine during this long pushing stage, and not the monitor.

The concept of "normalizing uniqueness", usefully rephrased in this book as "unique normality", came to me from watching midwives attend births and listening to their stories. They all knew "the rules", but they also seemed somehow to know when "the rules" didn't apply. They were always willing to stop and listen—to the woman, to the baby's spirit as well as its heart tones, to their own inner voice and to that of the mother. I saw and heard how often a birth that seemed "abnormal" by hospital standards could be perfectly normal by a woman's own individual standards and circumstances. And I learned about spontaneous synchronicity:

- a midwife suddenly puts on a wild CD when a caesarean seems imminent; she says, 'The heart tones are dropping – that means this baby needs to dance!'

- a husband reaches down during a moment of privacy to give his wife a clitoral orgasm during labour, or knows just when to kiss her and tell her she is magnificent

- a lit candle in the darkness, a group song, or a riotous joke changes the energy of the room and the labour to one of joy instead of tension

- instead of saying, 'Oh, you're still only four centimetres,' the midwife says, 'You're four centimetres – you are doing great! Your uterus is preparing, toning – fantastic! This may take a while, but once this toning stage is done, things will move really fast. This is the time to be patient, to move around a lot, to eat and drink to keep up your strength, to be in the water. All is well – there is no need to hurry this birth.'

- instead of saying, 'Oh no, you're at ten but your contractions have stopped, we'll have to restart them with pitocin (syntocinon),' the midwife says, 'Oh, delightful, you're at the "rest and be thankful" stage – your uterus just needs time to reshape around the baby, who is now really far down in the birth canal. So rest and be thankful for the break!'

The technocratic model needs no more defenders – it has plenty and their voices have long drowned out the kind of voices that speak in this book. We need to hear the voices that speak for such intangibles – that butterfly flapping its wings in the jungle – that can shift what a few people dare to call the 'energy' of the birth. We need to hear the voices that insist that the deviation can be the norm *for this woman and this baby at this time in this place*. A 'stalled labour' can be a very human and normal need for emotional release; a baby not breathing immediately can mean that the spirit is waiting to be called in, or that the baby needs more blood from the cord, or both! Such is holism in midwifery and birth – the recognition of emotion and spirit, the willingness to listen, and openness to the 'unique normality' you will find so wisely addressed in these pages.

Robbie E. Davis-Floyd
Austin, 2008

References

1. Betrán A, Merialdi M, Lauer J A, Wang, B-S, Thomas J, Van Look P, Wagner M 2007 Rates of caesarean section: analysis of global, regional and national estimates. Paediatr Perinat Ep 21:98–113

2. Etsuko M, Fumiko H In press, forthcoming 2008 Maternity homes in Japan: reservoirs of normal childbirth. In: Davis-Floyd R, Barclay L, Daviss B A, Tritten J (eds) Birth models that work. University of California Press, Berkeley and London

3. Davis-Floyd R, Davis E 1997 Intuition as authoritative knowledge in midwifery and home birth. In: Davis-Floyd R, Sargent C (eds) Childbirth and authoritative knowledge: cross-cultural perspectives. University of California Press, Berkeley, p 315–349. (Also available at www.davis-floyd. com)

4. Roncalli L 1997 Standing by process: a midwife's notes on storytelling, passage, and intuition. In: Davis-Floyd R, Arvidson P S (eds) Intuition: the inside story. Routledge, New York, p 177–200

5. Davis-Floyd R, St John G 1998 From doctor to healer: the transformative journey. Rutgers University Press, New Brunswick, NJ

6. Davis-Floyd R 2000 Global issues in midwifery: mutual accommodation or biomedical hegemony? Midwifery Today, March:12–17,68–69. (Also available at www.davis-floyd.com)

7. Davis-Floyd R, Cosminsky S, Pigg LS (eds) 2001 Introduction to daughters of time: the shifting identities of contemporary midwives, a special double issue of Med Anthropol 20(2/3,4):105–139. (Also available at www.davis-floyd.com)

8. Davis-Floyd R 2001 *La partera profesional*: articulating identity and cultural space for a new kind of midwife in Mexico. In: Davis-Floyd R, Cosminsky S, Pigg S L (eds) Daughters of time: the shifting identities of contemporary midwives, a special double issue of Med Anthropol 20(2/3,4):185–244. (Also available at www.davis-floyd. com)

9. Hodnett ED 2002 Pain and women's satisfaction with the experience of childbirth: a systematic review. In: The nature and management of labor pain: peer-reviewed papers from an evidence-based symposium, a special issue of the Am J Obstet Gynecol 186(3), part 2, March

Section **One**

Ways of seeing

CHAPTERS

From being to becoming: reconstructing childbirth knowledges

Soo Downe and Christine McCourt

1

Chapter contents

Introduction

The impetus for the work set out in this chapter was frustration with the near invisibility of normal physiological processes in Western approaches to childbirth. This included the apparent inability even to define 'normal birth', except as an absence of technical intervention. Thinking through the factors which have led to this point has given us the opportunity to share some of the insights and observations we have previously reported separately.[1-4] In the process, the synergy between our separate but connected areas of knowledge has become apparent to us. We hope that we have been able to make this clear in the account we give in this chapter.

In order to explain the conclusions at the end of the chapter, it is necessary to describe the recent history of some of the philosophies and theories that we feel have influenced current perspectives in the context of health. We also briefly describe the theories that are the basis of our proposal for new 'ways of seeing'.[5] We are aware that, in places, some of these accounts may seem to be very far from clinical practice, or from personal experiences of birth. Where we can, we have drawn theory–practice connections through reference to research based in practice.

In 1972, Archie Cochrane, then director of the Medical Research Council Epidemiology Unit, published a seminal book entitled *Effectiveness and Efficiency*.[6] He put forward the apparently simple view that 'all effective treatment must be free'. Its implication was revolutionary in that, by default, it proposed that ineffective treatment should not be free. This agenda has become central to political developments in health care in many countries worldwide since the early 1990s.

A problem arises, however, when we try to define and measure effectiveness. This is not merely a matter of asking 'does it work?' but, fundamentally, of deciding what should be evaluated, and how, and how the results should be interpreted. Who decides the nature of accepted knowledge? Even within

3

so-called 'hard' numerical, controlled studies, findings depend on a series of assumptions about what is to be studied, how the study is framed, what is seen as bias or 'noise' and how the findings are interpreted. All evidence is culturally bound and all is framed by the nature of the questions that are asked. As Ann Oakley pointed out: 'Science and knowledge are socially produced: that is, they are subject to the very influence of social processes and practicalities that their common-sense representations would dismiss as quite beyond their frames of reference' (p 335).[7] This has an impact on what is termed the 'authoritative knowledge' of health.[8,9] Such knowledge is characterized through its dominance and authority. This can be expressed at any level of a social system, usually through a combination of structural and explanatory power. It is generally so well established that it is difficult to question and tends to be taken for granted as right and proper, or even simply part of the natural order. At the extreme, powerful social groups may affirm the superiority of their way of knowing by associating it with established truths, such as with God or with nature. Jordan argues:[8]

> To legitimize one way of knowing as authoritative devalues, often totally dismisses, all other ways of knowing. Those who espouse alternative knowledge systems tend to be seen as backward, ignorant or naïve troublemakers … The constitution of authoritative knowledge is an ongoing social process that both builds and reflects power relationships within a community of practice. It does so in such a way that all participants come to see the current social order as a natural order, i.e. as the way things (obviously) are. (p 152)

With these observations in mind, we intend to examine the nature of childbirth knowledge (the 'epistemology' of childbirth) with particular reference to our understanding of normality. This chapter examines four aspects of current authoritative knowledge in childbirth: certainty, simplicity, linearity and pathology. We propose a new approach, based on uncertainty, complexity and the generation of well-being (salutogenesis). In presenting our case, we also make the claim that we need to see the world and the natural

processes within it from a cyclical and complex paradigm, rather than by the simple, linear model that underpins most of the current authoritative knowledge applied in health care.

The current childbirth paradigm

Certainty as a given

The kind of science that investigates ever more advanced technical solutions to human problems is arguably the fundamental guiding force in most 21st century societies. Although eco-warriors and anti-globalization campaigners seek to challenge this hegemony, it is firmly and deeply established. Health care is a prime example of the authority of this kind of science in our lives. This kind of authority is generally accepted by most members of a society, as it is taken to be the norm, but the issue of power is especially evident when the norms and certainties of applied health science are enforced legally on those who deviate from accepted practices. This phenomenon has been evident in US and UK cases where women who refuse caesarean section have been ordered by the courts to submit to surgery.[10,11]

The philosophical underpinnings of the approach to science used by the judge in such cases can be located in what has been termed 'enlightenment science'.[12] However, as we will illustrate, enlightenment science, paradoxically, also bore the seeds of scientific uncertainty. The enlightenment movement is identified by historians as having taken place in the 18th century in Europe. Bacon, Newton and Descartes were key thinkers influencing the science that developed in this period.[13] They were interested in understanding how the natural world and the phenomena within it worked. The analogy they used was that of the machine. This reflected their social context of rapid technical and industrial development. This model was characterized by simplicity and elegance. It offered a unified way of analysing all aspects of the natural (and human) world by reducing it to its constituent building blocks. It was believed that complex phenomena could be understood and explained by reducing them to these basic parts, and then by looking for the mechanisms through which they interacted. Newton hoped to use his theories to develop an overall, unifying explanation of the workings of this 'clockwork universe'.[14]

Hampson notes that this new science, which held that all previously believed 'truths' should be questioned, should have undermined the social certainties that had previously rested in traditional and religious ideas.[12] However, in an era of tremendous social and cultural change, societies of the time sought new certainties: as Capra wrote: 'as science seemed to establish itself on an impregnable basis of experimentally verified fact, doubt and confusion eventually gave way to self-confidence and the belief that the unknown was merely the undiscovered' (p 35).[14]

In contradiction to this desire by societies to find certainty, the 20th century philosopher Popper argued that science should proceed according to the principle of falsifiability. In his view, scientific knowledge should proceed incrementally, in an orderly fashion, by systematic testing of theories. Thus, 'truths' cannot be proven but only tested and falsified.[15] Such a philosophy of science does not appear to support the notion of certainty – quite the opposite in fact. However, writers such as Kuhn have shown that, although scientists may claim to operate according to Popperian principles, most scientific enquiry does not in fact follow this course.[16] He noted that research tends to proceed within what he called 'paradigms' of knowledge. These are the current accepted world views. There is considerable investment and security vested in working within the prevailing paradigm, and it is held tenaciously, even in the face of evidence that contradicts it. Kuhn wrote:[16]

Normal science, the activity in which most scientists inevitably spend almost all their time, is predicated on the assumption that the scientific community knows what the world is like. Much of the success of the enterprise derives from the community's willingness to defend that assumption, if necessary at considerable cost. (p 5)

This brings us back, then, to the example of legally enforced caesarean sections. The scientific community, almost in spite of its epistemological origins, has been adopted into a societal view of the certainty of science. This apparent certainty marks out the behaviour of individuals as acceptable or deviant, depending on the degree to which the behaviours fit with the scientific norms of the day, which implicitly also reflect moral and social norms.

Having very briefly explored the historical background to the relationships between science and health, it is not surprising to find that critical theorists in this area have claimed that the current paradigm of childbirth has been fundamentally based on the metaphor of the (female) body as a machine.[17] Metaphorically, from this perspective, research and practice rules tend to proceed on the basis that the machine is fundamentally faulty, and these faults can best be contained by setting strict 'quality control' rules within which the machine is known to function optimally. Behaviours and physiological processes outside of these parameters become, by default, pathologies. We discuss the role of pathology in current ways of seeing later in the chapter.

The implications of certainty

The currently held authoritative scientific and practice paradigm in most Westernized countries is based on the belief that the best, most certain evidence is that gained from research based on the study of specific elements of the system, with enough individuals to be fairly sure that the results can be generalized to whole populations. The ideal has been termed 'large trials with simple protocols'.[18] It is believed that this model increases certainty, and that the findings from such trials, if they are carried out well, should be applied wholesale to individuals.

In 1985, Bateson, a biologist, anthropologist and one of the founders of cybernetics, commented on the widespread assumption that generalizability to a population implies generalizability to each of the individuals in that population.[19] He described this tendency as a logical confusion between 'class' and 'individual'. He illustrated this point with the example of Brownian motion: molecules in boiling water. Although the boiling point of water can be reasonably accurately predicted, the point at which 'boiling' begins for a particular molecule cannot. Later in this chapter we will give several examples of ways in which this logical confusion has occurred in the implementation of 'evidence-based' practice in maternity care, where once a probability estimate of risk is established, a new protocol, such as timing of induction of labour for post-maturity, may be applied to all women, regardless of their individual characteristics.

One example of the way that the dominant paradigm of knowledge has come to override alternative views of the world is, then, the current interpretation of the concept of evidence-based medicine. We will set out the original philosophy behind this approach, and some specific clinical examples associated with it. We intend to illustrate the point that, while the concept of evidence has now become the underpinning feature of accepted knowledge in the health services, this only became possible after the original concept of evidence-based medicine as a fluid entity had been subverted by the wider professional demand for certainties.

Evidence-based practice and certainty

The pioneers of evidence-based medicine recognized that 'best practice' was an amalgam of good quality data with practitioners' skills and experience, and the individual service user's beliefs, knowledge and values.[20–22] As Jelinek points out, in arguing for a clinical approach to clinical trials: 'the randomised controlled trial … has to be balanced with other evidence of a biomedical, psychological and sociological nature: and with previous experience derived from both a core of relevant literature and of a personal or institutional base. It has to be applied to the individual patient as perceived by both patient and doctor' (p 86).[20]

This concept of best practice allows for fluidity in the interpretation of research, with individual variables and partnership between practitioner and client built in to the final clinical decision. However, the evidence-based medicine agenda as currently promoted in many countries is firmly rooted in certainty, with very little emphasis on the practitioner and the service user. This is illustrated by the very narrow definition of 'best evidence' that has been promoted within this field.[23]

The inexorable move towards a demand for maximum certainty has led to the creation of practice and clinical protocols in many countries that are written and adhered to as though the evidence were comprehensive, without limitations and equally applicable to all members of the population. Two examples will illustrate the point. The first is that of fetal auscultation policies during labour, and, specifically, the recommended time interval between periods of listening to the fetal heart.

Electronic fetal heart rate monitoring

For many centuries, midwives have listened to the fetal heart during labour intermittently. There does not appear to be any published evidence relating to the range of practice among midwives in terms of the interval between periods of auscultation, or to women's views of the acceptability of different monitoring intervals. However, it is clear from the personal clinical and birth experiences of one of us (SD), and from observation of the practices of midwives by both of us, that, where protocols allow for flexibility, this interval varies from irregular listening in every few hours or so to regular monitoring several times within the hour. Auscultation appears to become more frequent as labour advances, or if the midwife feels from other signs that there may be an impending problem with the labour or the baby. Such flexible practices appear to be more common during home births or in other out-of-hospital settings.[24] In contrast, in the context of the development of protocols for many aspects of labour in UK hospitals during the late 20th century, this flexible time interval was often standardized to every 30 minutes in the first stage of labour, and then after every contraction in the second stage.

Since the early 1990s, professional and governmental bodies across the world have responded to the accumulating evidence that labouring women and their babies, at least at the population level, may benefit from intermittent rather than continuous fetal monitoring in labour.[25–28] However, the main trial on which this evidence is based used an unusually intensive regimen of intermittent auscultation as the control for the intervention of electronic fetal monitoring. This involved listening in to the fetal heart every 15 minutes in the active first stage of labour, and more frequently in the second stage.[29]

The guidelines of national professional bodies cited above generally adopt a 15 (or 15–30) minute interval for auscultation in the first stage of labour, in contrast to preceding centuries of custom and practice. In the process, this practice is reified as the only safe way to undertake auscultation, despite the preceding decades of empirical evidence on less frequent regimens of monitoring. The frequency of the new regimen has made it very difficult to implement in many busy labour wards. Indeed, this is the rationale given by some practitioners for continuing with continuous electronic fetal monitoring.[30] This particular regimen is increasingly seen as mandatory and 'certain' because it is based on a trial, even if it is unachievable in actual practice. The issues of an individual practitioner's skills and knowledge, or a specific woman's beliefs and values and particular pattern of labouring, do not appear to feature widely in most formal protocols or guidelines in this area. Two specific points arise from this example. The first is that, even when there is evidence of an authoritative nature, according to the rules of 'normal science', it may not fit with the prevailing socio-cultural paradigm and set of beliefs around childbirth. This leads to non-adoption of the evidence. Secondly, in this case the 'normal science' rules were violated in the process of undertaking the research. The trial design compared continuous electronic fetal monitoring with an intensive pattern of intermittent monitoring which had not been previously evaluated for efficacy, acceptability or utility. Alternative patterns that were in common use at the the time the trial was conducted may have generated different results, one way or the other.

Induction of labour for post-maturity

Our second example is induction of labour for post-maturity. Based on the Cochrane review in this area,[31] benefits for populations of women and babies only begin to become clear after 41 weeks of gestation. Indeed, these advantages do not become really apparent until after 42 weeks of gestation. Rather than a clear cut-off point occurring, the balance of risks and benefits of induction shifts in a continuum over time. This shift follows an exponential curve, so the balance changes more rapidly as time goes on. Despite the recommendations that women be offered induction routinely after 41 weeks, anecdotally inductions for post-maturity are now routinely carried out in a number of settings and countries soon after the woman has reached 40 weeks of gestation. The routine nature of these practices are an example of Bateson's argument regarding logical confusion in interpreting probability statistics. This has occurred in parallel with rising rates of induction of labour, which, for example, were over 20% in the UK in 2003/4,[32] from around 17–18% between 1989 and 1993. Again, very little notice appears to be taken of the relationship between the practitioner and the woman, of the woman's skills and knowledge or, indeed, of the complexity of the relevant evidence. This raises serious questions about the application to individuals of population-level protocol or guideline-driven practices.

Rather than valuing certainty as illustrated above, it is possible to see science as a continuous process. Instead of taking a linear approach to evidence, in which we ask the question and we find the answer, such a paradigm sees science as an ongoing dialogue. In this case, evidence is a complex and fluid phenomenon, continually moving between developing and testing ideas. Before we come back to this possibility, however, we will examine the principle of simplicity, which is central to the experimental design of the randomized controlled trial.

Simplicity as a framework

Thinkers such as Descartes, Bacon and Newton aimed to develop theory that had simplicity. Bacon, for example, saw his method of experiment and induction as one that would offer 'an infallible method of distinguishing between truth and error' (p 36).[12] Newton built on this approach, aiming to identify simple basic principles that would allow generalization about the nature of the world: 'The beautiful simplicity of a single law which appeared to explain the operation of every kind of earthly and celestial movement was a triumphant example of the possibilities of the new learning' (p 37).[12]

Much research in the area of childbirth is based on this notion of simplicity. It also has resonance for practices that are regulated by protocols and guidelines. The assumption is that there is a straightforward cause–effect relationship in the physiology of birth. This can be found and codified if birth can be reduced to its essential components and then systematically examined. It is inherent in this paradigm that the single summary finding from the whole population of individuals in a trial can be directly and uniformly applied to the complex situations of individuals in practice, as we have discussed above. The promotion of large trials with simple protocols illustrates this simplicity-based approach. Additionally, this vision of knowledge assumes that clinical parameters are of overriding importance, in isolation from almost all other parameters that impinge on birth, such as social interactions and environmental impact, which may act independently and may also interact with clinical parameters in complex ways.

Randomization is used to get as close as possible to samples that are similar to each other and which represent the relevant population as a whole. This is intended to remove all possible sources of systematic bias, so that what is found in the samples can be said to hold true for that population. Randomization is used effectively to resolve the problem of achieving simplicity and control in experimental research involving people. In order to design an effective randomized controlled trial, simplicity is needed to achieve the required level of control. Control is crucial to ensure that the findings are not 'contaminated' by potentially confounding variables. This is particularly difficult to achieve with complex interventions, which are the very interventions that are often particularly relevant to maternity care. It requires considerable knowledge to be able to identify the nature of the intervention to be studied as well and to have the capacity to 'unpick' different aspects of an intervention. This is not always possible or desirable in complex systems, such as childbirth, where both input and outcome are influenced by an interacting 'net' of cultural, social, environmental, psychological and physiological factors.

Similarly, meta-analysis relies strongly on the principle of simplicity, as illustrated by attempts to control for heterogeneity in data synthesis. Examination of two particular meta-analyses within the Cochrane Library illustrates the difficulties of operating on the principle of simplicity in a complex environment.

An overview of trials of antenatal support interventions with a primary outcome measure of reduction in low birth weight includes interventions as diverse as antenatal classes (of various types), home-based support and peer and professional support, in a wide range of cultural and health service contexts.[33] The studies measured a range of different, although overlapping, outcomes. Few of the trials studied in depth the degree to which women perceived the intervention to be supportive, despite a body of psychological research suggesting that perception of support is a key measure.[34,35] Similarly, the Cochrane meta-analysis of position in labour summarizes any position that is not supine as 'upright'.[36] The physiological variability between trials using the lateral position and those using squatting is not explored in the analysis.

The problem of interpretation without attending to potential underlying variables is neatly illustrated by the published accounts of so-called 'active management of labour'.[37,38] This highly prescriptive approach originated at the National Maternity Hospital in Dublin. Active management comprised a range of elements, including monitoring, augmentation of labour and constant midwifery support. A review of published accounts of the system in the mid-1990s suggested that active management could reduce emergency caesarean section rates , but that the most effective ingredient of the package was probably continuous support for labouring women.[39] In practice, however, the findings of the original work were interpreted as suggesting that the surveillance and intervention elements of the package were the most important aspects to implement. It is of interest that more recent data from the home of active management in Ireland, published in 2004, indicate a sharply rising caesarean section rate among nulliparous women.[40] Both the tendency to adopt the technical aspects of the package over the social ones, and the trend to rising caesarean rates are not surprising in the context of what has been termed the 'technocratic' paradigm of childbirth currently prevailing across most of the world.[41] Although evidence from trials of continuing support in labour[42] has been used to challenge the prevailing interpretation of active management of labour, practices in many labour wards continue to favour a simplistic, technocratic implementation.

Bateson argued that seeking the simplest, most elegant explanation that will cover the known data (parsimony) is an obligation of science.[19] However, he also noted that reductionism becomes a problem if the simplest explanation is seen as the only explanation. Although many writers in this field, even those publishing in the medical journals, have begun to question the framing of issues in terms of certainty and predictability,[43] the telling factor which indicates where the beliefs of the current system lie is the allocation of resources. As we have indicated, large, preferably multicentre trials and meta-analyses head the list of 'best evidence' in all the standard lists. Big trials are not funded unless they are powered for a single primary outcome. Subanalysis is written off as 'data trawling' since it is always possible for researchers to find some significant difference, purely by chance, with a large number of measures. Knowledge that is generated by hands-on experience, by messy interactions with people and with events, and by intuitive understandings and decisions[44–46] is dismissed as being biased or unscientific. The term 'noise' is used to describe anything in the environment or context that is not defined as part of the issue of interest.[47] These elements are dismissed as confounding variables.

Linearity of thinking

Linear thinking is particularly characteristic of certain cultural/religious philosophies. Christianity and Judaism, for example, provide views of history and time that have a clear beginning, a line of development and a clear endpoint (such as Judgement Day). Other religious philosophies, such as Buddhism or Hinduism, have more cyclical views. Such basic cultural concepts and philosophies have been shown by historians and anthropologists to have profound effects on the way enquiry and knowledge are framed.[48,49] Reflecting on this, Hampson writes: 'scientific evidence can only answer the questions that scientists think fit to ask' (p 21).[12] Examples of linear thinking include the interpretation of Darwin's theory of evolution, which saw the development of *Homo sapiens* as a process of orderly change (despite its basis in random mutation) towards a higher evolutionary point, and 19th century European liberal economics, which sought continual progress through competition.

It is not surprising then that such concepts of time and of progress also frame Western medical thought. The standard interpretation of Friedman's work on definitions of normal progress of labour is a particularly clear example of this.[50] Although Friedman did not necessarily intend his work to form the authoritative account of 'normal' progress in labour, his findings, and those of subsequent researchers in this area,[51] have become seminal in modern obstetrics. However, we suggest that this classic work has involved unexamined assumptions about the linearity of physical time and physiological processes of birth. Friedman undertook his research with women who laboured in a particular hospital setting in South Africa. Although the findings were then tested in other hospitals, the work has never been undertaken for births out of hospital. Given the emphasis in hospitals on time as the principal delineator of progress,[52–54] studies of physiological processes in such settings run the risk of providing the answer to the wrong question. These findings are about typical progress of labour in a hospital, and in a particular cultural context, rather than the physiology of labour in women labouring spontaneously. Friedman's curve does allow for differential rates of progress at different stages. However, the interpretation of his findings, and the development of action and alert lines for labour, has led to the creation of powerful beliefs about normal progress in labour.

The socially situated nature of these beliefs can be illustrated by the changes in norms of labour duration given in successive obstetric textbooks. While in 1962, Lennon's text described normal labour as lasting up to 24 hours, by 1980 standard texts such as *Obstetrics Illustrated* described labour as lasting up to 12 hours in a primigravida or 6–8 hours in a parous woman.[55,56] In neither case was any supporting evidence given for these firm statements, as was usual until recently in textbooks, but they clearly reflected both the voice of authority and the norms of practice of their time. This phenomenon has also been reported by one of us in a chronological review of midwifery textbooks.[57] Many hospital protocols specify the number of centimetres of cervical dilation per hour a woman's cervix should progress before intervention should be considered, with little allowance for physiological variation or plateaux in progress. The irresistible nature of these beliefs is illustrated in a series of recent studies of the progress of labour, which sought to escape the rigidity of post-Friedman definitions by using the assessments of nurse-midwives in hospitals deemed to be more relaxed in their approach.[58,59] While the interpretation of the data generated allows slightly slower cervical dilation per hour than in the prior standard definitions of progress, the authors still propose that cervical dilation increases regularly hour by hour. This is in contradistinction to the clearly variant progress evident in Friedman's curve itself.

These findings stand in stark contrast to anecdotal accounts of midwives undertaking home births. Such stories report an ebb and flow of labour, which may take days rather than hours and which moves on in increments rather than in a smoothly linear process.[60] These accounts allow for the possibility that 'progress' is influenced by a range of emotional, spiritual, psychological and environmental factors as well as factors such as parity and previous birth history.

Positivist approaches to knowledge rest on the view that direct, simple cause–effect relationships can be established, in the manner of logical operations, as in the example of support in labour given in Figure 1.1.

However, this notion of cause and effect is not very efficient when real-life research encounters complexity. The model where A, operating on B, leads to C begins to break down unless it can cope with the kind of 'noise' mentioned above. This 'noise' may be the individual practitioner's skills and attitudes, the culture of an organization, the efficiency of administration systems or any number of factors that actually influence the nature of care delivery. The context of practice becomes a problem to be dealt with because it does not conform to the philosophical models inherent in the formal evidence base. Even the issue of complexity in the physiological process of labour is not accommodated well in such a model. We will come back to the issue of linearity later in the chapter when we discuss alternative approaches that may take us closer to an understanding of normality in childbirth.

Pathology as pivotal

The central place of pathology in the current childbirth paradigm is underpinned by assumptions of certainty, and by the primacy of risk, as we have discussed. Concepts of risk are discussed in more detail in Chapter 7. From an economic perspective, it is clear that where health is framed by a constant expectation of danger, there is money to be made in providing investigative, preventative or curative products to counteract the risks. The largely hidden, unacknowledged and unaccountable influence of markets such as the pharmacological, biotechnological and 'hi-tech' equipment industries on our everyday construction of health risk is an element in the promotion of a pathological perspective.

As we note above in the context of clinical trials, the evidence for the central place of pathology in mainstream beliefs about childbirth is most clearly indicated in the budget allocated to it. This spending

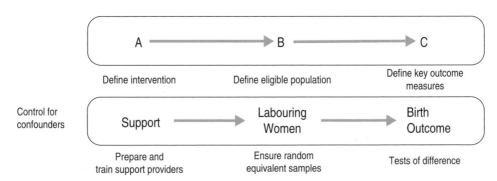

Fig 1.1 • Logical operations: support in labour.

can be seen in clinical risk systems, in insurance premiums and in the widespread application of equipment and treatments that were originally designed to maximize 'safety' for the very few who are truly at high and imminent risk of serious pathology if an intervention does not take place.

This emphasis is also evident in the standard outcome measures used in intervention-based research in childbirth. Most published studies utilize short-term measures of clinical mortality and morbidity, such as rates of caesarean section, depression, anxiety, back pain, tiredness and urinary incontinence in the mother, and perinatal mortality or morbidity in the baby. Aside from breastfeeding uptake or, occasionally, satisfaction or quality-of-life scores, positive experiences are usually not accommodated, except as the absence of morbidity or mortality.

It may be argued that there is no point in assessing wellness, since it does not need to be treated, and therefore it is not of interest to health services. However, this very argument illustrates a pathological paradigm. If health and well-being is only defined as what is left over after illness is dealt with, then illness becomes the defining characteristic of health care. Such an approach ignores the possibility that understanding well-being may be the key to minimizing illness. In terms of childbirth, such an approach may also render the potential benefits of physiological labour and birth invisible. In fact, even in the context of 'normal' birth, the outcome measures proposed by at least one authoritative UK body included maternal death and incontinence.[61] Subtle, positive longer-term outcomes, such as capacity to parent or maternal and infant well-being, are rarely measured in routine assessments of care delivery.

Having expressed our view that many randomized controlled trials operate on the basis of maximizing certainty, we also acknowledge that the use of confidence intervals, and of sensitivity analyses in economic studies, indicates that ideas of uncertainty do feature in the authoritative knowledge of mainstream health research. Unfortunately, as we have already discussed, this is not generally translated from the trials to evidence-based medicine as it is applied in maternity unit protocols or to individuals. In the next section of this chapter, we present an alternative way of seeing. We suggest that we cannot begin to understand 'normal childbirth' without reframing some of our basic assumptions about knowledge in general. We also note that some of these alternative ideas are beginning to feature in medical publications, particularly where the focus is general practice and community care.[62]

Alternative ways of seeing

Uncertainty

In the previous section, we discussed the importance of certainty as a goal of modern science. We noted that certainty arose from 'enlightenment' ideas about seeking general explanatory scientific theories, based on mechanical metaphors. As long ago as the 18th century, scepticism regarding the new certainties of enlightenment science was developing, partly influenced by contact with different cultures. Hampson cites the philosopher Kant, who, in his *Critique of Pure Reason* published in 1781, argued that empirical knowledge could convey information to a human observer not about things as they existed (noumena) but only as they were perceived (phenomena).[12] The observer imposes his or her perceptions of the dimensions of space and time onto the object. Anthropologists began to develop the argument that the way in which the world is perceived is a product of mental processes, and of interactions with the environment, which are, at least partly, culturally and socially shaped.[48] This theoretical perspective was echoed a century later in the theories of relativity and thermodynamics. These ideas presented a significant challenge to assumptions of certainty in science.[14] While physics may seem to be very far away from normal birth, the insights gained from these new areas are relevant to human understanding of all phenomena, including biological processes. Capra has explored this area in detail,[14] and we summarize some of his insights next.

Maxwell's laws of thermodynamics represented an important shift in concepts of nature from those that pertained previously. While his first law described the principle of conservation of energy, the second described its dissipation (such as by movement producing heat). This implied a shift from order to disorder and led to the concept of entropy (that all matter breaks down over time). Einstein's relativity and quantum theories built on this work. The new capacity to observe subatomic particles was also of importance. In keeping with a mechanical model of the universe, particles had always been thought of as 'matter' or 'things'; the new theory proposed that particles might be better understood as forms of energy and relationships. Electrons, for example, were understood to be in a continual state of flux, sometimes with the properties of waves, sometimes of particles. This observation led to Heisenberg's 'uncertainty principle' and to Bohr's 'complementarity principle', which argued that the properties of particles are only definable and observable through their interaction with other systems.

The implication of the new subatomic physics was that certainty was replaced by probability, or the notion of tendencies rather than absolutes: 'we can never predict an atomic event with certainty; we can only predict the likelihood of its happening'.[14] Equally, the implication was that the properties and behaviour of things are better thought about in terms of systems and relationships rather than as individual components that can be examined separately. This directly contradicts the mechanistic model we explored above, and it implies that a subject such as normal birth needs to be looked at as a whole rather than by its parts. We discuss this further in the section on complexity.

If this approach is accepted, cause and effect need to be approached in a very different way. In particular, the role of the individual and relationships within the system must be taken into account. As we have noted, cross-cultural theory within anthropology proposed that the world is experienced and understood differently by different individuals according to the environmental, social and cultural shaping of that experience. Similarly, quantum and relativity theory in physics proposed that the consciousness of the observer is a part of and necessary to the whole. To do the experiment is to become part of it. Consciousness influences what is observed and the types of question asked influence the answers that can be obtained. This challenges the basic notion of an objective, certain and value-free science.

When we turn to the implications of this paradigm shift for our understanding of health, it becomes clear that the benefit or harm of an intervention for an individual can only be established with reasonable certainty by identifying and taking into account all the relevant 'noise'. This includes environment, carer attitudes, skills and beliefs, and the expectations of the woman and her family. Similarly, the appraisal of research evidence needs to consider the concepts, attitudes and roles of the researchers and how these may have framed or influenced the process of generating evidence. Such an approach may seem to be impossibly open-ended and complex. However, it is exactly the approach set out in the original proposals for evidence-based medicine described at the beginning of this chapter. In this version, best practice is a constructed position, dependent on the interactions between the practitioner, the research evidence and the service user; it will be different for each separate set of circumstances. Interpretation of these variables depends on the weight given to the potential factors involved by the individuals concerned. Since it is likely that all the risks and benefits relative to an intervention will never be established for populations, let alone for individuals, and that research produces probabilistic statistical findings, decisions must be made in a state of relative uncertainty. As David Sackett and his colleagues state: 'Diagnosis is not about finding absolute truth, but about limiting uncertainty ...' (p 92).[22]

There are a number of techniques that have been proposed for use in clinical practice to address these issues. These include likelihood ratios for diagnostic tests[22] and Bayesian techniques.[63–65] Both these approaches are based on finding out what the current state of evidence might be before adding in the results of a new trial or test. In the case of the likelihood ratio, the pre-test probability that an individual has a certain disease is estimated, based on their circumstances, the clinician's expertise and the evidence. A clinical test is undertaken, and the findings are put alongside the pre-test probability to estimate the likelihood that the individual does indeed have the condition being considered. In Bayesian theory, so-called 'priors' are established to find out the consensus about an intervention before a further study is undertaken. These priors can be established by groups of stakeholders, including service users. They can then be moderated by data arising from formal investigation, whether the data are generated from a strictly controlled randomized trial of sufficient size or not. This approach depends on recalculations of relative risk and sensitivity analyses after a new study or other piece of evidence is added to the prior probability.

The value of these methods of interpreting data lies in the fact they do not depend on black and white acceptance or rejection of a null hypothesis. They can give far more information to an individual than simply that based on aggregated population-based data. They also explicitly accept the fact that most researchers, and most users of research, have strong views about an intervention, and they bring this to their interpretation of new data.

To examine the issue of interpretation further, we want to explore another phenomenon. This is the issue of the time it takes to implement formal evidence into practice. The first example is of a technique that has been examined over many years and many trials, but which is still not well accepted or established in many hospitals. This is auscultation in labour for well women and babies. We have discussed the evidence in this area earlier in the chapter. However, there are recent examples of single trials that have led to widespread changes on the ground, even before authoritative guidelines from august bodies have been produced. The Term Breech Trial is a case in point.[66] A multicentre audit of practice in the sites where the trial was run, undertaken two years after the results were published, indicated that the vast majority had instituted the findings of the trial wholesale.[66,67] This is despite the findings in the original study that the advantages of caesarean section were less evident in some sites taking part in the study than in others, and also despite the warning of the authors of the current Cochrane review in this area: 'The data from this review cannot be generalised to settings where caesarean section is not readily available, or to methods of breech delivery that differ materially from the clinical delivery protocols used in the trials reviewed …'.[68] In this case, it seems that the evidence arising from the Term Breech Trial was so convincing, so certain, that changes were made immediately, worldwide, across disparate groups of individuals and without attention to the health-care setting, practitioners'

variable skills and knowledge, and women's beliefs and values or the impact of resource issues on how care is delivered. It is not clear if this change has persisted following publication of the two-year follow-up data which demonstrated that, taking account of deaths and neurodevelopmental delay from the point of randomization to two years after birth, there were no differences between the two groups: while mortality was higher in the vaginal birth group, neurodevelopmental delay was higher in the caesarean section group.[69]

What is the explanation for the difference in implementation of formal evidence between the two areas of practice? In each case, the studies seem to have been carefully designed and implemented. Why has one approach been so resistant to change and the other so amenable?

There are probably a number of possible explanations, from the economic to the technical. However, it seems likely that a good case could be made for suggesting that this response is based on belief systems, which, in turn, can be located in the cultural norms of post-industrial societies. At root, many if not most doctors, midwives, managers and birthing women believe that electronic fetal monitoring must be good for babies, as it provides apparently objective technical data. In addition, many if not most of us do not believe that women can birth breech babies spontaneously and safely, as this is an uncommon, and therefore, we assume, an abnormal/pathological position for the fetus to adopt. Prior beliefs in both the utility of cardiotocography and in the efficacy of caesarean section for breech babies are so strong that they continue to override the accumulating evidence against the belief in the former and rapidly accommodated the evidence for caesarean section in the latter. This may be seen as a case against the use of the creation of prior hypotheses as part of 'evidence', as recommended in Bayesian theory, since they can give credence to what may be unfounded certainties.[70] However, the advantage of using something like Bayes' theorem in interpreting evidence is that it makes researchers and practitioners face up to the role of belief. As Merry and colleagues state: 'Bayes' theorem provides the key to the ways in which beliefs should fit together in the light of changing evidence

… [it allows us] to establish rules and procedures for … disciplined uncertainty accounting (while maximizing utility) …'.[71]

In the use of such theory, priors could be constructed for population-based evidence, with input from a variety of views and beliefs, including those of lay commentators. They could also be constructed in clinical practice, with the input of both the practitioner(s) concerned and the individual childbearing woman. Such 'disciplined uncertainty accounting', if we were to formalize it, may reveal a number of profound flaws in our current approach to birth. Its use would allow us to acknowledge the relative uncertainties of applying formal research to individuals. While all good-quality evidence is valid in this construction of knowledge, one trial with simple protocols, or even an infinite number of such trials, cannot give us certainty of acting in the context of any single individual. Such trials can only give us more or less support for our beliefs. Very convincing trials may even change our beliefs, as in the case of the Back to Sleep studies.[72,73] As Salsburg states:[74]

There is no 'correct' (approach). Scientific reasoning consists of attempts to fit the complexities of reality into models useful for the organisation of observations … some fit for the time being until we can find one that fits better, or until the lack of fit begins to trouble us. But we must always recognize that we fit our observations to very arbitrary models, and we must be prepared to abandon a model if it leads to nonsense.

Acknowledging uncertainty leads us to question some current accepted views about the nature of normal birth. As discussed in Chapter 4, the commonly quoted definitions tend to include specific features, such as gestation, position of the fetal head and length of labour, as prerequisites for 'normality'. However, issues of relativity, uncertainty and belief systems begin to suggest that the absolutism of these kinds of approach may be misleading. They may be a factor in the nonsense of our apparently headlong rush to intervene in large numbers of labours that would otherwise progress physiologically if left alone. This leads us to explore alternative ways of approaching the problem, through theories of complexity and chaos.

Complexity and chaos

A solution to the dissonance between the evidence claims of much of the current research in health and health care, and its apparent lack of application to individuals, may lie in the very heart of quantitative knowledge, namely quantum physics. This profoundly 'scientific' branch of physics is fundamentally linked to observations that the natural systems of the world are not simple and predictable, but complex and chaotic.

Theories of complexity and chaos arose simultaneously in a number of fields. The terms are often used interchangeably, though some maintain that chaos is a function of the non-linearity, or non-periodic pattern, of complex systems. The meteorologist Edward Lorenz is credited with the crucial first insights into 'deterministic non-periodic flow' in the early 1960s.[75] The rapidly expanding theoretical and mathematical developments in complexity and chaos have influenced fields as diverse as management theory and cardiac regulation.[76,77] However, a number of authors have cautioned against oversimplistic generalization of the seductive post-modernist aspects of multiplicity and connectivity that are expressed in these theories. Carol Haigh, writing from a nursing perspective, sees the misuse of chaos theory as being particularly prevalent within nursing research and philosophy.[78] She cautioned that application of the chaos construct is not relevant without a thorough understanding and use of the mathematical underpinning of the theories. While we accept her thesis to some extent, we depart from her apparent rejection of the potential for the insights of complexity and chaos to provide new ways of seeing health at the macro level. We agree, however, that applied research in this area will need to pay attention to the mathematical and statistical tools that have been developed to support research from this perspective.

Carol Haigh alluded to a number of nursing theorists in her critique of the use of chaos theory. As we have noted above, primary-care practitioners have also published accounts of complexity in practice.[62,79] However, only very recently have a small number of researchers begun to engage with the potential of this approach for understanding childbirth.[79-81] The rest of this section sets out some of the central tenets of complexity theory and provides some initial insights into how it could be applied in the context of childbirth.

The power of complexity theory lies in the observation that events are profoundly interconnected. The concept of a simple linear process is replaced with the metaphor of a web or network of interconnections. It therefore challenges the assumption that there is a one 'right' way of doing things for everyone, and all we have to do is to find it and then stick to it. Rightness becomes 'problematized', because we are usually basing our judgement on only one part of the story. Take the professional insistence on laying all babies on their face to prevent inhalation of vomit until more recent evidence has persuaded us that this practice is linked to higher rates of cot death for some babies. We still do not know which babies benefit from the new approaches and which may be disadvantaged. Complexity holds that, even if we have good trial data for populations, we cannot know many of the wider long-term consequences of implementing such a policy, or any other such policy (such as auscultation every 15 minutes in labour, widespread implementation of midwife-led units or caesarean section for babies presenting by the breech).

The phenomenon of connectivity is formally termed 'sensitive dependence on initial conditions'. It has been brought to the popular imagination through the concept of the 'butterfly effect': the idea that 'a butterfly flaps its wings in the jungle and there is a hurricane in New York'. This suggests that small changes within systems may achieve large effects while large changes may achieve small effects.[79] While the example may sound overly romantic, the point is that any simple input into a dynamic system, such as the weather, an organization or a labouring woman, will have consequences that are not linear but which bifurcate – that is, a + b = c & d, b + c = e & f, b + d = g & h and so on ad infinitum. Figure 1.2 sets this out graphically. The diagram is generated from a computer set to track changes in a chaotic system (such as the weather or heart rate patterns). It is clear that the way the system progresses is, at first, predictable: it is a straight line. However, at a certain point, the system reaches a moment when it tips from this smoothly linear progression into a so-called 'chaotic region'.

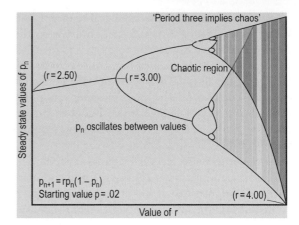

Fig 1.2 • Bifurcation diagram.

It may go one of two ways at this point and then, quickly, the divisions (or bifurcations) happen again and again, until they become so frequent that the system becomes chaotic and unpredictable.

What is apparent is that, although the way the individual paths divide may seem to be random and chaotic, the overall pattern is regular (as in Bateson's example of Brownian motion and the boiling point of water molecules). There is order in the chaos. This is determined by the connections between and the overall connectivity of the wider system. This reverses the notion in positivistic science that the parts determine the behaviour of the whole.

So, to take an extremely simplified example, a woman who is 'overdue' and who is told that this is dangerous for her baby and she should accept induction (or who is fed up and wants induction) has an emotional response to the news, which has neurohormonal consequences. This responsive neurohormonal state provides an unpredictable basis for receiving prostaglandin. The effects of the prostaglandin interact with her emotional state and her feelings of loneliness if her chosen companions are not there, or relaxation if they are. Her unpredictable response to pain interacts with her unknown physiology to create an unpredictable physiological response to the prostin gel … and so on. While the overall pattern (the labour proceeds and the baby is born) may be predictable, the interacting elements and process that produce this outcome are not simple.

In opposition to this physiological reality, labour and birth are currently managed in a framework that seeks to bind these essentially complex and relatively unpredictable processes into ever tighter constraints to ensure certainty. This clash of realities carries potential dangers on the physiological, emotional, spiritual and psychological level, for both mother and baby. Some of these consequences are explored in other chapters in this book.

Beyond the issue of constraining unpredictable processes, complexity theorists indicate that change as opposed to stasis is an indication of an effective dynamical system, and that: 'complex adaptive systems adapt to, and on, the edge of chaos ... Systems in the complex region ... can adapt most readily ...'.[71] This means that systems that show unpredictable behaviour are those most likely to be healthy, and to innovate. The metaphor often given here is of a heart in persistent sinusoidal rhythm – the pattern is smooth and highly predictable at both the macro and the micro level. It often indicates pathology. In contrast, a healthy heart produces a clear pattern of activity at the macro level, but shows wide variation and unpredictability at the micro level. This indicates its capacity to adapt dynamically to changing situations and stressors within and outside of the body. Applying this thinking to labour seems to imply that it is at the time when labour is at its most complex, its most unpredictable, its least controllable, that the maternal and infant system can most easily make the necessary changes in so-called 'phase space' to move from one aspect of labour to another: to make a 'phase transition'.[79] It may even imply that if systems such as labour are not allowed to progress to the edge of chaos, the body cannot make the dynamic changes necessary to accomplish essential phase transitions. Ilya Prigogine, Nobel Prize winner in the area of quantum physics, talked of this as 'from being to becoming' in the context of quantum mechanics.[82] It is also termed a *far-from-equilibrium state*. This is not necessarily a negative concept. It is in far-from-equilibrium states that the most positive changes to systems can occur. This does not mean states that are fundamentally out of control. It does mean states that do not conform to obvious and predictable patterns. They are subject to the phenomenon called the 'strange attractor'. James Gleick describes the process by which David Ruelle and Floris Taken came to this concept (p 132–4),[75] which they saw as a phenomenon that pulls processes and organisms out of the edge of chaos and into a new more stable phase space.

An example of the strange attractor at work in labour may be transition. This is a time when the rhythm of labour changes pace, when many women feel themselves to be in an unfamiliar place, and when their requests and pleas can be interpreted as demanding a 'fix', rather than support for the adjustment needed. If women are supported through transition, it moves from an apparently chaotic state into the calmer more organized space of spontaneous bearing down, or to the so-called 'rest and be thankful' phase. Such states in labour are within the pull of the 'strange attractor', which may be a hormonal cue, a function of the practitioner's technological or physiological outlook or any number of other interconnected factors: '[the state of] ... "far from equilibrium" ... allow(s) an alternative attractor to define a new context for the system ...'.[83] The actual attractors in operation remain to be discovered by formal research.

Complex systems have emergent properties. Sweeney and Griffiths understood emergence to be 'the phenomenon by which new properties arise through the complex interactions and connectivity of lower order processes' (p 42).[79] This implies that the sum of the functioning of parts considered separately is seldom equal to the functioning of the whole. Ackoff gave the example of constructing a car to illustrate this: 'if you picked the best parts from a range of vehicles to make up a supercar you may well find it doesn't work at all'.[84] This is because the whole is dependent on interactions of parts. As Merry states: '... behaviour can be predicted by studying how elements interact and how the system adapts and changes throughout time ... the complex system cannot be understood by reducing it to its parts' (p 58).[71] However, raising the possibility that birth is a complex adaptive process raises the possibility that we can begin to understand it in a different and possibly more meaningful way in the future. This work has still barely begun.

Applying complexity: from linearity to cycles of knowledge development

This complexity theory way of seeing may seem to be seductive but ultimately useless. If labour is seen as being so incredibly complex, how can it ever be understood? Luckily, one of the current theories of complex adaptive systems is that they may be underpinned by simple rules. This may seem to be counterintuitive. The classic example of the flocking behaviour of computer generated birds (termed 'boids') may make it more understandable. Observed casually, the way birds flock in the sky seems to be completely random or non-predictable and yet it forms a pattern. However, as Sweeney and Griffiths note,[79] three simple rules (derived originally from studies of chemical reactions, and modelled on the computer generated 'boids') may explain the ability of this apparently chaotic behaviour to produce patterns. These are:

1. Maintain a minimum distance from other boids.
2. Match the velocity of the other boids in the neighbourhood.
3. Try to move towards the perceived centre of the flock.

Running a computer program based on these rules results in apparently random flocking behaviour that, nevertheless, exhibits underlying if complex patterning. It is of interest that the rules describe the dynamic nature of the relationship between each boid and the next. They are not reductive to the parts of the flock, but descriptive of how the parts fit together. This emphasizes the importance of connectivity in complex systems.

The observation that simple rules of relationship may help in describing the behaviour of complex systems offers the potential for understanding a phenomenon such as transition in labour without recourse to exhaustive description of every influence upon it. If similar rules of connectivity could be identified that encompass the wide range of normal-but-not-average variation in pregnancy and labour, we may be in a position to begin to move away from rules of practice that only describe a narrow band of the 'average' normal.

Building on the connectivity described by complexity and systems theorists, an alternative

to the linear view of scientific progress is that the process of knowledge development is essentially cyclical, as in Figure 1.3. Science works through cycles of observation and inductive thinking, theory development and testing, reflection and evaluation. Effective research proceeds by raising new and more informed questions as much as by seeking to provide answers. Analogies can be drawn between this approach and the operation of complex feedback mechanisms. The specific graphical example given in Figure 1.4, again related to social support in labour, may serve to illustrate the point.

Based on the arguments we have set out above, we assert that even the most apparently simple interventions in childbirth are framed by (and, crucially, dependent upon) the 'noise' of beliefs, skills and values. In claiming this, we are not suggesting that linear models, or indeed randomized controlled trials, do not have an important and powerful role in research. They work within certain parameters. What we do suggest is that they form important links within a wider cycle of knowledge development. We also suggest that even this cyclical view must be considered as taking place within complex systems. It does not necessarily proceed in an orderly manner, from lack of knowledge to enlightenment. As Bateson argues: 'all you have is the hope of simplicity, since the next fact may drive you to the next level of complexity'.[19] This implies a shift in thinking away from the notion of the randomized controlled trial as the 'gold standard' of evidence for medicine, to the notion of the trial as an important but partial aspect of the evidence base for care. To be effective, experimental research needs to build on considerable prior knowledge, much of which will need to be developed using a range of methodologies and taking into account a range of considerations. Its findings will need to be interpreted in the light of knowledge of the wider system of which it forms a controlled part.

In 2000, the UK Medical Research Council published guidelines for research on what it saw as the special case of overtly 'complex' interventions, such as the introduction of multicomponent systems.[85] While this is valuable, it does not take into account the possibility that the majority of the unanswered questions in health-care provision

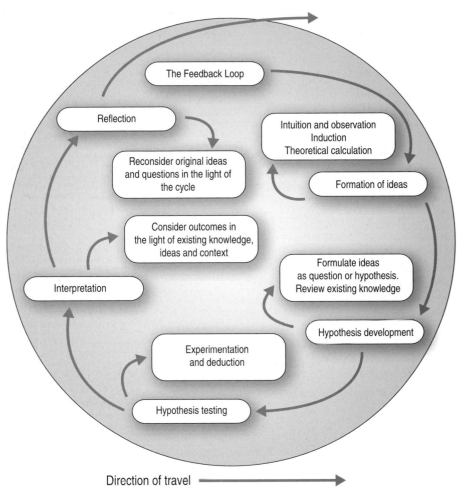

The Feedback Loop

Reflection

Intuition and observation
Induction
Theoretical calculation

Reconsider original ideas
and questions in the light of
the cycle

Formation of ideas

Consider outcomes in
the light of existing knowledge,
ideas and context

Formulate ideas
as question or hypothesis.
Review existing knowledge

Interpretation

Hypothesis development

Experimentation
and deduction

Hypothesis testing

Direction of travel

Fig 1.3 • Science/knowledge development as a cycle.

and policy entails complexity, in the sense we are discussing. In order to examine the feasibility of taking this approach in practice, we turn next to a discussion of systems theory as a model for ways of encapsulating complexity in research, practice and care provision.[86] According to this theory, cause and effect involves uncertainty and contingency. Contingency means that effects are dependent on the situation, may be influenced by a range of factors and are, therefore, never absolutely predictable. Additionally, an action may have unintended as well as intended consequences. Again, key advocates of evidence-based medicine allow for this when they note that the 'best' evidence is always provisional, not certain. Instead of a linear relationship between

cause and effect, this approach rests on the kind of web of connections, or connectivity, identified by complexity theorists. Systems analysis has played a major role in the thinking in economics and business modelling, and in more obviously scientific disciplines such as climatology.

To look at how this could be relevant to the understanding of normal birth, we want to look in detail at Hodnett's work on labour support. In reporting on this body of work to a conference on research in the area of normal childbirth, Hodnett noted how she had come full circle in her thinking. Her research career started with the question, based on her experience as a labour nurse, 'why do some women go out of labour after hospital admission?'.

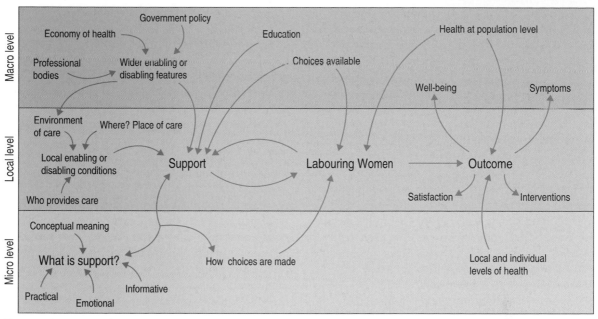

Fig 1.4 • Simplified example of influences on input and outcome in relation to social support and labouring women.

Through a series of classic trials and overviews of trials, which were based in positivist linear thinking and which were very well designed according to these tenets, she investigated the importance of the continuing presence of a support nurse in labour, seeing this as the active ingredient in preventing the problem of stalled labour, and its potentially adverse consequences. Despite nurses' perceptions of improved awareness and ability to provide support in her latest trial, following in-depth training,[87] the intervention was found to make no difference to almost all the outcomes assessed. To understand this paradox, Hodnett found herself returning to her original question about the environment of care: why, given the systematic review evidence on the effectiveness of labour support, did labour support apparently make no difference in practice in this trial? 'Bottom line: it's the environment. I've come full circle.'[88]

In acknowledging the contextual influences in this study, and in a subsequent Cochrane review of home-like settings for place of birth,[89] Ellen Hodnett and her colleagues have begun to incorporate the integral effect of context and 'noise' in trials of complex health interventions. Beyond

this lesson from complex adaptive systems thinking comes another insight from emergence. Wilson and colleagues make the following claim: 'health can only be maintained (or re-established) through a holistic approach that accepts unpredictability and builds on subtle emergent forces with the overall system'.[83] Accepting this claim would allow us to move away from trying to understand and categorize every aspect of variation as potentially pathological. We could then spend our time trying to see how the system works as a whole for each individual. The next section picks up this possibility in the specific context of salutogenesis.

Salutogenesis

We have discussed above our claim that current systems of health care are rooted in pathology. This is despite the pronouncement by the World Health Organization that health is a state of well-being.[90] Outside of clinical research, there have been a number of psychological and sociological studies of the nature of well-being. Within the maternity services, however, as we have noted, most outcome measures are focused on morbidity.

We wish to propose that practice, research and policy development in the maternity services should instead be framed by the concept of salutogenesis, or the generation of well-being. This term was coined by an American researcher named Aaron Antonovsky in 1979.[91] We do not propose that all elements of Antonovsky's approach should be taken up. However, in order to set the framework for our application of the concept, we set out the basic principles of his thesis below.

Antonovsky developed his initial theories while researching survivors of Holocaust concentration camps. He expected to find high levels of pathology and social disintegration. However, to his surprise, he found that some survivors had high levels of optimism and social success. This phenomenon caused Antonovsky to ask the question: 'how is it that some people survive such terrible experiences apparently completely intact emotionally and spiritually, and others disintegrate entirely?'. His further studies indicated that the answer lies in connections: in the connectivity between individuals, their experience and their social histories. In this sense, the concept of salutogenesis differs markedly from other well-being theories, or, for example, concepts of mastery or self-efficacy, which see the essence of well-being in self-empowerment.

Antonovsky challenged the current biomedical discourse, arguing that: 'A salutogenic orientation, concerned with overall health, pressures one to think in systems terms … it leads one to seek to understand and deal with all the entropic [disorder-promoting] forces and … negentropic [order-promoting] forces …' (p 115).[92] In the same paper, he goes on to pose the following fundamental question: 'We are all familiar with the concept of a risk factor. Can we not think of the concept of a salutary factor?' (p 116).

As can be seen, Antonovsky's theories fit well with the complex, uncertain systems-orientated approach we have set out in the preceding sections. His philosophy opens the door to turning the concept of risk systems on its head. Rather than starting with a long list of conditions and social situations that rule women out of having a physiological birth, maybe in a stand-alone unit or at home, the idea of positive or order-promoting forces allows a woman to bring salutogenic aspects of her clinical, emotional, social,

spiritual and family history to the table. For example, a woman who has a family history of prolonged gestation or long labours may not be entering the realms of pathology when her pregnancy reaches the 42nd week, or her active labour has gone on for 10 hours with only small apparent signs of progress, but with mother and baby coping well. A woman with a previous history of a stillbirth following a premature labour may be ideally suited to have her baby in a free-standing unit if she feels that, emotionally, this is one way to heal the trauma of her past experiences, and she is now at 38 weeks of gestation. A well-controlled diabetic may do better relaxed in the care of midwives she knows than tense in a highly monitored environment with highly skilled carers she does not know. All these situations may maximize the opportunity for normal birth. Some researchers suggest that maximizing normal birth may even have unlooked-for consequences on maternal and, therefore, infant biochemistry and neurohormones.[93–95] Indeed, in his 1979 publication, Antonovsky was beginning to explore connections between his work and psychoneuroimmunology in adults. A 1999 German review of Antonovsky's own work and that of researchers associated with it demonstrated that the field appeared to be under-researched at the time.[96] A more recent review of nearly 500 studies, published in 2006, indicated associations between the so-called sense of coherence construct and perceived health across a range of population groups.[97] This was particularly striking for psychological well-being. The evidence was less clear for physical health.

Antonovsky proposed that individuals who score highly on the sense of coherence (SOC) construct tend to experience high levels of well-being, with a strong sense of positive health, even in apparently extreme circumstances. The SOC equates somewhat to the psychological concept of 'buffering',[98] but it is more than simply a protective barrier. It has three components: meaningfulness, manageability and comprehensibility:

1. Meaningfulness: the deep feeling that life makes sense emotionally; that life's demands are worthy of commitment. It is essentially seeing coping as desirable.
2. Manageability: the extent to which people feel they have the resources to meet the demands, or feeling that they know where to go to get help.

3. Comprehensibility: the extent to which a person finds or structures their world to be understandable, meaningful, orderly and consistent instead of random and unpredictable. Paradoxically, a strong sense of coherence appears to help individuals cope with chaos and uncertainty when they do encounter it.

Antonovsky held that the development of the sense of coherence is a product of infancy and childhood. He believed that if a sense of coherence was not well developed by the time an individual was a young adult (and, more precisely, before they reached their 30s), it was unlikely to develop further in later life. He emphasized that the components necessary for its occurrence included personal and familial elements, and community and societal factors.[91] He also held that societies (at least within small groupings) could exhibit a sense of coherence. This perspective reverberates with concepts of community capacity and social capital, which are gaining credibility in policy circles in a number of countries.[99]

We feel that the fundamental components of salutogenesis as proposed by Antonovsky are potentially powerful factors in optimum childbearing. We also concur with the overall concept of salutogenic well-being as the product of a complex personal and societal interaction, and with the reformulation of health care and health research towards a way of seeing that is salutary as opposed to pathogenic. However, we diverge from Antonovsky's view that a sense of coherence is largely fixed by the time of early adulthood. We contend that major life-changing events, such as childbirth, could have a profound effect, and that this, in turn, can have an impact on the social capital necessary to promote a positive sense of coherence in others, including children, the wider family and local communities.

One clear practice-based example of our contention is that of the La Paz project in Brazil. Brazil is a country with extremely high caesarean section rates. A recent population-based study in Sao Paulo state found rates of 32.9% in the public sector and 80.4% in the private sector in 2001–2003.[100] Levels have been high for at least a generation. In 2001, a collaborative group of Japanese and Brazilian researchers reported on a project that set out to make changes in practice with a view to influencing ways of birth in one particular Brazilian hospital.[101] Prior to the implementation of changes, women were in labour without privacy or companionship, and with routine pharmacological and technological intervention. Before starting the project, the researchers asked the local community what the most important health issues were. Childhood diarrhoea was at the top of the list. The implementation phase took two years. It involved simple changes, like installing curtains round labour beds for privacy, allowing companions for the women in labour and making the rooms warmer. At the end of the two years, members of the community were again asked what the most important health issues were for them. While childhood diarrhoea was still seen to be important, normal birth was at the top of the list. Beyond this, the researchers note: '"Project Luz" has given many women the feeling of strong confidence in a safe delivery and child rearing … leading to self-transformation, which empowers them profoundly. This … raises their concerns about society, their lives, and motivates their participation in community activities and development.' (p S1).[101]

While a sense of coherence was not assessed in the Project Luz study, there are elements of manageability, meaningfulness and comprehensibility in the above account. Beyond this, there are issues of social capital. The value of positive and respectful birth, then, may have implications for societal well-being. Again, these issues remain to be explored in the future.

As an example of a systems approach that is rooted in a salutogenic philosophy, the Ontario Women's Health Council (OWHC) of Canada took a conscious decision to look at positive (salutogenic in Antonovsky's terminology) factors in childbirth, by investigating units with low rates of caesarean section as opposed to those with high rates, in order to understand what made things go right.[102] The 12 characteristics identified in the four units studied included pride in a low caesarean section rate, one-to-one care in labour and belief that birth was a normal process. As noted above, one of us (SD) has previously discussed the potential of a salutogenic way of seeing as both a way of maximizing the potential for optimum birthing and an outcome measure for birth.[2] This use of the concept, in synergy with acknowledgement of connectivity, would allow for the design of birth settings and of supportive care that consciously maximizes a sense of coherence in the birthing woman. Some aspects of this are pursued further in Chapter 3. Such changes to the way of doing birth would not privilege either technological or physiological approaches. Instead, they would acknowledge that each woman and her baby enter pregnancy, childbirth and the postnatal period with a unique set of circumstances and 'initial conditions' in the complexity theory sense. In this context, the woman, baby and caregiver would be partners in a dynamic process, in which the mother feels emotionally as well as physically safe.

Salutogenesis gives us a new framework for understanding women's experiences of labour. It permits us an understanding of how we can base maternity care and research in this area on promoting positive well-being as a primary approach, with the identification and treatment of pathology as a component rather than a driver. Such an understanding can extend beyond individuals to systems and organizations, as is illustrated in the Brazilian and Canadian studies described above. This way of seeing may also maximize the contribution of childbearing women to the social capital of their community, as was evidenced in La Paz. This potential remains to be evaluated.

Implications of the new way of seeing for normal birth

As we said at the beginning of this chapter, the impetus to examine the sometimes rather obscure ideas and theories set out in the preceding sections arose from the difficulty one of us (SD) found in trying to define and understand 'normal birth'.[1,2,57,103,104] Throughout this book, various authors have examined aspects of normality and, in Chapter 4, Beverley Beech and Belinda Phipps offer a useful account of different definitions in use currently. Our understanding of the nature of normality has been profoundly influenced by the theories we have explored, and by the new

framework of complexity, uncertainty, non-linearity and salutogenesis that we propose for health care in general, and for childbearing in particular. While Ann Oakley's discussion of birth as a normal process is relevant to our thinking in this area,[105] it is the brief discussion of 'normalizing uniqueness' by Robbie Davis-Floyd and Elizabeth Davis that has captured our imagination.[60] The discussion takes place in the context of an examination of intuition in midwifery knowledge and home birth. The authors state: 'The midwifery normalization of uniqueness must be understood in the context of the technomedical pathologization of uniqueness' (p 165).[60] Their chapter sets out numerous examples of midwives' responses to uncertainty, to connectivity in labour, to sensitivity to initial conditions and to recognition of edge-of-chaos, far-from-equilibrium and phase states. Examples are cited where the woman's sense of coherence is illustrated. Cyclical, non-linear patterns of care, support and decision making are illustrated. These conceptual terms are not used in the chapter, and neither author makes reference to the theories we have expounded above. However, in their exposition of a midwife's 'intuitive' response to the 'unique normality' of labour, our theories appear to come together. Davis-Floyd and Arvidson[46] address the topic of intuition in depth and from a range of disciplinary perspectives, but it has rarely been explored rigorously in the midwifery literature. In a meta-synthesis of literature on maternity care expertise, intuition emerged as a component of what was termed 'enacted vocation'.[106] The authors did not see intuition as mysterious, but, following Benner,[107] as a process that is: 'built on the knowledge, understanding and experience that precedes the intuitive leap' (p 136).[106]

This seems to describe a non-linear way of thinking, with a high level of dynamic connectivity between knowledge, understanding and experience. Expert practitioners with this orientation are likely to approach normal birth with an appreciation that it is a dynamic and non-linear process. In this construction, each woman's labour is unique to her and her baby, and to the interaction and connectivity between her personal and familial history, her biophysical processes and those of her fetus, the environment in which she labours, the attitude and response of the caregiver(s) and a multitude of other factors.

We are left, then, back in what appears to be some confusion. If we cannot define normality in precise terms, how can we measure and quantify it? Are we really saying that everything is relative, and that high rates of intervention and morbidity, and low rates of well-being, are acceptable?

No, we are not taking this position. Our stance is that well-being is maximized by a salutogenic approach to birth, in which a sense of coherence in the woman, baby and family is maximized. It is likely that, for most women, this outcome is promoted by maximizing the possibility of physiological birth, while optimizing the experience of necessary intervention for the few who need it, whether this need is clinical, psychological, emotional or spiritual. The promotion of the conditions for physiological birth is best achieved by the recognition of flexible definitions of normality, understood in the context of uncertainty, non-linearity and complexity. We believe that this recognition of the 'unique normality' of each woman should be a fundamental midwifery skill, and it should be recognized and supported by other health professionals and the health-care systems within which caregivers operate.

Conclusions

As described by Rose,[108] the preferred philosophical stance for the underpinning science of normal birth is that which is generated from 'hand, brain and heart'. In an Egyptian context, this has been reinterpreted as 'skilled help from the heart'.[109] Without this understanding of the complexity of birth, the uncertainty of our knowledge in the area and the salutogenic potential of childbearing, we approach normality with very limited vision.

We believe that our exploration in this chapter of the recent history of scientific thought and of theories from fields as far apart as physics and psychology has been a positive move towards optimizing birth.[110] What we are advocating is not a rejection of science but a movement on from the 'art or science?' dichotomy. Science needs to be reclaimed from the narrow, positivist construction that has effectively dominated health research and the evidence-based health movement to date, and the artistry of clinical practice (in midwifery and obstetrics) needs to be reconstructed as a legitimate skill for dealing with contingency. In the process, we may come to acknowledge what most expert practitioners know: clinical artistry and science are not as distinct as we have tended to assume.

Perhaps we can learn something by looking back at Mendel's work on inheritance. Mendel was a monk, scientist and gardener. His studies, which formed the foundation for modern genetic theory, were virtually overlooked in the 19th century, perhaps because they did not fit the paradigm of his time and society. Mendel combined careful extended observation, intuition, inductive and deductive theory development and experimental testing. His work was rooted in the tacit knowledge of gardening, a complex ecological system, yet he was able to use theory to identify fundamental simple principles within that complex system. Research, by contributing to the development of knowledge, by providing evidence of various kinds and as part of decision making for better health care, could be seen in a similar way.

We recognize that our proposal that childbirth should be framed by the concept of 'unique normality' is currently more of a manifesto than a reality. We are grateful to the many thinkers whose ideas and theories we have used as building blocks for our proposals. We hope that you, our readers, will find something of interest in what we have said, and that it will inspire you to explore further this fascinating and crucial topic, normal birth.

References

1. Downe S 2000 A proposal for a new research and practice agenda for birth. MIDIRS Midwif Digest 10:337–341

2. Downe S 2006 Engaging with the concept of unique normality in childbirth. British Journal of Midwifery 14(6):352–356

3. McCourt C 2005 Research and theory for nursing and midwifery: rethinking the nature of evidence. Worldviews on Evidence-based Nursing 2(2):1–9

4. Beake S, McCourt C, Page L 1998 The use of clinical audit in evaluating maternity services reform: a critical reflection. J Eval Clin Pract 4:75–83

5. Berger J 1990 Ways of seeing. Penguin, London

6. Cochrane A L 1972 Effectiveness and efficiency: random reflections on health services. Nuffield and Provincial Hospitals Trust, London

7. Oakley A 1992 Social support and motherhood. The natural history of a research project. Blackwell, Oxford

8. Jordan B 1993 Birth in four cultures: a cross-cultural investigation of childbirth in Yucatan, Holland, Sweden and the United States. Waveland Press, Champaign, IL

9. Davis-Floyd R E, Sargent C F 1997 Childbirth and authoritative knowledge; cross cultural perspectives. University of California Press, Berkeley, CA

10. Weaver J 2002 Court ordered caesarean sections. In: Bainham A, Day-Sclater S, Richards M (eds) Body lore and laws. Hart, Oxford

11. Samuels T-A, Minkoff H, Feldman J et al 2007 Obstetricians, health attorneys, and court-ordered cesarean sections. Womens Health Issues 17(2): 107–114

12. Hampson N 1968 The enlightenment. Penguin, Harmondsworth

13. Gribben J 2002 Science. A history. Allen Lane, London

14. Capra F 1983 The turning point: science, society, and the rising culture. Fontana, London

15. Popper K 1959 The logic of scientific discovery. Harper and Row, New York

16. Kuhn T S 1970 The structure of scientific revolutions. University of Chicago Press, London

17. Martin E 1989 The woman in the body. Open University Press, Milton Keynes

18. Yusuf S, Collins R, Peto R 1984 Why do we need some large, simple randomized trials? Stat Med 3:409–420

19. Bateson G 1985 Mind and nature. A necessary unity. Fontana, London

20. Jelinek M 1992 The clinician and the randomised controlled trial. In: Daly J, McDonald I, Willis E (eds) Researching health care: designs, dilemmas, disciplines. Tavistock Routledge, London, p 76–89

21. Sackett D, Rosenberg W, Muir Gray J et al 1996 Evidence based medicine: what it is and what it isn't. Br Med J 312:71–72

22. Sackett D L, Straus S E, Richardson W S et al 2002 Evidence based medicine. How to practice and teach EBM. Churchill Livingstone, Edinburgh

23. National Institute for Health and Clinical Excellence (UK) 2007 The guidelines manual 2007: Chapter 7. Online. Available: http://www.nice.org.uk/page.aspx?o=422950 (accessed 13 August 2007)

24. Duff M, Winter C (In press) The progress of labour. Orderly chaos? In: McCourt C (ed.) Time and childbirth. Berghahn, Oxford

25. Royal Australian and New Zealand College of Obstetricians and Gynaecologists 2006 Intrapartum fetal surveillance clinical guidelines, 2nd edn. Online. Available: http://www.ranzcog.edu.au/publications/womenshealth.shtml#IFSG (accessed 13 August 2007)

26. National Institute for Health and Clinical Excellence (UK) 2001 Inherited clinical guideline C. Electronic fetal monitoring: the use and interpretation of cardiotocography in intrapartum fetal surveillance. Online. Available: http://guidance.nice.org.uk/CGC (accessed 13 August 2007)

27. Society of Obstetricians and Gynaecologists of Canada 2002 Fetal health surveillance in labour (Part II). Online. Available: http://www.sogc.org/guidelines/index_e.asp#Obstetrics (accessed 13 August 2007)

28. Alfirevic Z, Devane D, Gyte G M L 2006 Continuous cardiotocography (CTG) as a form of electronic fetal monitoring (EFM) for fetal assessment during labour. Cochrane Database Syst Rev, Issue 3. Art. No.: CD006066. DOI: 10.1002/14651858.CD006066

29. Macdonald D, Grant A, Sheridan-Pereira M et al 1985 The Dublin randomized controlled trial of intrapartum fetal heart rate monitoring. Am J Obstet Gynecol 152:524–539

30. Walker D S, Shunkwiler S, Supanich J et al 2001 Labor and delivery nurses' attitudes toward intermittent fetal monitoring. J Midwifery Womens Health 46:374–380

31. Gülmezoglu A M, Crowther C A, Middleton P 2006 Induction of labour for improving birth outcomes for women at or beyond term. Cochrane Database Syst Rev, Issue 4. Art. No.: CD004945. DOI: 10.1002/14651858.CD004945.pub2

32. Department of Health 2005 UK statistical bulletin. NHS maternity statistics, England: 2003–04. Online. Available: http://www.dh.gov.uk/en/Publicationsandstatistics/Publications/PublicationsStatistics/DH_4107060 (accessed 13 August 2007)

33. Hodnett E D, Fredericks S 2003 Support during pregnancy for women at increased risk of low birthweight babies. Cochrane Database Syst Rev, Issue 3. Art. No.: CD000198. DOI: 10.1002/14651858.CD000198

34. Mander R 2001 Supportive care and midwifery. Blackwell, Oxford

35. McCourt C 2003 Social support. In: Squire C (ed.) The social context of childbirth. Radcliffe Medical Press, Oxford

36. Gupta J K, Hofmeyr G J, Smyth R 2004 Position in the second stage of labour for women without epidural anaesthesia. Cochrane Database Syst Rev, Issue 1. Art. No.: CD002006. DOI: 10.1002/14651858.CD002006.pub2

37. O'Driscoll K, Meagher D 1980 Active management of labour. Clinics in obstetrics and gynaecology. Saunders, London

38. O'Driscoll K, Foley M, MacDonald D et al 1984 Active management of labour as an alternative to cesarean section for dystocia. Obstet Gynecol 63:485–490

39. Thornton J G, Lilford R J 1994 Active management of labour: current knowledge and research issues. Br Med J 309:366–369

40. Foley M E, Alarab M, Daly L et al 2004 The continuing effectiveness of active management of first labor, despite a doubling in overall nulliparous cesarean delivery. Am J Obstet Gynecol 191(3):891–895

41. Davis-Floyd R 1994 The technocratic body: American childbirth as cultural expression. Soc Sci Med 38: 1125–1140

42. Hodnett E D, Gates S, Hofmeyr G J et al 2003 Continuous support for women during childbirth. Cochrane Database Syst Rev, Issue 3. Art. No.: CD003766. DOI: 10.1002/14651858.CD003766. pub2

43. Kernick D 2002 The demise of linearity in managing health services: a call for post normal health care. J Health Serv Res Policy 7:121–124

44. Schon D A 1983 The reflective practitioner. Basic Books, New York

45. Benner P, Tanner C A, Chesla C A 1996 Expertise in nursing practice. Caring, clinical judgement and ethics. Springer, New York

46. Davis-Floyd R, Arvidson P S 1997 Intuition: the inside story. Routledge, New York

47. Edwards A, Elwyn G, Hood K et al 2000 Judging the 'weight of evidence' in systematic reviews: introducing rigour into the qualitative overview stage by assessing signal and noise. J Eval Clin Pract 6:177–184

48. Bloch M 1967 From cognition to ideology. In: Ritual, history and power. Selected papers in anthropology: London School of Economics Monographs on Social Anthropology No. 58. Athlone Press, London

49. Thompson E P 1967 Time, work-discipline, and industrial capitalism. Past Present 38:56–97

50. Friedman E A 1978 Labour: clinical evaluation and management, 2nd edn. Appleton-Century-Crofts, New York

51. Studd J W, Philpott R H 1972 Partograms and action line of cervical dilatation. Proc R Soc Med 65:700–701

52. Frankenberg R (ed.) 1992 Time, health and medicine. Sage, London

53. Simonds W 2002 Watching the clock: keeping time during pregnancy, birth, and postpartum experiences. Soc Sci Med 55:559–570

54. McCourt C (ed.) In press. Time and childbirth. Berghahn, Oxford

55. Lennon G G 1962 Diagnosis in clinical obstetrics. John Wright & Sons, Bristol, p 196

56. Garrey M M, Govan A D T, Hodge C et al 1980 Obstetrics illustrated, 3rd edn. Churchill Livingstone, Edinburgh

57. Downe S 1996 Concepts of normality in the maternity services: application and consequences. In: Frith L (ed.) Ethics and midwifery: issues in contemporary practice. Butterworth Heinemann, Oxford, p 86–103

58. Albers L L, Schiff M, Gorwoda J G 1996 The length of active labor in normal pregnancies. Obstet Gynecol 87:355–359

59. Albers L L 1999 The duration of labor in healthy women. J Perinatol 19:114–119

60. Davis-Floyd R, Davis E 1997 Intuition as authoritative knowledge in midwifery and home birth. In: Davis-Floyd R, Arvidson P S (eds) Intuition: the inside story: interdisciplinary perspectives. Routledge, New York, p 145–176

61. Troop P, Goldacre M, Mason A et al (eds) 1999 Health outcome indicators: normal pregnancy and childbirth. Report of a working group to the Department of Health. National Centre for Outcomes Development, Oxford

62. Kernick D 2006 Wanted – new methodologies for health service research. Is complexity theory the answer? Fam Pract 23(3):385–390

63. Cornfield J 1969 The Bayesian outlook and its application. Biometrics 25:617–657

64. GRIT Study Group 2003 A randomised trial of timed delivery for the compromised preterm fetus: short term outcomes and Bayesian interpretation. BJOG 110(1):27–32

65. Hazen G B, Huang M 2006 Large-sample Bayesian posterior distributions for probabilistic sensitivity analysis. Med Decis Making 26(5):512–534

66. Hannah M E, Hannah W J, Hewson S A et al 2000 Planned caesarean section versus planned vaginal birth for breech presentation at term: a randomised multicentre trial. Term Breech Trial Collaborative Group. Lancet 356:1375–1383

67. Hogle K L, Kilburn L, Hewson S et al 2003 Impact of the international term breech trial on clinical practice and concerns: a survey of centre collaborators. J Obstet Gynaecol Can 25:14–16

68. Hofmeyr G J, Hannah M E 2003 Planned caesarean section for term breech delivery. Cochrane Database Syst Rev, Issue 2. Art. No.: CD000166. DOI: 10.1002/14651858.CD000166

69. Molkenboer J F, Roumen F J, Smits L J et al 2006 Birth weight and neurodevelopmental outcome of children at 2 years of age after planned vaginal delivery for breech presentation at term. Am J Obstet Gynecol 194(3):624–629

70. Kempthorne O 1969 Commentary on Cornfield J 1969 The Bayesian outlook and its application. Biometrics 25:649

71. Merry U 1995 Coping with uncertainty: insights from the new science of chaos, self-organization and complexity. Praeger, Westport, CT

72. Department of Health 1993 Report of the Chief Medical Officer's Expert Group on the sleeping position of infants and cot death. HMSO, London

73. Willinger M, Hoffman H J, Hartford R B 1994 Infant sleep position and risk for sudden infant death syndrome: report of meeting held January 13 and 14, 1994, National Institutes of Health, Bethesda, MD. Pediatrics 93:814–819

74. Salsburg D 1990 Hypothesis versus significance testing for controlled clinical trials: a dialogue. Stat Med 9:201–211

75. Gleick J 1998 Chaos: the amazing science of the unpredictable. Vintage, London

76. Lissack M R 2003 Chaos and complexity – knowledge management? Online. Available:http://www.leader-values.com/content/detail.asp?ContentDetailID=47 (accessed 29 August 2007)

77. Pikkujamsa S M, Makikallio T H, Sourander L B et al 1999 Cardiac interbeat interval dynamics from childhood to senescence: comparison of conventional and new measures based on fractals and chaos theory. Circulation 100:393–399

78. Haigh C 2002 Using chaos theory; the implications for nursing. J Adv Nurs 37:462–469

79. Sweeney K, Griffiths F 2002 Complexity and healthcare, an introduction. Radcliffe Medical Press, Oxford

80. Winter C 2002 Assessing the progress of labour: orderly chaos. MSc Thesis, South Bank University, London

81. Gross M M, Drobnic S, Keirse M J 2005 Influence of fixed and time-dependent factors on duration of normal first stage labor. Birth 32(1):27–33

82. Prigogine I 1987 From being to becoming: the new science of connectedness. Bantam Dell, New York

83. Wilson T, Holt T, Greenhalgh T 2001 Complexity science: complexity and clinical care. Br Med J 323:685–688

84. Ackoff R L 1980 The systems revolution. In: Lockett M, Spear R (eds) Organisations as systems. Open University Press, Milton Keynes

85. Medical Research Council Health Services and Public Health Research Board 2000 A framework for development and evaluation of RCTs for complex interventions to improve health. MRC, London

86. O'Connor J, McDermott I 1997 The art of systems thinking. Thorsons, London

87. Hodnett E D, Lowe N, Hannah M E et al, for the Nursing Supportive Care in Labor Trial Group 2002 Effectiveness of nurses as providers of birth labor support in North American hospitals: a randomized controlled trial. J Am Med Assoc 288:1373–1381

88. Hodnett E D 2002 Comments made during keynote address: Is the hospital culture a major risk factor for abnormal labour and birth? The research evidence. First Normal Birth Research Conference, University of Central Lancashire, Preston, UK, 29 September 2003

89. Hodnett E D, Downe S, Edwards N et al 2005 Home-like versus conventional institutional settings for birth. Cochrane Database Syst Rev, Issue 1. Art. No.: CD000012. DOI: 10.1002/14651858.CD000012.pub2

90. World Health Organization 1992 Basic documents, 19th edn. WHO, Geneva

91. Antonovsky A 1979 Health stress and coping: new perspectives on mental and physical well-being. Jossey-Bass, San Francisco

92. Antonovsky A 1993 The implications of salutogenesis: an outsider's view. In: Turnbull A P, Patterson J M, Behr S G et al (eds) Cognitive coping: families and disability. Brookes, Baltimore, MD, Ch. 8

93. Soloman A 1985 The emerging field of psychoneuroimmunology: advances. J Inst Adv Health 2:6–19

94. Chirico G, Gasparoni A, Ciardelli L et al 1999 Leukocyte counts in relation to the method of delivery during the first five days of life. Biol Neonate 75: 294–299

95. Gitau R, Menson E, Pickles V et al 2001 Umbilical cortisol levels as an indicator of the fetal stress response to assisted vaginal delivery. Eur J Obstet Gynecol Reprod Biol 98:14–17

96. Bengel J, Strittmatter R, Willmann H 1999 What keeps people healthy? The current state of discussion and the relevance of Antonovsky's salutogenic model of health. Online. Available: http://www.bzga.de/bzga_stat/pdf/60804070.pdf (accessed 13 August 2007)

97. Eriksson M, Lindstrom B 2006 Antonovsky's sense of coherence scale and the relation with health: a systematic review. J Epidemiol Community Health 60(5):376–381

98. Grote N K, Bledsoe S E 2007 Predicting postpartum depressive symptoms in new mothers: the role of optimism and stress frequency during pregnancy. Health Soc Work 32(2):107–118

99. Lin N 2001 Social capital. Cambridge University Press, Cambridge

100. Kilsztajn S, Carmo M S, Machado L C Jr et al 2007 Caesarean sections and maternal mortality in Sao Paulo. Eur J Obstet Gynecol Reprod Biol 132(1):64–69

101. Misago C, Kendall C, Freitas P et al 2001 From 'culture of dehumanization of childbirth' to 'childbirth as a transformative experience': changes in five municipalities in north-east Brazil. Int J Gynecol Obstet 75:S67–S72

102. Ontario Women's Health Council 2000 Attaining and maintaining best practices in the use of Caesarean

section: an analysis of four Ontario hospitals. Report of the Caesarean Section Working Group of the Women's Health Council. Online. Available: http://www.womenshealthcouncil.on.ca/English/page-1-361-1.html (Accessed 30 August 2007)

103. Downe S 1994 How average is normality? Br J Midwifery 2(7):303–304

104. Downe S, McCormick C, Beech B L 2001 Labour interventions associated with normal birth. Br J Midwifery 9:602–606

105. Oakley A 1993 Birth as a normal process. In: Oakley A (ed.) Essays on women and health. Edinburgh University Press, Edinburgh, p 2

106. Downe S Simpson L, Trafford K 2007 Expert intrapartum maternity care: a meta-synthesis. J Adv Nurs 57(2):127–140

107. Benner P 1984 From novice to expert: excellence and power in clinical nursing practice. Addison-Wesley, Menlo Park, CA

108. Rose H 1983 Hand, brain, and heart: a feminist epistemology for the natural sciences. Signs: J Women Culture Soc 7:73–90

109. el-Nemer A, Downe S, Small N 2006 'She would help me from the heart': an ethnography of Egyptian women in labour. Soc Sci Med 62(1):81–92

110. Cragin L, Kennedy H P 2006 Linking obstetric and midwifery practice with optimal outcomes. J Obstet Gynecol Neonatal Nurs 35(6):779–785

The role of pain in normal birth and the empowerment of women

2

Nicky Leap and Tricia Anderson

Chapter contents

And a woman spoke, saying, Tell us of Pain.
And he said:
Your pain is the breaking of the shell that encloses your understanding.
Even as the stone of the fruit must break, that its heart may stand in the sun
So must you know pain.[1] (p 82)

Introduction

Where it is unavoidable, pain can be transformed into something usable, something which takes us beyond the limits of the experience itself into a further grasp of the essentials of life and the possibilities within us … This insight illuminates much of the female condition, but in particular the experience of giving birth. (p 158)[2]

The authors of this chapter embraced the opportunity to co-write about the role of pain in labour. We are both enthusiasts regarding each other's work and writings in this area; we share a passionate belief that how we approach the business of being with women in pain in labour is the most central tenet of 'keeping birth normal', with potentially profound consequences for women and babies. Living on opposite sides of the world, we suspected that to share writing would involve 'bouncing ideas off each other' through the ether, in a process far more stimulating and creative than the lonely business of solo writing. And so it turned out to be. We have included a range of literature and styles of writing in this chapter. This is an attempt to engage the reader in a lively debate about the complexity and potentially far-reaching consequences of the experience of labour pain for women in terms of how they feel about themselves and how they negotiate the world around them:

To have experienced birthing pain offers the possibilities of self-knowledge, knowledge of our limitations and capabilities, knowledge of new life: birth, death and rebirth. As we birth our children, we in a sense, birth ourselves. We are mothers, like our mothers, and our daughters after us. (p 103)[3]

This chapter enables the voices of midwives interviewed by one of us (NL)[4] to be heard. The words of ten midwives from the United Kingdom, Canada, Australia and Holland are woven *in italics* throughout the text. These midwives were invited to participate in a qualitative study on midwives' attitudes to pain in labour because all of them had experience of attending women giving birth at home. It was presumed that they would have interesting ideas about how to answer the challenge: 'Why would you *not* routinely offer all women pain relief in this day and age? Why on earth would you let women suffer the barbaric pain of childbirth when we have the ultimate form of pain relief in the form of epidurals?'. Such questions form the basis of this chapter as we explore the role of pain in labour in relation to the midwife's role of 'keeping birth normal'. We shall explore the culture of 'pain relief' versus the culture of 'being with women in pain in labour' and will include a short overview of how, in the Western world, we arrived at a situation where pain relief and birth in hospital became synonymous with notions of choice and women's rights.

Background

An overview of relevant literature provides some background to the context in which we shall be exploring these issues. Lesley Page[5] highlights the fact that midwives on both sides of the world face the same challenges in trying to reduce high intervention rates and offer women the opportunity of sensitive continuity of care. In Western countries, the use of pharmacological pain relief in labour has continued to rise in the face of this focus on choice and woman-centred care and in spite of research that raises concerns about the potential morbidity of pharmacological pain relief.

Epidurals and narcotics: evidence causing concern

In recent years, considerable concern has been raised about rises in obstetric intervention rates and the potential public and psychological health impact of rates of intervention above those that are indicated by current evidence.[6–9] The use of epidural anaesthesia is directly linked to the increased morbidity associated with interventions, and questions have been raised about the potential iatrogenic risks of this form of pain relief in terms of prolonged labour, instrumental vaginal birth and caesarean section.[9–13] There is also widespread concern about the use of narcotics in labour, such as pethidine. Longer labours, and harmful effects upon the mother's birth experience,[14,15] can be coupled with the potential compromise to the baby, including difficulties initiating breastfeeding.[16] An important message for pregnant women is that, while narcotics induce sedation, they are usually ineffective in terms of pain relief.[14,17]

These potential side effects of pharmacological pain relief, particularly the effects on the baby, are of concern both to women and health professionals.[7] These concerns are a source of motivation for women from a range of socioeconomic backgrounds, who choose to give birth in situations (such as birth centres or at home) where obstetric analgesia is not an option.[18] There are, however, concerns that these women are not always supported well by midwives in this choice,[19] with many more women using pain-relieving drugs than had wished to.[20]

Practice regarding epidurals, narcotics and elective caesarean section varies greatly regionally, between different maternity units and according to practitioner employment status,[21] with particularly high rates in the private obstetrics sector (see Ch. 5).[6] Variations often appear to be related to institutional cultures or professional opinion rather than population factors or individual women's choices.[21] In particular, the rise in elective caesarean section rates has been apportioned to women making choices that help them deal with uncertainty and the fear of pain in labour.[22]

Encouraging evidence

On a positive note, there is strong evidence that continuity of caregiver throughout pregnancy, labour and birth reduces the amount of pain relief women have during labour and increases their satisfaction with their maternity care.[23] In addition, women who have continuous support from a female caregiver during labour are less likely to use pharmacological pain relief and are more likely to have a spontaneous vaginal birth.[24] While there is some evidence from trials that acupuncture and hypnosis may be useful in reducing labour pain,[25] strong evidence is emerging that women find immersion in water a useful tool in the first stage of labour,[26] particularly as an alternative to Syntocinon augmentation when progress is slow.[27] These issues are explored in more detail by Walsh in Chapter 10 of this book.

Women's views of pain in labour

Women have identified that their experience of childbirth is enhanced by both midwifery support to enable them to cope with pain in labour, and access to different ways of reducing or relieving pain.[28–30] However, effective forms of pain relief are not necessarily associated with greater satisfaction with the experience of birth.[31,32] Indeed, in several studies, women who had epidurals reported lower satisfaction rates than those who experienced pain.[20,28,33]

A large study carried out in the UK in 2000 repeated a survey that was carried out in 1987 in order to study the inter-relationships between women's expectations and experiences of decision making, continuity, choice and control in labour and psychological outcomes.[20] Women were more likely to feel satisfied with their experience of labour if they had had a spontaneous vaginal birth; had been able to make choices about pain relief; felt good about the way they responded to pain; had one midwife throughout labour; and if they had *not* had an epidural.[20] When comparisons were made with the findings of the 1987 study, there was a significant increase in women hoping to have an epidural and feeling very worried about pain. The use of epidurals for pain relief had increased: for primiparous women, from 19% to 59%, and for multiparous women, from 4% to 23%. Many more women, however, had used pharmacological pain relief than had wanted to. There was an increase in women reporting feeling 'frightened', 'powerless' and 'helpless', particularly primiparous women who had epidurals, and a decrease in women feeling 'confident' and 'involved', notably among multiparous women who had epidurals.

Anxiety about pain has been shown to be a strong predictor of negative experiences during labour, lack of satisfaction with birth and poor emotional well-being.[20] Interactions between midwives and women, about pain in labour and choices that women may make, do not always fully address these factors and are often dominated by a mechanistic and medicalized understanding of the meaning of childbirth and of pain.[34] This is reflected in recent studies in Nigeria where women reported childbirth as extremely painful, and identified that they would have liked obstetric analgesia had it been available.[35–37] The underlying belief system of the researchers in such studies is that labour pain should be relieved as a woman's right. This drives the questionable process of asking women to score their pain in labour and the potentially misleading and simplistic questioning of women regarding their inability to access obstetric analgesia.

Although almost all women will describe the pain of labour as extremely severe, regardless of the use of analgesia, those who use non-pharmacological methods of pain relief are less likely to complain of unbearable pain.[28] Culturally diverse groups of women have described childbirth as a difficult, yet empowering, experience leading to a sense of achievement and feeling of pride in their ability to cope with intense pain.[29,30,38]

A review of the literature relating to women's memory for labour pain identified that, although memories of labour pain can evoke intense, negative reactions in 'a few' women, memories are more likely to give rise to positive consequences relating to coping, self-sufficiency and self-esteem.[39] For many women, the confidence they gain from coping with pain in labour is associated with a positive birth experience.[40]

The experiences around pain appear be more important to women than the level of pain per se,[21] particularly in terms of how the experience impacts on their lives as new mothers.[30] Measuring women's sense of self-esteem and achievement following childbirth is fraught with difficulty, and more qualitative research is needed to give women a voice about their experiences of pain in labour and the effect this had on their lives.

Midwives 'working with pain' and facilitating normal birth: exemplary practice

An evaluation study of the Albany Midwifery Practice, a community-based midwifery practice composed of self-employed midwives working in the National Health Service (NHS) from King's College Hospital, London, demonstrated outcomes warranting further investigation.[41] In spite of working in an area of high socioeconomic deprivation, this midwifery group practice has been particularly successful in facilitating normal pregnancy and birth and continuity of carer. When compared to other midwifery group practices at King's, the Albany practice had lower rates of intervention, and significantly lower use of pharmacological pain relief (69% of Albany women did not use any pharmacological pain relief compared to 18% in the other midwifery group practices). On being asked if they felt adequate pain relief was offered, significantly more Albany women said no pain relief was required. The researchers suggested that one explanation for this difference might be the development of confidence in women who were able to develop a personal relationship with their midwives. The need for further research to explore women's perspectives was highlighted and this is currently being undertaken in a range of studies at King's College, London.

The Albany midwives work in a case-load practice model that has consistently demonstrated improved outcomes related to the promotion of normal birth and home birth through high levels of continuity of carer; antenatal groups based on story telling; birth talks at home at 36 weeks and decision making about the place of birth during labour.[42,43] Data collected by the Albany Midwifery Practice for the year 2006 (unpublished) showed that 82% of the 210 women who were attended by Albany midwives had a spontaneous vaginal birth. Of these, 174 women, 93.6%, chose no analgesia, 2.6% used Entonox and 3.4% chose to use epidurals. It is possible that strategies used by the Albany midwives to encourage women to labour without using pharmacological pain relief may have psychological, public health and financial benefits. Anecdotal evidence suggests that currently, in most maternity units, midwives are more comfortable talking about 'pain relief' than they are engaging with women around the notion of 'coping with pain'.

The culture of Western maternity care and 'pain relief'

There is no doubt that the pain of labour is central to women's experience of childbirth. There is also no doubt that the attitudes of birth attendants have a profound effect on the choices women make regarding how they deal with that pain. In spite of its potential to decrease the chance of normal birth, the choice of an epidural in labour tends to be seen as a woman's right in Western society. It is only one step away from that other choice increasingly embraced by some in the quest for certainty: elective caesarean section – referred to seductively as the 'vaginal bypass', the modern woman's way to ensure a 'honeymoon vagina'.

Midwives report accusations of 'cruelty' if they encourage women in pain to hold out for a normal labour without pharmacological pain relief. In such a culture, there is clearly a need to find a way to articulate the role of pain in promoting normal birth that makes sense to women and to our colleagues. This is not necessarily easy. Any argument has to acknowledge that such a notion runs directly counter to the dominant ideology of the culture of Western childbirth in the 21st century. Furthermore, although it is assumed that the high levels of endogenous opiates such as beta-endorphins and dynorphin in pregnant and labouring women's bodies play a role in affording women 'hypalgesia',[44] there does not seem to be any published evidence explaining the intricate role of pain in relation to the complex neurohormonal cascades that promote physiological birth and pain relief for women.

Labour as a rite of passage

The publications of childbirth theorists, and women's accounts of the role of pain in relation to feelings of empowerment, are an important contribution to the literature that informs this subject. According to Robertson:[45]

Submission to the all-consuming and overwhelming nature of birth and the weathering of the inherent pain is an empowering process for a woman, and one that should not be denied unless critical for her own well-being or that of her baby. (p 88)

The notion of triumph associated with giving birth is directly associated with pain, altered states of consciousness and privacy, as these women's accounts testify:[3]

… the deep significance of the momentous quality of the pain … As we are surrounded by the deep sense of inwardness, we are forced to recognise our independence, our loneliness, and our selfhood, to be conscious of our own existence. This actual self-consciousness exposes us to our wholeness, our strengths and our endurance. (p 101)

The spiritual aspects of labour pain which this quote suggests are explored in more detail in Chapter 3.

The pain of labour is constructed by Kelpin as an expression of the 'narrow gateway leading to release in the expanse of life' (p 101).[3] The release she describes with the birth of her baby is given the significance of change from 'self as world' to 'baby as world' where a new pain comes with the awe of focusing on a new being. She quotes Phyllis Chesler (p 281)[46] – 'Being born with motherhood is the sharpest pain I've known' – and uses words like 'relief', 'disbelief', 'joy' and 'exhilaration' to describe the excitement and poignancy of her new baby's presence (p 102).[3]

Davis-Floyd provides a useful analysis from an anthropological perspective of giving birth as a rite of passage, in which the experiencing and triumphing over pain is an essential component.[47] She explains that a rite of passage is a series of rituals designed to transport an individual from one social state (in this case, non-mother) to another (mother). These rites are culturally determined and designed to convey important societal values and meanings that the individual then incorporates into her new role.

It was about the best thing I ever experienced. I was totally amazed. The labour was like I had died. I had just died. The minute she came out, I was born again. It was like we'd just been born together.[48] (p 135)

If society wants mothers to be strong and fearless and able to fight for the well-being of their young, these qualities need to be experienced as part of their rite of passage. If, on the other hand, society wants mothers who are passive and biddable, then the rite of passage needs to be reconstructed to be passive. Labour experienced with epidural anaesthesia is just such a process which conveys strongly to the mother that her body can function without her and offers her little potential for transformation.

A rite of passage, explains Davis-Floyd, has three phases: *separation* (in which the individual leaves behind his or her previous state); *transition* (in which the individual is neither one thing nor the other); and *reintegration* (in which the individual is accepted and incorporated into society in a new state). An essential feature of the transition state is a liminal phase, which is characterized by individuals being in a malleable, vulnerable state as they experience and then incorporate at a deep level the changes needed within themselves to take on their new social status. The experience of labour, which involves experiencing pain, provides the liminal phase for the transition to motherhood. If there is no resolution, no triumph – if the woman's pain is taken away by someone else – then the new mother is left in a state of limbo which can have long-lasting effects:

I had a caesarean too. That was forty years ago – imagine! … and you know, I've never gotten over it. I still remember that mask coming down over my face, and I still feel as angry as I did then, when I woke up. Those people took my birth away from me. I don't know why and I don't know how, but I've never felt the same about myself since.[47] (p 40)

As Gill Gribble writes in her moving poem 'Motherhood' of her experience of caesarean section, there is often a sense of something lost or missing: it is 'the strangest feeling, to be a mother without childbirth'.[49]

Pain and the power of birth

Before exploring the issues raised above any further, we offer a cameo that Tricia wrote early one morning in a particularly impassioned moment when contemplating writing this chapter:

If you are privileged enough to have witnessed a woman giving birth unaided in a place she has chosen, what will you have seen?

You will first have been in awe of her strength. Her thighs stand strong and mighty like those of a warrior as she stands, sways and squats to find the best position to ease her baby out. Then you will hear the deep primal cries she makes as she does her work, sounds that come not from her throat but from her belly as she grunts and moans and roars with her exertion: sounds seldom heard except in the most uninhibited of love-making. Maybe you will notice the glistening river of mucus tinged with blood and waters that run down her thighs unheeded: she is beyond noticing such things, moved as she has done into another plane of existence. And then finally perhaps you will be struck by her beauty: her face softened with the flow of oxytocin, her eyes wide and shining, her pupils dark, deep and open. And you will think – for how could you not; why, what a phenomenal creature is a woman.

But you will only have seen this astonishing sight if you have understood that if you disturb her in her work, she will be thrown off course. Like a zoologist, you must first learn how to behave; how to sit quietly and patiently, almost invisible, breathing with her, not disturbing her mighty internal rhythm. And you will see that the pain of her labours seldom overwhelms her.

Nature would not have organised labour to be intolerable. It is man in his wish to control all he surveys that has oppressed labouring women by making them labour in the most tortuous and fiendish environment he could construct. Let us bring them into harsh rooms with bright lights. Let us make them lie on their backs on hard narrow beds. Let us tether them to machines so they cannot move. Let us make them stay silent and make no noise with their pains. Let us expose their most private parts and threaten them with cold steel. Let us make them push their babies upwards, against the pull of the earth. Let us monitor and measure and chart every move that they make. Let us swab them and wipe them, and prod them and poke them, and irritate and confuse them and frighten them as much as we can.

In these conditions labour swiftly becomes unbearable and pain relief becomes a woman's only hope. Get me some pethidine, give me an epidural, cut it out of me, anything, make it stop, please help me …

This is not the natural cry of a woman in labour bringing a child to birth, although if you have only ever witnessed childbirth in a medicalised setting you might be forgiven for thinking so. This is the screaming plea of a tethered animal in pain. Her only hope for salvation in her cell lies in the anaesthetist who numbs the pain and the obstetrician who, finally, makes it stop. The midwives – the prison guards: what of them? They have no real power here. They can do no more than slip an extra ration in for a favoured prisoner; at best buy an hour or two of time.

Feminist perspectives

Is it ineptitude? Is it a misguided but well-meant attempt to help, to save lives? Or is it part of an age-old conspiracy – the latest chapter in a history of control, oppression and denigration of the innate reproductive power of women that has been going on for thousands of years?

Rich's explanation for this phenomenon is that men fear women's mysterious powers and they desire to control and contain the uncontrollable, thus maintaining their patriarchal authority.[2] In a historical analysis of women in power and history, De Reincourt writes that, in prehistorical times,[50]

Every evidence points to the fact that men stood in awe of the female, as he did of all natural phenomena – storms, lightening, earthquakes, volcanic eruptions. Weak, relatively defenseless, and more or less isolated in small scattered groups, yet increasingly capable of abstract thought, primitive man was afraid of nature's mysterious displays of grandiose power. In exactly the same way, he stood in awe of the mysteries of gestation and childbirth because they were natural manifestations of creative power. (p 17)

He explains how, over the centuries, man has constructed elaborate rites and rules to control and constrain that creative female power; both in limiting women's sexual activities (but not his own) to within marriage to ensure paternity, and in confining childbirth to foster female weakness and dependence.[50]

Davis-Floyd also concluded that the ritual use of high technology in pregnancy and birth denies the creative power of women. She offers many examples of how the rituals of technocratic birth deprive women of their 'cosmic significance as birth-givers, transformed in the transformation of giving birth into mere machines to be manipulated and repaired' (p 286).[47]

Feminists have argued that pain relief in labour may have far-reaching negative emotional and psychological consequences for women in terms of rendering them passive in a gendered world:[2]

[Analgesia and anaesthesia] … a new kind of prison for women – the prison of unconsciousness, of numbed sensations, of amnesia, and complete passivity … a dangerous mechanism which can cause us to lose touch not just with our painful sensations but with ourselves. (p 158–159)
As long as birth – metaphorically or literally – remains an experience of passively handing over our bodies to male authority and technology, other kinds of social change can only minimally change our relationship to ourselves, to power and to the world outside our bodies. (p 185)

In this analysis, midwives who freely offer pain relief to women in normal labour can ultimately be seen both as agents and products of patriarchal oppression, fostering as they do the notion of woman as weak, unable to cope and dependent.

Attitudes to pain relief in the past

Pain is never the sole creation of our anatomy and physiology. It emerges only at the intersection of bodies, minds and cultures.[51]

The attitudes of caregivers in labour are always a product of their particular 'bodies, minds and cultures'.[51] Any historical (herstorical) analysis of the role of pain in labour needs to bear this in mind. However, a quick romp through 'herstory' inevitably 'rings a few bells' in terms of considering attitudes and contested meanings of pain that still resonate today.

In Judeo-Christian societies, the notion of women paying for Eve's sin in bringing about the fall of man in the Garden of Eden – 'In sorrow shalt thou bring forth' (Genesis 3:16) – persisted from the 5th century AD until the 1600s, when scientific enquiry began to reconceptualize pain as part of 'nature'. Until that time, the pain of childbirth was likened to the suffering of men in war and was seen as both punishment and redemption; crucial processes for ensuring divine ordination and life's continuity. Any person who tried to take away this pain was therefore in potential danger of being seen as evil by the church. However, in parallel with this antagonism to unacceptable approaches, there was a wide range of officially sanctioned interventions to help women in labour cope with pain. These included support from other women, and herbal remedies, which were in general household use for comfort and ailments in most cultures. There is evidence that soporific sponges dipped into fluids like hemlock, mandragora or ground ivy were used. Also sanctioned were amulets, semi-precious stones, manuscripts, magic girdles and the Christian liturgy.

Before childbirth belonged to medicine, it belonged to women.[52] (p 68)

With very few exceptions, throughout the world, women have always asked other women to be there alongside them to give them comfort and confidence when they give birth. In 17th century England, women prepared a careful list during pregnancy of invited female guests who would be there to support them during labour and in the six weeks following birth. As soon as labour began, the woman's husband would be sent out to round up these women, a process known as 'nidgeting'. Thereafter he would be banned from the birth room until six weeks after the birth when the woman would resume her wifely duties, having undergone the Churching of Women service – a Christian ritual of thanksgiving and purification. The support team would arrive for the labour with victuals, including an alcoholic beverage akin to mead, to sustain them through the labour. Some say that the origin of the word 'gossips' derives from the ritual sipping of this beverage ('Godsips'); others say that these women were siblings of God ('Godsibs') in their important role. The midwife or 'gracewife' played a different role. She was not part of the support group and was the only person allowed to touch the woman's genitals.

In many other societies, similar rituals of support exist to this day, involving women who attend labour and stay with the woman afterwards, relieving her of all her household duties and childcare while she establishes breastfeeding to ensure the survival of the infant.

As the positivistic scientific approach to life gathered momentum – in Europe from about 1600 – moral or religious interpretations of pain faded and permission was granted to the notion of 'pain relief'. During the 19th century in the Western world, humanitarian ideals gave a platform to concerns about pain and suffering, paving the way for acceptance of the development of analgesia and anaesthesia in childbirth.

The notion of a systematic approach to 'pain control' in labour begins in Edinburgh with the experimental work of James Young Simpson in the 1840s.[53] In 1847, Simpson administered diethyl ether to facilitate the forceps birth of a baby whose mother had a deformed pelvis. This occurred a few weeks after the first public demonstration of the use of ether for surgery by William Thomas Green Morton, a Bostonian dentist. Simpson was the pioneer of obstetric anaesthesia; he is also remembered for his infamous dinner parties, where friends and colleagues were invited to try out his latest anaesthetic drugs and, with the great man himself, frequently ended up under the table, unconscious (p 12).[53]

Despite suspicion and doubt expressed by his medical colleagues, Simpson strongly advocated for the acceptance of obstetric anaesthesia. Concerns about safety and risks, accusations that such techniques were 'meddlesome' and questions concerning the notion of pain as an important

component of healing are all strikingly familiar. In the face of such concerns, Simpson continued to use anaesthesia and sing its praises without offering proof of its safety other than claims that he had not 'observed any harm whatever to either mother or infant', but that he had seen 'no small amount of maternal suffering and agony saved by its application'. He attacked any colleagues who expressed concerns as inhumane and 'professionally cruel'.

In the late 1800s, the invention of the hypodermic syringe and the isolation of morphine and codeine from opium, plus the introduction of inhalation analgesia, or 'twilight sleep', led to a new array of pain relief methods. Simpson's medical colleagues were increasingly convinced that women were vulnerable creatures who needed rescuing from the torture of labour and giving birth. With our modern understanding of the subtle endocrinology of labour, we now see how the mere presence of Simpson and his male colleagues in the childbirth room might have contributed to that impression.

Davis-Floyd points out how anaesthesia is also a very effective way of removing the sexual aspects of birth. Women's natural sexuality at this time was seen as a 'devilish temptation to righteous men', and women who enjoyed sexual intercourse were considered deviant.[47] Poovey also highlights the new medical professions' fear of female sexuality in childbirth during this era,[54] and it is easy to see how the sometimes overtly sexual behaviour of a labouring woman, in particular her spontaneous vocalizations and secretions, would be very disturbing to the sensibilities of Victorian medical men. Sedate that woman immediately!

Debates and concerns about the advisability of analgesia and anaesthesia in terms of safety and possible physical and psychological consequences have changed little since Simpson's day. The 'danger of drugs and the social value of pain' versus 'the preservation of meaning in childbirth in the absence of pain' continue to be hotly debated issues.[53]

The notion of heroics in terms of saving women from pain is a theme in medical discourse around pain in labour. However, in the late 19th century, women themselves began to voice an interest in pain relief during labour. Inspired by Queen Victoria and Fanny Appleton Longfellow, feminists in the UK and USA increasingly demanded the right to manage the pain of labour with drugs. They confronted obstetricians and governments in aggressive campaigns for the right of all women to use opioids and inhalation analgesia in childbirth. The move away from birth at home is directly linked to women's wishes to access pain relief in all its technological splendour, alongside health professionals' increasing belief system that pain relief and hospital birth are an appropriate, even necessary, choice.

The ongoing, vigorous campaign by middle-class women for pain relief was dented to some extent in the 1930s and 1940s by Grantly Dick-Read who linked fear to pain in childbirth and claimed that: 'healthy childbirth was never intended by the natural law to be painful'. The front cover of the 1957 edition of Grantly Dick-Read's *Childbirth Without Fear* boasts sales of over 250 000 and features a quotation that reads: 'Into a world where pain and fear are rampant this book brings a message of hope'.[55]

Grantly Dick-Read's books inspired the early 'natural childbirth' movement. Vestiges of his philosophy can be seen in many of the present-day writings of those who question the medicalization of childbirth, in particular the routine offering of 'pain relief' to women in labour.

What we're doing isn't so terribly different from what people like Grantly Dick-Read were doing back in the 1930s. I mean, they were saying to women, 'You can do it. It's OK ... And that whole fear–tension–pain thing makes a lot of sense, and whether women feel secure and how that affects their experience of pain ... and the attitudes of midwives antenatally will have a profound effect. If you can build up confidence in women that they can definitely get on and do this, then I think they will.

Modern readers of Dick-Read's work may find the florid writing style of this early childbirth guru off-putting. His support of the eugenics movement would be unacceptable today. However, there is no doubting the sincerity of his awe of childbearing women. His belief in the potential of childbirth to make a difference to the way people carry out their lives may resonate for some at this time of world crisis:[55]

Many women have described their experiences of childbirth as being associated with a spiritual uplifting, the power of which they have never previously been aware. I have witnessed this so often and been profoundly impressed by the inexplicable transfiguration of women at the moment of their baby's birth, that I have been led, as usual, to ask: Why is this? It is not sentimentality; it is not relief from suffering; it is not simply satisfaction of accomplishment. It is bigger than all those things ...
The philosophy of childbirth is in the reality of its spiritual manifestations and the incomprehensible miracle of its mechanism – familiarity with its natural performance directs our minds to a closer understanding of human nature and conduct ... For my own part, I stand in awe and utter humility before a woman with her newborn babe. There is so much to see and learn in her presence, so much that I am unable to understand or to explain, so much that makes me aware of the limitations of my own ability. It may be that amongst my colleagues there are those who feel the same. Childbirth is not a physical function. The drama of the physical manifestations has blinded observers to the truth – the birth of a child is the ultimate phenomenon of a series of spiritual experiences, from fantasy to fact and from fact to fiction ...
The powers of physical destruction are established. If the peoples of this world are to survive there will be a gigantic philosophical revolution. Armageddon is of the mind; ordinance of spiritual forces in the great conflict will emerge from childbirth and mother love. The full significance and magnitude of this supreme human function must not be neglected or belittled by the subjective materialism of modern science. (p 10–12)

In comparing Dick-Read's philosophy with that of Simpson, we can see the contesting beliefs driving what can be summarized as two contemporary paradigms. On the one hand, the ideology of promoting normal birth encourages us to think in terms of 'working with pain', rather than trying to take it away. On the other hand, we have the dominant paradigm of 'pain relief', which is reinforced by neo-liberal concepts of individualism and informed choice.

The 'pain relief' paradigm

In my training I was led to believe that you had to do everything you could to alleviate the pain. You knew it was there for a purpose, but you were taught that it was so unpleasant for the woman that the most important thing was to try and get rid of the pain so that she could labour normally.

The 'pain relief' paradigm can be characterized as a set of attitudes, values and practices incorporating the following features and beliefs:

- A paternalistic system where practitioners want to be 'kind' and make full use of 'the benefits of modern technology'.
- A conviction that 'in this day and age, no woman should have to suffer the 'barbaric' pain of childbirth'.
- The personal discomfort experienced by practitioners around being with women in pain.
- The practitioners' crucial role and responsibility to inform women of all the options for pain relief so that they can make an 'informed choice'.
- Women who are having first babies rarely manage without pharmacological pain relief, even if they say they want to avoid it during their pregnancies.
- The disadvantages and risks of pharmacological pain relief are far outweighed by the benefits of pain relief.
- The 'natural childbirth' lobby are responsible for making women feel guilty and a sense of failure when they choose pain relief.

The 'pain relief' approach is evident across all settings, but it is particularly obvious in Western labour wards or so-called delivery suites, where the pressures of lack of continuity of care (not knowing women), staff shortages, hierarchical structure and medical dominance impact heavily on the working lives and attitudes of all staff:

I have seen women coping well with pain in hospital but it's much harder to facilitate that there. If women come to me saying that they want a hospital birth, it's an area I find really difficult to facilitate choice around because

I have an agenda that it'll work better at home.

Tricia uses the metaphor of disturbing animals in labour to encourage urgent consideration of the drastic effects of routine hospitalization of women for birth.[56] She hypothesizes a situation where all cats are interrupted in labour and taken to brightly lit, noisy, modern laboratories where they are attached to monitors and probes, subjected to scrutiny by strange technicians who constantly come in and out with clipboards. The technicians' conclusions that 'cats do not labour very well' leads to the invention of machines to improve their labours and monitor their kittens' oxygen levels, pain killing drugs and tranquilizers, and more drugs to make labour become regular and stop it slowing down. She concludes: '… in that modern laboratory – which is of course a modern maternity unit – childbirth is in a mess' (p 65).[56] The links between disruption in labour and an increase in pain relief, and complications due to hospitalization, have also been explored by Robertson (p 20),[57] Helman (p 203),[58] Kitzinger[59] and Morse & Park.[60]

Midwives have commented on how the fear of pain on the part of practitioners is exacerbated in hospital units by the particular type of noises that can be heard when women in labour are frightened or distressed, or when their contractions are artificially intensified by infusions of synthetic oxytocin:

It's a panic, it's a scream and it's different from the noise they make when they're working with their bodies … Oh it's a horrible noise. It sounds like someone's being murdered … you don't hear that sound when you know women. You don't hear it at home births. That awful kind of scream and it really goes right through me.

Susan Taylor eloquently describes the difference between natural, normal pain and the abnormal pain of an augmented labour from the mother's perspective in her short poem entitled 'Oxytocin'.[61]

Oxytocin

The electric pump clicks,
Drip fed through that meter,
by clear plastic tubes
and a needle jammed into my vein,
this is not my body's pain.

It did not rise like breath
or the fierce arched rainbows
I have imagined.

From a burning bush,
it spreads like a forest fire,
with me in front of it,
running.

There are reports of midwives telling women to make less noise in case they frighten other labouring women and in order to conserve their energy.[62] It seems that this discomfort around the noise of pain can extend to the noise of normal labour, as identified by this midwife:

You can come out of a room where you were with someone who was making a lot of noise and they say, 'What's going on in there?' Like it's something abnormal. 'Can't you do something about that?' and you say, 'She's fine, I think she's nearly there.' And they say, 'God, I hope she has the baby soon, she's making a dreadful racket' … So that's where the 'Room 11's nicely sedated' comes in. It's about the midwife needing not to have to deal with someone else's pain, someone else's expression of pain.

In training hospitals where the majority of women have epidurals, many students are rarely exposed to drug-free labours and so the 'pain relief' paradigm is perpetuated:

I think the majority of midwives don't actually see that many women in labour that aren't under the influence of one drug or another. I've seen a lot of women in labour who haven't had drugs and I think I've learnt a lot about the sort of variation of how women cope with it. But I think if you haven't seen that, it's very difficult to know what 'normal' might be, and it might be very frightening then.

In a culture that promotes individualism and 'choice in childbirth', it is seen as part of the midwife's role to offer what has been described as 'the menu' of pain relief methods on offer.[4] This is a hierarchical menu (see Box 2.1) which can be offered in reverse order, depending on the ideology of the person offering it. Midwives tend to start with offering an array of 'non-pharmacological methods' with

Box 2.1

The pain relief menu (not a comprehensive list)

1. Methods you control yourself: water, changing positions, moving around, vocalizing, breathing techniques, relaxation, psychoprophylaxis, music
2. Methods with your chosen attendant: heat packs, massage, breathing techniques, counting, chanting, labour coaching, hiring a doula
3. Complementary therapies: herbs, homeopathy, acupuncture, acupressure, reflexology, hypnotism, biofeedback machines
4. The TENS (transcutaneous electrical nerve stimulation) machine
5. Entonox (inhalation of nitrous oxide)
6. Subcutaneous injections of sterile water in your back
7. Pethidine (or any equivalent injection of an opiate)
8. Epidural anaesthesia

relative confidence and comfort. They then work their way down through the menu in the name of 'informed choice', explaining the 'pros and cons' of each method, citing research evidence and women's experiences. In this process, they may attempt to mask the fact that their enthusiasm wanes in direct proportion to the menu's increasing dependence on technology, with its concurrent risks of surgical birth and ensuing complications. They do this in an effort to allay any feelings of guilt that women might suffer as a result of 'resorting to pain relief'. The menu presented thus ends with the most effective method of all, the epidural. Some practitioners, in particular doctors, may start offering the menu with the epidural and work their way through other options with decreasing conviction. Whichever way the menu is presented, the messages are clear:

You can try all of these things. Each method has its own merits and disadvantages. There may well be one method that suits you – pain is after all a highly individual thing – but, if you cannot cope, the epidural is there as the ultimate promise of pain relief. You don't have to be a martyr.

Insinuated in the offering of the menu is that, with few exceptions (usually those who have had babies before), women *will* need something to cope with the pain of labour.

The search for control

The embracing of pain relief is part of the desperate search to remain 'in control' during labour, as losing control is seen as the very worst that could happen to a woman, almost worse than dying.[63] In Tricia's qualitative study of women's experiences of the second stage of labour, women's predominant fear was that of being 'out of control'. Yet, paradoxically, in order to give birth women need to 'let go'. The women in Tricia's study (who laboured without opiate or epidural analgesia) described entering an altered state of consciousness involving a separation of mind and body, facilitated by endorphin release, which enabled their minds to let go and their bodies to be in control.[63] In this sense, there was no loss of control. The midwife was crucial to this process. By being competent, trusted and familiar, quiet and calm, supportive and unobtrusive, the midwife provides a safe anchor that enables the woman to enter this state of separation and thus retain control. 'The midwife keeps you safe going through all that', said one respondent.[63] The participants' sense of triumph and achievement on giving birth normally was strong. Yet most modern maternity services are organized in such a way that women are not able to develop a trusting, secure relationship with the midwife who will care for them in labour, and thus women are not able to use this natural, physiological coping strategy. In the uncertainty of not knowing who will be with you in labour and not knowing whether they are trustworthy, the security of a pain relief menu with the ultimate offer of an epidural is very appealing. Only then can you be 'certain' that the deepest fear – that of a public, humiliating loss of control in front of strangers – will be avoided.

The 'working with pain' paradigm

The characteristics of the 'working with pain' paradigm include the following attitudes and beliefs:

- Pain plays an important role in the physiology of normal labour.
- Women can cope with the pain of normal labour.
- There are long-term benefits to promoting normal birth in terms of women's experiences and lives.
- The offering of pharmacological pain relief to a woman when she is in pain is irresistible to her and associated with reducing the chances of normal labour.
- The genuine need for pain relief is associated with abnormal labour.
- Pain is a stimulator of endogenous opioids which are part of the hormonal cascades that promote normal birth.
- The midwife's role is to reduce stimulation to the senses to facilitate endorphin release.
- The expression of pain gives clues to progress.
- An understanding of the concept of normal pain helps midwives to sit back and deal with their own discomfort around pain.

If I think the labour's going well and the woman is experiencing what I would call 'normal pain' – which of course is debatable to some people – then I think I'm happy to sit and wait and not want to take the pain away.

The concept of 'normal' and 'abnormal' pain can be seen as a key to understanding the paradigm of working with pain. Midwives will often describe situations in home birth settings where, if a woman is 'climbing up the wall' with pain, one of two things are happening: she is either in transition or she is in early labour with a baby in an awkward position:

I remember the director of the Dutch Midwifery School telling me that for a normal birth, there is always normal pain. And it's the art of the midwife to discriminate whether this is normal or abnormal pain. If it's abnormal pain … there is something really pathological going on. In Holland where everything is divided into physiology/pathology, normal/abnormal, the need for pain relief is abnormal. I was taught in midwifery school that once a woman starts to scream and yell, you the midwife should be happy.

For many midwives, it may be their experience of attending births at home that teaches them the full impact of the notion of normal and abnormal pain:

Since I've been involved in home births, I've hardly seen a woman crying out for pain relief in use this in class!

early labour unless there's a really big positional complication and I've never seen a woman with a baby in a normal position and a normal labour with good contractions not able to deal with it … Once I felt I understood the difference between normal and abnormal pain, I began to think that it was important, sometimes a critical part of appropriate treatment of abnormal labours, to provide generous chemical pain relief, and that chemical pain relief wasn't necessary for normal labour.

The rationale for not offering pain relief is often based in listening to feedback from women after they have given birth and gaining confidence that their expressions of pain do not necessarily warrant immediate attention in terms of pain relief – even when they are pleading for an epidural in transition, as in this situation:

Of course I did talk to her afterwards and what she said was interesting. Bear in mind that she was very clear when we got to hospital that she wanted an epidural – 'I know I wrote down that I didn't want one, but now I really do'. What she said to me afterwards was: 'I didn't want an epidural. That wasn't what I was saying. What I wanted was something magic that no one had ever thought of before that you were going to invent right then to make it all better. But I didn't really want an epidural … It was an expression of my pain. I'm really glad that the relationship we had meant that you could interpret what I was saying'.

Afterwards, I'm still emotionally and physically wrecked and they've moved on completely. It's like, through a fog they can remember the time they were pleading for an epidural but they've moved on. So that's been significant for me just in terms of women's ability to recover or move on or have a different agenda in a very short space of time. And that's given me enormous confidence to … just be there … and not see pain as long-term damage.

Theories about the purpose of pain in labour also play a part in developing a rationale for 'working with pain' as identified in Box 2.2, and in the following quotations from the midwives' explanations of these theories:

Box 2.2

Theories about the purpose of pain in labour

- Pain as pure physiology
- Pain stops women and allows them to find a place of safety to give birth
- Pain marks the occasion
- Pain summons support
- Pain develops altruistic behaviour towards babies
- Pain heightens joy
- Pain is the transition to motherhood
- Pain gives clues to progress
- Pain reinforces the triumph of going through labour
- Pain is a trigger of neurohormonal cascades

Pain as pure physiology

When you think of the process involved, when you think that the woman has to get the baby from within to the outside, it's not surprising that there's some discomfort and pain.

Pain stops women and allows them to find a place of safety to give birth

So that women aren't in the middle of Safeways – which isn't a safe place to be – dropping their baby out. They have to get to a safe place. So they have these pains knocking on the door.

Pain marks the occasion

There is such an incredibly huge enormous thing about to happen that somehow you just can't do it by turning outwards and laughing and joking. You have to do something that's equally as enormous to yourself, something that you wouldn't normally be doing, a behaviour pattern that you wouldn't normally be assuming. It's like pulling everything out isn't it? Just getting hold of everything inside so that you can do that incredible transition into having a baby.

Pain summons support

It's a big transition to becoming a mother. All these big transitions in life, like also death, need love and attention to help you deal with them.

41

And pain relief – especially epidurals – it takes away her feeling and in doing so deprives her of enough love and attention.

Pain develops altruistic behaviour towards babies

Pain triggers a complex interplay of hormones and chemical changes together with a social adaptation ... it helps to stabilise and awaken the instinct that you have to care for this baby for 20 years.

Pain heightens joy

The ability to feel both joy and pain seems pretty central to our being here and, to hide behind Newtonian physics, I would say that every action has to have an opposite reaction. You have to have some experience of pain for the experience of joy and pleasure to have meaning.

Pain as the transition to motherhood

Pain takes us through that transition from being pregnant and growing a baby to the end product. I know it's a cliché talking about journeys and needing to go through it, but I think we do need to go through it.

The expression of pain: clues to progress for women and midwives

The way women are behaving, the way they respond to contractions – that doesn't just mean the noise – will give us an indication of where they are in labour ... that's part of the skill of midwives who don't routinely use drugs to control pain. If you're relying on un-drugged feedback from women, you get very good input, don't you, as to what's going on.

The triumph of going through pain

Women feel proud of themselves because they've done something very big ... like running a marathon, a huge sense of achievement.

Pain as a trigger of neurohormonal cascades

I think there's some sort of mechanism which enables women to cope with gradually increasing pain. I think we have to subscribe to this because we see it all the time, don't we? I think contractions get stronger and more painful, but not necessarily harder to deal with. So therefore there has to be something making that happen. I'm not sure if that's what's making her do the 'turning the eyes off bit' ... but I don't know what an endorphin is. It doesn't really matter.

The key is that sort of letting go, withdrawal thing. You see it and immediately you think, 'Ah good!' Yes, I see it as related to endorphins and I talk to people about facilitating endorphin release – you know: relaxation, comfort, and environment, feeling safe – all those kinds of things.

A midwifery approach to being with women in pain

In order to promote normal birth, with all its important ramifications for women, we may need to begin by finding a new way to talk to pregnant women about labour pain. Instead of moving straight to 'the menu', we may do well to begin with a message to the woman that, given the right environment and circumstances, she will be able to cope with the pain of normal labour; she will find her inner resources with the aid of her body's own internal 'opiates', which in turn will trigger and interplay with the hormonal cascades that promote strong contractions and normal birth.

I say to women, 'If you go into labour spontaneously at term and you have a baby in the right position and you're in a place where you feel safe, you're not going to be sent more pain than you can deal with. I believe it. I really believe it. And this might sound cocky, but I also think that by saying it and repeating it, we make it possible for women to do it. What's missing in antenatal care for women in our culture is that completely accurate confidence building reinforcement of their own ability to actually have a baby ... And the attitudes of midwives will have a profound effect. If you can build up confidence in women that they can definitely get on and do this, then I think they will. I suppose

I see it as our responsibility sometimes to believe in women when they don't believe in themselves. It's a protection against all that conditioning.

Often all that is necessary is to start a conversation acknowledging that most women are fearful of pain in labour. For a woman having a first baby, or for a woman who has only ever experienced Syntocinon-induced contractions, it can be illuminating to describe the nature of contractions in normal labour: the 'fierce arched rainbows that rise and fall like breath'.[61] Such descriptions could include the following components: emphasizing that contractions rarely last more than a minute; describing the building and fading of intensity and then the magic break between contractions where there is no pain; noting the fact that, as they get stronger and last longer, her body will produce more pain-killing hormones to help her cope. Such information often changes the ways in which women approach labour. The information may go a long way to promoting confidence that she will be able to cope with this pain. Strong reassurance that the midwife is trustworthy, that she will guard and watch over her throughout and that she will keep her safe may also remove much of the fear.

Arguably, we would do well to move away from the idea that women need to engage in the training programme of their choice in order to increase their chances of normal birth:

There are some women who've been trained or who have decided that they're going to fix their gaze on X's face or whatever, but I think that's a training thing. I did it myself when I had babies. But I think, left alone, women will be – and are – completely able to do it themselves and go right into their own depth of resources. And they don't look out at all, they don't look at you except to open their eyes and plead for a Caesarian or something in a panic moment when they're in transition ... I think a woman who's not desperate and who's coping, she'll disappear completely from connection with you. She becomes disconnected from her environment and from her carers or friends or whoever is supporting her, and she's in her own little space. It's like being in a bubble really ... and you as the midwife can only sit and watch and really admire, I suppose, how it works and what's going on.

Conclusion

Within the framework and context of modern parlance of choice and empowerment, we shouldn't forget that there is a place for professional interaction – for goodness sake, women need midwives and if we didn't have a clearly defined role in all of that then we wouldn't be needed. And I think some of that is to maintain a space of authority and knowingness. And I think the circle's going to turn back to midwives seeing themselves as being very important to the relationship, only from a very different perspective. But all this 'one-to-one' and 'know your midwife' – midwives don't even know themselves, and the whole nature of the relationship is framed on intimacy and knowing.

Most people will agree that to offer a labouring woman 'pain relief' when she is in pain in labour will be irresistible to her. Women often say that, when in pain, they would have accepted anything offered to them in the name of 'pain relief'. They describe relying on the midwife's belief that they 'could do it' when they didn't believe in themselves and say that this made a difference to the whole experience.

Midwives working in diverse settings share an understanding of the concept of 'working with pain'. However, it often feels as though we are swimming against the tide when the majority of women in Western countries expect some form of 'pain relief' in labour. We may need to be unashamedly persuasive in articulating the advantages of promoting normal birth and the role of pain within this if we are to convince many of our colleagues and women who expect to work their way through 'the menu' of pain relief. The relief of pain has its place in abnormal labours – those particularly long and hard labours, most often associated with malpositions. But to offer women in normal labour pain relief is to deny them their transformation and their triumph,[29,30] and to ultimately diminish them, both as strong women and as mothers.

Meanwhile, for those women who are clear that they want to give birth without the aid of drugs, there is a new possibility in the offing. Increasingly we are seeing a birth attendant, not unlike the 'Godsip', who is being promoted, particularly in the

USA, as an 'evidence-based' strategy to improve birth outcomes. A thriving private industry is growing in response to women's identified wish to hire this person who meets the pregnant woman in her home; gets to know her; works with her on preparing for birth; guarantees to be there with her in labour and to work with her to avoid drugs and promote an empowering experience of labour and giving birth. In the postnatal period, she visits the new mother at home, offers practical support and helps her establish breastfeeding.

The doula movement is gaining momentum in a climate where many women cannot get this service from midwives and where they cannot be sure that whoever they start with in labour will stay with them, or even have a philosophy of not offering 'pain relief'. In some cases, hospitals start to employ doulas to help staff the overstretched birthing units. There is plenty of sound evidence, including that arising from randomized controlled trials, that doulas are a 'cost-effective intervention', improving outcomes for women and their babies.[24] As a non-professional, the doula is a lot less threatening in the turf wars of childbirth than the midwife. Her allegiances are clearly with the woman. She also costs less to employ.

The questions have to be asked. Where does the midwife employed by the hospital fit in relation to the doula in the future? If maternity services are not reorganized soon to offer the certainty and support of a known and trusted midwife, will her role be to look after those women who bypass labour pain and reach instead for the 'certainty' and 'control' of the epidural and the elective caesarean?

Postscript

We finish this chapter with the unedited transcript of part of an interview with the well-known Dutch midwife, Beatrijs Smulders, who participated in Nicky's study, *A Midwifery Perspective on Pain in Labour*:[4]

The pain is really your friend in labour. In these big transitions in life the pain is coming to help you. And that is such a different concept of pain, that pain is your friend instead of your enemy. It's the same as in big emotional problems. The pain actually helps you when you're grieving … If you really dive into the pain, then finally the pain in someone becomes sweet. If you don't go through this pain, it becomes sour, you lose feeling and you get cut off from life.
I think the purpose of pain is to get the cascade going. From the moment the labour starts you have this self-reinforcing system of prostaglandins, oxytocin, endorphins and many more … it's like an avalanche. Once the snow starts to roll, the process is self-reinforcing and it has to go on and on and on. The uterus has to get more and more powerful, powerful, powerful, stronger, stronger, stronger … and when the baby's born the process stops immediately, the avalanche has fallen down and then there's silence. And if you take away the pain – some people are naïve enough to think that you can take away pain – but if you take away one thing, then you change the whole thing. One of the big aims of pain is to get the avalanche rolling. And very often you see that if you take away the pain, the avalanche stops in the middle of its rolling and the birth just doesn't get underway.
Pain's part of it and women just know in Holland that pain never traumatises. What is traumatising is when the midwife or obstetrician is not nice. They blame the pain if they felt not listened to.

References

1. Gibran K 1993 The prophet. Heinemann, London

2. Rich A 1977 Of woman born: motherhood as experience and institution. Virago, London

3. Kelpin V 1992 Birthing pain. Qualitative health research. In: Morse J (ed.) Qualitative research. Sage, London, p 93–103

4. Leap N 1997 A midwifery perspective on pain in labour. MSc Thesis, South Bank University, London

5. Page L 1997 Impressions of midwifery in New Zealand and Australia. Birth Issues 5:5–7

6. Roberts C L, Tracy S, Peat B 1999 Rates for obstetric intervention among private and public patients

in Australia: population based descriptive study. BMJ 321:137–141

7. Johanson R, Newburn M, Macfarlane A 2002 Has the medicalisation of childbirth gone too far? BMJ 324: 892–895

8. Department of Health 2004 National service framework for children, young people and maternity services. Department of Health, London

9. Kotaska A J, Klein M C, Liston R M 2006 Epidural analgesia associated with low-dose oxytocin augmentation increases caesarean births: a critical look at the external validity of randomized trials. Am J Obstet Gynecol 194:809–814

10. Lieberman E, O'donoghue C 2002 Unintended effects of epidural analgesia during labor: a systematic review. Am J Obstet Gynecol 186:S31–S68

11. Hunt S 2003 The epidural: a barrier to 'natural' birth? Pract Midwife 6:42–46

12. Mander R 2004 Failure to deliver: ethical issues relating to epidural analgesia in uncomplicated labour. In: Frith L, Draper H (eds) Ethics and midwifery, 2nd edn. Books for Midwives, Oxford, p 57–73

13. Anim-Somuah M, Smyth R, Howell C 2005 Epidural versus non-epidural or no analgesia in labour. Cochrane Database Syst Rev, Issue 4. Art. No.: CD000331. DOI: 10.1002/14651858.CD000331.pub2

14. Bricker L, Lavender T 2002 Parenteral opioids for labour pain relief: a systematic review. Am J Obstet Gynecol 186:94–109

15. Hunt S 2002 Pethidine: love it or hate it? MIDIRS Midwif Digest 12:363–365

16. Heelbeck L 1999 Administration of pethidine in labour. British Journal of Midwifery 7:372–377

17. Olofsson C, Ekblom A, Ekman-Ordeberg G et al 1996 Lack of analgesic effect of systematically administered morphine or pethidine on labour pain. Br J Obstet Gynaecol 103:968–972

18. Hodnett E D, Downe S, Edwards N et al 2005 Home-like versus conventional institutional settings for birth. Cochrane Database Syst Rev, Issue 1. Art. No.: CD000012. DOI: 10.1002/14651858.CD000012.pub2

19. National Childbirth Trust 2005 Are women getting the birth environment they need? The 2005 Better Birth Environment Survey. National Childbirth Trust, London

20. Green J M, Baston H A, Easton S C et al 2003 Greater expectations: The inter-relationships between women's expectations and experiences of decision making, continuity, choice and control in labour, and psychological outcomes. Summary report. Mother and Infant Research Unit, Leeds

21. Hodnett E D 2002 Pain and women's satisfaction with the experience of childbirth: a systematic review. Am J Obstet Gynecol 186:S160–S172

22. Silverton L 2001 Why women choose caesarean section. RCM Midwives Journal 4:328

23. Hodnett E D 2000 Continuity of caregivers for care during pregnancy and childbirth. Cochrane Database Syst Rev, Issue 1. Art. No.: CD000062. DOI: 10.1002/14651858. CD000062

24. Hodnett E D, Gates S, Hofmeyr G J et al 2007 Continuous support for women during childbirth. Cochrane Database Syst Rev, Issue 3. Art. No.: CD003766. DOI: 10.1002/14651858.CD003766.pub2

25. Smith C A, Collins C T, Cyna A M et al 2006 Complementary and alternative therapies for pain management in labour. Cochrane Database Syst Rev, Issue 4. Art. No.: CD003521. DOI: 10.1002/14651858. CD003521.pub2

26. Cluett E R, Nikodem V C, McCandlish R E et al 2002 Immersion in water in pregnancy, labour and birth. Cochrane Database Syst Rev, Issue 2. Art. No.: CD000111. DOI: 10.1002/14651858.CD000111.pub2

27. Cluett E R, Pickering R M, Getliffe K et al 2004 Randomised controlled trial of labouring in water compared with standard augmentation for management of dystocia in first stage of labour. British Medical Journal 328:314

28. Chamberlain G, Wraight A, National Birthday Trust Fund (Great Britain) et al (eds) 1993 Pain and its relief in childbirth: the results of a national survey conducted by the National Birthday Trust. Churchill Livingstone, Edinburgh

29. Halldorsdottir S, Karlsdottir S I 1996 Journeying through labour and delivery: perceptions of women who have given birth. Midwifery 12:48–61

30. Lundgren I, Dahlberg K 1998 Women's experience of pain during childbirth. Midwifery 14:105–110

31. Dickenson J E, Paech M J, McDonald S J et al 2003 Maternal satisfaction with childbirth and intrapartum analgesia in nulliparous labour. Aust N Z J Obstet Gynaecol 43:463–469

32. Heinz S D, Sleigh M J 2003 Epidural or no epidural anaesthesia: relationships between beliefs about childbirth and pain control choices. J Reprod Infant Psychol 21:323–333

33. Morgan B M, Bulpitt C J, Clifton P et al 1982 Analgesia and satisfaction in childbirth (the Queen Charlotte's 1000 Mother Survey). Lancet 2(8302):808–810

34. Olsson P, Jansson L, Norberg A 2000 A qualitative study of childbirth as spoken about in midwives' ante- and postnatal consultations. Midwifery 16:123–134

35. Olayemi O, Adeniji R A, Udoh E S et al 2005 Determinants of pain perception in labour among parturients at the University College Hospital, Ibadan. J Obstet and Gynaecol 25:128–130

36. Imarenglaye C, Ande A 2006 Demand and utilisation of labour analgesia service by Nigerian women. J Obstet Gynaecol 26:130–132

37. Kuti O, Faponle A 2006 Perception of labour pain among the Yoruba ethnic group in Nigeria. J Obstet Gynaecol 26:332–334

38. Callister L C, Khalaf I, Semenic S et al 2003 The pain of childbirth: perceptions of culturally diverse women. Pain Manag Nurs 4:145–154

39. Niven C, Murphy-Black T 2000 Memory for labor pain: a review of the literature. Birth 27:244–253

40. McCrea H, Wright M E, Stringer M 2000 Psychosocial factors influencing personal control in pain relief. Int J Nurs Stud 37:493–503

41. Sandall J, Davies J, Warwick C 2001 Evaluation of the Albany Midwifery Practice: final report. Nightingale School of Midwifery, King's College, London

42. Reed B 2002 The Albany Midwifery Practice (1). MIDIRS Midwif Digest 12:118–121

43. Reed B 2002 The Albany Midwifery Practice (2). MIDIRS Midwif Digest 12:261–264

44. Bonica J 1994 Labour pain. In: Wall P, Melzack R (eds) Textbook of pain. Churchill Livingstone, Edinburgh, p 615–641

45. Robertson A 1994 Empowering women: teaching active birth in the 90s. ACE Graphics, Sydney

46. Chesler P 1979 With child: a diary of motherhood. Thomas Y Crowell, New York

47. Davis-Floyd R 1992 Birth as an American rite of passage. University of California Press, Berkeley, CA

48. Lewin E 1985 By design: reproductive strategies and the meaning of motherhood. In: Homans H (ed.) The sexual politics of reproduction. Gower, London

49. Lichy R, Herzberg E 1993 The waterbirth handbook. Gateway, Bath

50. De Reincourt A 1983 Woman and power in history. Honeyglen, Bath

51. Morris D 1991 The culture of pain. University of California Press, Berkeley, CA

52. Wilson A 1990 The ceremony of childbirth and its interpretation. In: Fildes V (ed.) Women as mothers in pre-industrial England. Routledge, London, p 68–107

53. Caton D 1999 What a blessing she had chloroform: the medical and social response to the pain of childbirth from 1800 to the present. Yale University Press, New Haven, CT

54. Poovey M 1986 Scenes of an indelicate character: the medical treatment of Victorian women. Representations 14:137–168

55. Dick-Read G 1957 Childbirth without fear: the principles and practice of natural childbirth, 3rd edn. William Heinemann, London (first published 1942)

56. Anderson T 2002 Out of the laboratory; back to the darkened room. MIDIRS Midwif Digest 12:65–69

57. Robertson A 1996 The pain of labour. Midwif Today 37:19–42

58. Helman C G 1990 Culture, health and illness, 2nd edn. Butterworth-Heinemann, Oxford

59. Kitzinger S (ed.) 1987 Giving birth: how it really feels. Victor Gallancz, London

60. Morse JM, Park C 1988 Homebirth and hospital deliveries: a comparison of the perceived painfulness of parturition. Research in Nursing and Health 11: p 175–181

61. Taylor S 1990 Oxytocin. In: Palmeira R. In the gold of flesh. Poems of birth and motherhood. The Women's Press, London

62. McCrea B H 1996 An investigation of rule-governed behaviours in the control of pain management during the first stage of labour. DPhil Thesis, University of Ulster, Northern Ireland

63. Anderson T 1997 To the ends of the earth and back: women's experiences of the second stage of labour. MSc Thesis, University of Surrey, Surrey

Birth and spirituality

Jennifer Hall

Acknowledgement: Meg Taylor co-wrote this chapter in the first edition, but due to ill health has been unable to contribute to its revision.

Chapter contents

Introduction

During the 20th century, over 1200 studies investigated the connection between religious belief and health.[1] Many have shown a positive relationship between having religious faith and aspects of health, although the quality and methodology of some of the studies have been questioned. In recent years, there has also been an increase in book publications relating spirituality to different health disciplines.[2-12] There is a clear indication from this literature that spiritual issues are thought to be relevant in relation to health care. However, despite some authors addressing the spiritual aspects of midwifery and childbirth,[7,9] this work is limited, with the focus of care, education and research generally being applied to the physical, emotional and social issues experienced by women and midwives within the maternity services.[5] Since this chapter was first published, a few papers have been written related to the field. It appears there is limited research being carried out specifically on spiritual issues by midwives, though it is known that PhD studies are in progress in Australia, Hawaii and the UK (personal communication). This apparent lack of interest in spiritual care at the beginning of life is surprising considering the wealth of literature and understanding of spiritual need among those who give care to the dying. The purpose of this chapter is to explore some of the issues of spirituality and spiritual care in relation to the normality of childbirth and to encourage discussion about how midwifery practices may include these issues in the future.

Holistic concepts in midwifery regulations

In recent years, the aim to provide holistic care, to regard the individual as 'whole' and 'complete', has been part of midwifery and nursing culture. The implication of this is that a person is to be regarded at least as a combination of physical, emotional and spiritual aspects.[12-14] Others suggest this should also include intellectual and social aspects (Fig. 3.1).[2] However, Goddard has argued that this potential separation into parts may be in itself reductionist, and that it conflicts with the need to care for people as a whole.[15]

Davis-Floyd suggested that the aim to give holistic care may be too great a challenge in institutions that are technologically orientated.[16] Yet, the philosophical expectation of the International Confederation of Midwives[17] is that 'Midwifery care is holistic in nature, grounded in an understanding of the social, emotional, cultural, spiritual, psychological and physical experiences of women and based upon the best available evidence' and 'Childbearing is a profound experience, which carries significant meaning to the woman, her family and the community'. Further: 'Midwifery care promotes, protects and supports women's reproductive rights and respects ethnic and cultural diversity'.

It is clear from this worldwide philosophy for midwifery practice that spirituality is regarded as important for women and their families and subsequently for their carers. This implies that those who train midwives will know what spirituality and spiritual need are, how they can be assessed and implemented and how they should be taught.[18]

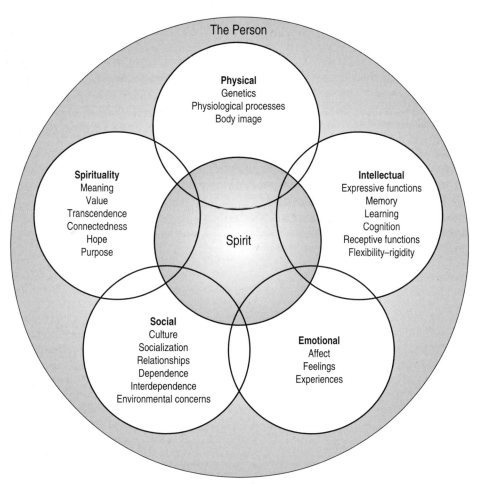

Fig 3.1 • The five dimensions of the person. From Swinton,[2] modified with permission from Beck, Rawlins and Williams Mental Health Psychiatric Nursing (Mosby 1988).

What is the nature of spirituality?

If spiritual issues in relation to childbirth are to be explored, carers require an understanding of what they are. It is often assumed that religious belief is necessary as a foundation for spirituality and, therefore, those without religious beliefs may be disregarded as having no spiritual experiences or needs. This is reflected in methods of assessment and history taking in maternity care, where such questions are limited to finding out the religious denominations of the women, rather than taking time to assess the nature and depth of their beliefs.[19-21] Clarke[22] indicates that the spiritual nature of those with religious beliefs should not be ignored, and Swinton[23] argues for religious and non-religious spirituality to be approached separately. In contrast, Totton suggests that spirituality and religious practice are quite different.[24] He distinguishes the two by stating that spirituality always involves an enlightenment practice:[24]

> ... not just a theory or belief but a technique or a set of techniques, aimed at creating some sort of change in persons ... The shift that is attempted can be described and conceptualised in many ways. But perhaps all the practices I am considering might agree that it involves a radical lessening of anxiety: a profound relaxation which follows from a reappraisal of our situation as human beings. (p 131–132)

This shift within a person can sometimes be tumultuous and has been labelled *spiritual emergency*.[25-27]

Totton's emphasis may be exclusive of those who are unwilling to engage in such practice.[24] A more inclusive approach to spirituality may be one that focuses on each person's experience. If we are to regard each person in the terms of wholeness and completeness, as indicated by the principles of holistic care, there is potential for a spirit in all humans and the expression of this aspect of life may come in many forms. In establishing the links between the physical, emotional and spiritual aspects of a person, McSherry argued that 'spirituality pervades all dimensions of one's existence in a meaningful and intricate manner, whether there is a conscious

awareness of this or not'.[4] He further indicated that the spiritual dimension of a person's life exists even if the person's intellect or psychological abilities are not functioning. Dombeck suggested that 'the spiritual issues in a person's life are at the core of all other issues' and, as a consequence, 'small changes in one's spirit can affect radical change in all aspects of one's life'.[28] This is demonstrated in Swinton's model (see Fig. 3.1),[2] which illustrates the interdependence of five dimensions of the person and the spirit.

The root of the word spirit is the Latin word *spiritus*, meaning breath, and the Greek word for breath, *pneuma*, is reference to the soul; Burkhardt & Nagai-Jacobson enlarged on this to state 'The soul animates all that we are and do'.[8] The spirit is viewed as 'the expression of the self that is within us all'.[29] It is clear that this implies a need to understand the considerable complexity in the relationship of spirituality to people's lives. It could be asked then how credible it is even to attempt to produce a definition that covers every belief, non-belief, religion, culture, gender, creed, ethnic group or social situation.

Examination of the studies on spiritual issues in relation to health care show that the definitions contain many similar elements that could be associated with spirituality within a person and in the provision of spiritual care (Boxes 3.1 and 3.2).[5] A question arises whether evidence of one of these elements is sufficient to define spirituality or whether a number of them have to be present in order for a person to be thought of as 'spiritual'.[5] How anyone expresses spirituality will be affected by their social, cultural and historical background.[30-34] Definitions of spirituality have tended to be vague, illustrating the

---

Box 3.1

Elements of spirituality identified from health research

- Transcendence
- Searching for meaning and purpose
- Belonging and connecting
- Relational aspects
- Self-awareness
- Hope and faith
- Creativity

Box 3.2

Elements of spiritual care identified from health research

- Recognizing value and acceptance of each person
- Giving support/having presence
- Self-awareness
- Understanding
- Openness/intuition
- Willingness to help others to find meaning
- Counselling skills
- Love and compassion

Box 3.3

Suggested characteristics of feminine spirituality

- Caring
- Compassion
- Non-violence
- Power to 'create and nurture life'
- Unity with 'Mother Earth'
- Wholeness
- Intuition
- Suffering as a source of strength
- Attention to detail
- Faithfulness
- Listening
- Selfless giving
- Adaptability to people
- Encouraging love
- Story-telling
- Establishing connecting relationships

(Accumulated from Burkhardt & Nagai-Jacobson,[8] Tucakovic,[40] King[41])

problem of frameworks that aim to be inclusive of everyone.[35,36] They tend not to address adequately the relation of spiritual issues to a person's bodily and emotional functioning.

Most studies into spirituality do not distinguish between men and women in the populations investigated.[5] It is not known to what extent gender is relevant in shaping spirituality, though women are reported to have greater tendency toward spiritual connection and faith than men.[34] Some women have argued that women's spiritual experiences have been viewed from a patriarchal perspective.[32,37,38] Gender stereotyping should, of course, be avoided,[39] but some writers have attempted to suggest characteristics of spirituality that may be specifically applicable to women (Box 3.3). While intuitive knowledge has been suggested to be a specifically feminine trait,[40–44] it is not exclusive to women, and Swinton commented that 'intuition and feeling form a significant aspect of the ways in which human beings make sense of large parts of their experiences'.[2] The culture of modern health care requires evidence-based knowledge, and intuition does not lend itself easily to quantification. There is a risk that the contrast of the unquantifiable with the medical paradigm may lead to further gender stereotyping, with intuition written off as specifically feminine and evidence of women's difficulty in reasoning.[45] Women's spirituality may also be viewed in relation to the hormonal cycles that women experience. It has been claimed that these cycles may lead to women being more open to the 'intuitive, unplanned and nonrational, leaving room for the unexpected'.[8] Rather than a deficit in

reasoning, which has to be compensated for, this could be seen as an advantage.

If we are to apply an awareness of spirituality to women and their families, it is necessary to engage in a women-centred approach, with each person treated as an individual and their needs and aspirations addressed accordingly.[5] It may also be advisable to stop trying to research spirituality as a separate entity, and instead to research people's lives as they are, recognizing their complexity and seeing spirituality as part of the whole of their existence.[28]

Spirituality and childbirth

How can spirituality be placed within the context of normal childbirth and what are the implications for all those who are part of this experience? Despite the evidence cited above that spiritual care is inscribed in midwifery philosophy,[17] it is rare to find detailed explorations of this concept in frameworks of care, or within educational programmes.[46] However, the spiritual nature of the midwifery role remains in many cultures[47] and, historically, in the developed world, midwives were involved in giving spiritual care to women during labour.[48,49] It has been suggested that they learnt to avoid drawing attention to their role in spiritual matters to ensure professional survival when the powerful Christian church tried to suppress non-standard spiritual approaches, and when medical practice and research was often male dominated.[50] At that time, to be a midwife was to be seen as influential and powerful.[48]

This perception, and the role of midwives, has changed since the large-scale move of birth into hospitals throughout the world. Rising caesarean section rates worldwide reveal the extent to which birth has become entrenched in a biomedical model.[16,51,52] Furthermore, the social structure in which women in the developed world live has become far more complex. Technological advances have had a profound psychosocial impact on attitudes affecting women's perception of birth. The speed and range of new technologies have contributed to an intolerance of delay and a sense that much that was previously seen as beyond human control can and should be manipulable. To some extent, it is now an 'instant' world, where the expectation is to have what is desired immediately, with as little waiting as possible. Instant access to information and communication via the Internet and cable and satellite television has increased the amount of choice at the touch of a button. Such altered expectations have subsequently changed the expectations of the women who enter the maternity services. Their potential tolerance for 'waiting', for appointments or even the birth of a baby, may be lowered. The increased use of antenatal investigations and ultrasound techniques has opened a window to women of the potential earlier relationships with their unborn and fears of not achieving 'perfection'. The expectation of a positive experience may be raised. The excessive use of technology to speed up all aspects of birth exacerbates a pre-existing tendency to separate carer and the person being cared for, as the carer focuses more on the machine. This creates a disconnection between women and their carers.[16]

It has been suggested by some psychologists that one of the major psychological tasks of pregnancy is first to identify with and then to distinguish oneself from the baby.[53] Some modern technological developments, such as mobile phones and text messaging, may impact on this by reducing one's ability to tolerate separation and delayed gratification. The sociological issues raised here may reflect a culture of fear that pervades society and the lack of trust in oneself and in each other.[54] Concomitant fear of natural processes will impact on women's attitudes to giving birth. The nature of this fear and the associated risk women experience when coming to give birth are explored later, but recognizing the need to understand the background culture of each woman is helpful in introducing the concept of spirituality. Mainstreaming this aspect of care will need a major change in the philosophical approach to birth by women, by midwives and by other carers, in order to encourage recognition of spiritual need. However, if caregivers are to accept that birth is a normal, natural, creative, physiological process and that a woman needs to be cared for in a holistic, woman-centred way, they must recognize her personal understanding of her spiritual needs and aspirations. Once this is acknowledged, it is possible to see how the elements identified in Boxes 3.1 and 3.2 could be applied to the care of pregnant and labouring women.

Effect of spirituality on mothers

Richards highlighted birth as being 'one of the most powerful forces on earth and certainly the most powerful that can occupy a human body'.[55] When women tell their birth stories, some women do so in the language and framework of a spiritual experience,[56,57] using terms such as 'holiness' and 'miraculous'.[6,38] The reality of experiencing pregnancy and motherhood may provide the opportunity for discovering personal significance and growth, which may, in turn, be regarded as a spiritual event.[6,57–65] It is suggested that for those with religious belief, the birth experience may bring them closer to the Higher Being they believe in. For example, Baumiller stated: 'Bringing a new person into the world for whom one has responsibility must cause a great feeling of closeness with God and the infinite love that is co-creating a human being whose destiny is in God's and her hands'.[66] The personal value women place on the unborn may also have implications for their views of the sacredness of the birth event.[29]

Do all women have a spiritual experience during birth? If so, do some women not recognize the phenomenon when they experience it? Can women who have an inherently technologically managed birth still regard it as an opportunity for spiritual growth? Birth as an event is full of symbolism and ritual behaviours[30,67–69] and has the potential to be life changing. The implication from this is that a woman cannot go back to the way she was before she gave birth. In many cultures, birth is regarded as a rite of passage, a time when a woman moves from one social state to another. She may also move from one spiritual state into a state of greater awareness.[6] A number of individual issues may influence the meanings a woman gains from her childbirth experience. These could be culture, age, parity, personal experience and religious faith or spiritual beliefs.[63] The depth and richness of this experience will be dependent on her background and previous life challenges, as well as on her beliefs.

The development of a search for meaning and purpose in life appears to be a significant element within a person's spiritual experience. In Klassen's study of religious women in America who gave birth at home, she established that they gave meaning to home as the place of birth, their bodies as the basis of new life and their pain as the trigger of physical and spiritual power.[6]

Pain as a spiritual experience

Nicky Leap and Tricia Anderson explore the concept of pain in labour in some depth in Chapter 2. In this section, we concentrate on the spiritual dimension of pain in labour. The women cited in Klassen's study[6] chose to give birth at home, away from the technological environment of hospital, and were generally willing to experience the pain of labour as a source of growth. The pain coexisted with a sense of pleasure in feeling the sensations and power of the birth, and the satisfaction of being able to endure the labour. Elsewhere, the pain of childbirth has been described in terms of being positive and 'normal'.[70] Some women perceive that the intensity of labour pain gives meaning to the transition to being a mother.[71] For those women with a religious belief, the sense of openness may lead to a greater closeness to their God.[5] The inability to escape from the power of the pain has been described as being 'useable' leading 'beyond the limits of the experience itself'.[61] Taylor took this further by relating it to the

closeness of the experience to the boundaries of death: 'To give birth one needs to go through the pain of labour, to survive the darkness and the fear, which is the fear of death. To go through this easiest requires acceptance, an opening to the experience, which is also an opening of the cervix'.[65]

If the meaning of the pain is so intense and deep, it is perhaps not surprising that some are fearful of experiencing such opening of themselves. They may seek to have the pain removed from them by analgesic or anaesthetic means. There is a delicate balance between pain relief interfering with the natural process of labour and the relief of pain that enables a woman to regain her personal level of control.

In order to be so wide open in the emotional and spiritual sense as well as physically, to be so totally vulnerable, a woman requires a place of safety. She needs to feel safe within her physical environment and with the people with her if she is to be able truly to let go of who she is and open herself up to what she will become. Odent described this as a 'period when the mother behaves as if she is "on another planet" cutting herself off from our everyday world and going on a sort of inner trip'.[72] To be able to establish such a change in a level of consciousness requires the woman to trust the carers who are with her and for the carers to understand that this is part of the process of a normal labour. There is a paradox here in that women need to have sufficient control of their own labour to be able to feel safe enough to lose total control. Some women ensure this place of safety by finding methods of putting themselves in situations where they can avoid 'being interfered with' by the midwives: for example in a birthing pool where they can float away from the side.[73] The degree of safety will be enhanced if the woman and her caregivers have had an opportunity to build up a relationship with each other before the event, but it will be hindered if the birth attendant does not have knowledge of the normal physiological processes of birth or tries to control the situation to meet her own needs.[16,72] Caregivers need understanding of the rhythms and breathing patterns women experience within a normal physiological labour and the 'letting go' of power and control to the woman's body. For some of the women in Klassen's study, this control was experienced as submission of themselves into the hands of a Higher Power in relation to their belief.[6] Consequently, some women's decisions regarding care in labour may be directed by their religious beliefs. These decisions could include refusal of analgesia, rejection of interference in the timing of labour, such as by induction, or refusal to agree to operative delivery or blood transfusion.[30,74]

Place of birth

For some women, the only sacred, safe space where they can truly let themselves go is their own home; for others, a spiritually safer environment will be a hospital. For both, there will be a need for privacy and security within the environment.[72] The environment will need to be 'right' for the woman to feel free to practise the ceremonies for labour related to her religious or spiritual beliefs. This may not be easy in hospital. For those couples of Jewish faith within Sered's study, the ceremonies were carried out before going into hospital.[68] This demonstrates the difficulties associated with institutional acceptance of religious ritual, even in societies where religious faith is central and highly visible. Rituals that women in labour may wish to use to convey faith may include chanting, music, prayer, use of candles and specific care of personal hygiene or ritual hand washing. However, such women may find that they will encounter barriers to their use within hospital settings.[5] Some women in Klassen's study felt 'the religious aspects of the birth were best respected in the home'.[6] How they then observed these practices were personal to them. In Kahn's unequivocal view, a spiritual experience of birth in a hospital environment is not possible.[75] However, anecdotally, women speak of the spiritual experiences taking place within hospitals and it has also been suggested that women can prepare their own space spiritually within a hospital setting when they enter the room, or by 'absent visualization' if they have been able to visit the labour rooms before the birth.[76]

Risk and safety

The choices that women make for their labour will be related to their concepts of risk and safety and their level of fear.[6,56,60,77–79] Furedi stated that 'The

term risk refers to the probability of damage, injury, illness, death or other misfortune associated with hazard. Hazards are generally defined to mean a threat to people and what they value'.[54] For women coming to labour, there is a definite threat to their integrity physically and emotionally, and to the value they place on themselves and their unborn child. Being on the borders of life and death, they take the risk of not knowing whether they will survive intact. The reality of the pain and the raw power of the birthing process lay women bare, placing them in touch with their real selves. Yet for each person involved in the birth process, including the woman, partner, midwife and medical team, the sense of risk and safety will be individual to them, and it may be different from the others who are there. If a woman regards the technological environment of a hospital as safer, then that is the better option psychologically for her. Partners may feel more safe within the home, but many would feel safer in hospital. Some midwives may prefer the different sense of safety that a home birth offers while others prefer hospital-based environments. This can lead to stress and conflict within the woman if she senses she is not being supported in her views. It is to be recognized that those with religious faith may have concepts of risk and fear that are embedded in trust in a Higher Power,[6] but this will also be dependent on their personal levels of fear and anxiety.

Some theorists consider that the Western world is currently entrenched in fear.[54] Fear is a normal, human reaction, available for the safety and protection of ourselves. To be fearful in dangerous situations is sensible and normal. However, fear that becomes all-encompassing and all-enveloping may lead to emotional and physical paralysis in people's lives. The alleviation of fear could also be regarded as a spiritual need, given the potential of fear to prevent an individual from reaching personal fulfilment, from finding meaning and purpose within a situation, of preventing connecting relationships, of taking away hope. Watson defined spiritual emergencies as 'critical, experientially difficult stages of profound psychological transformation involving one's entire being'.[26] According to this definition, birth could be regarded as a potential spiritual emergency as there is a positive potential for change: there is also a chance of devastation. Richards stated that fear of pain and of childbirth itself is further perpetuated through the effect of cultural, religious, gender and societal influences.[55] Psychiatrists have recently defined a pathological condition of tocophobia,[80] though it has been challenged as to whether this is actually a 'normal' reaction to a traumatic event.[81] There are currently inconsistent results from studies investigating whether the increase in caesarean sections in recent years may be related to women's fear.[82,83]

The evidence surrounding fear in labour is increasing and suggests that it may prevent labour from starting, increase the amount of pain experienced and lead to higher rates of operative deliveries, especially elective caesarean section. In addition, there would seem to be a greater chance of pre- or post-term delivery, restriction in growth of the baby or asphyxia at birth.[80,84–90] If the aim is to increase the chance that women will birth normally, it is clear that there is a need to address the concept of fear, both within individuals and culturally within societies. Potentially, midwives may alleviate these fears by being known carers and by developing effective communication, including effective listening, in particular asking the right questions. They could help the woman to find meaning and purpose in the situation by assisting her in understanding where her fears are coming from and in facing them.[91] They could provide an opportunity to pray or find support from her religion if this is what she wants. The last point is demonstrated in Klassen's study, where the women were able to turn to resources beyond themselves or within their religious community to ease their journey.[6] Women need to address their fears before they move into labour, perhaps before they even embark on pregnancy. Midwives and other professionals should be aware of the possibility of fear, provide opportunities for women to talk about their fears and to acknowledge that this activity is part of the process of providing care.

Most midwives are women, and as such have either given birth or have the potential to do so. They are, therefore, vulnerable to the same fears regarding childbirth as their clients. Also, as women, they carry cultural fears: all of us have grown and developed in the body of a woman and experienced women as mothers at a time when we have been vulnerable in earliest infancy. According to psychoanalytic theory, this makes women the objects of powerful unconscious feelings, both positive and negative. If women are to approach birth from a spiritual perspective, which requires them to be open and accepting of uncertainty, they will demand a level of support from their birth attendants that can accommodate this.[92]

Relationships and spirituality

Creating and forming relationships is valuable in itself. For a pregnant woman, it could become an important aspect of her spiritual journey. By the time she has reached labour, she will have had the time of pregnancy, of being challenged by the concept of having a new person growing inside her. This is described as a 'mysterious union' where the woman and her unborn baby are as one, but two separate human beings.[60] Rubin argued that the child cannot be independent from the way the mother is or how she behaves.[59] Her own boundaries of where she ends and the baby begins may have been confused, merged together within her psyche. She may also have experienced the mystery of giving love to an unborn child and perceiving love received in return. Rubin's study of women's maternal experience suggested that a woman demonstrates the action of giving of herself by the act of birth through letting go of her 'physical, mental and social self', with the aim of giving the child to her partner first, then to the rest of her family and subsequently to society.[59] A different study examining the experiences of women of Jewish faith demonstrated that many women felt that it was the development of their relationship with their new baby that gave them a spiritual experience rather than the process of the labour.[68] There is some limited evidence suggesting that the mother's negative perception and inability to integrate the experience psychologically may lead to difficulties with early attachment with her new baby.[93] The intensity, power and empowerment of experiencing normal birth may have a positive effect on the relationship with her child. The sense of having 'gone through something' together, of having been in touch with the creation of birth may subsequently increase the depth of the relationship. Odent has explored this further in his claims that oxytocin is the 'hormone of love'.[72] He also wrote about the 'fetus ejection reflex', which occurs in women who are able to be upright in labour, and who have an adrenaline rush prior to birth. This process induces the infant to be more alert at birth, thus encouraging eye contact and mutual bonding. This is a physical manifestation of the psychological and spiritual aspects of the love relationship, indicating the depth of the intertwining of all parts of a human being and the need for wholeness for this relationship to develop.

Being able to form relationships that are 'connecting' has been seen as particularly spiritually significant to women.[42] These may be made through a relationship with God or 'Ultimate Other' or, in more secular terms, through a sense of self, in connection with history and the future, nature or other people.[42] During birth, women may wish to establish some or all of these connections as part of their spiritual experience. Some women have written of their identification with other women's experiences as they give birth, describing being on a continuum with all women who have given birth before and will do after.[53,56,57 61,64,75,94] The relationship with a woman's own mother may also be significant here and it may be a spiritual context that leads a woman to make contact with her mother around birth.[5] Baumiller stated that there is a particular bond that develops because of the sharing of knowledge about the birthing experience: 'A woman's mother often becomes an even more special person in a daughter's life because now they too know'.[66] Conversely, the birth may have a detrimental effect of revealing hidden negative feelings towards the baby's grandmother.[53,61,95] Further difficulties may arise where a woman has two perceived mothers, for instance in adoption.[53,62] It may only be speculated how this effect could manifest in women born as a result of infertility treatments.[5] Hampton's study of the birth experiences of 20 adoptees identified these women as lacking a sense of 'belonging', which resulted in the need for a majority to search for their natural mother during pregnancy or shortly after birth.[62] Those who were able to find her before the birth were helped by the knowledge, while those who did not felt disadvantaged. This implies that the opportunity and capacity of being able to connect with a woman's natural mother is significant

to the birthing experience, psychologically and spiritually.[5]

Many participants in a study of women's self-development identified childbirth as the most important learning experience in their lives and linked the creative nature of birth with an increased depth of understanding of their creative abilities.[96] An investigation of the development of maternal identity establishes that '… childbearing requires an exchange of a known self in a known world for an unknown self in an unknown world'.[59] The act of birth may thus be seen as a peak experience in women's lives,[60] with the survival of pain seen as part of the process of achieving the appropriate depth of self-knowledge. Such depth of connection with self in childbirth may be a key aspect of a woman's spiritual growth as it establishes the person she really is and places her in a totally vulnerable and open position.

Some women may experience a connection with the earth and nature during pregnancy,[57,97,98] or desire to spend time outside in labour, to feel sand or grass under her feet or to smell nature through flowers or woody odours.[56] Others may be particularly drawn to water: to be close to, to swim in, to labour in or to give birth in.[72] Odent highlighted the 'mysterious power of water on the birth process', and stated 'Water, as a symbol, helps humans to feel secure in a great variety of circumstances'.[72] Such desire for security may be another indication of the spiritual nature of the whole process.

A woman's relationship with her partner will also be of significance during the birth process. There are accounts of men describing the wonder of the beauty and creation inherent in childbirth, and some may feel a spiritual experience themselves despite being an 'outsider'.[56] There is evidence that some women develop a new connecting relationship with their partner during the birth as they change from being a couple to a family.[64] It is important for the woman to feel that the birth supporters will also enhance her birth experience and not detract from it. Both Gaskin[56] and Klassen[6] have given examples of how unwelcome people present at the birth can prevent the woman from giving birth effectively. It is a challenge to midwives to be able to recognize if someone's presence or interference is effectively preventing the woman's ability to 'flow' in labour, especially without having formed a relationship with the woman prior to the labour. There have been continued discussions whether men should be totally excluded from birth rooms because of the 'feminine' nature of the act. In some cultures it is not normal for a man to be present, where birth is the exclusive role of women within the society. Where it is the social norm for male partners to be present, it is feasible to expect that the birth may be a spiritual experience for the men as well as the women. However, they will be carrying their own perceptions of risk and fear, and conflict will arise if this is at a different level to that of the women. How much a man trusts the other carers within the situation and how much he trusts the woman's body to be able to give birth will have an influence on his own understanding and fear within the situation. His own concepts of value and worth will also be important, as well as the strength of his love and care towards his partner. Within some religious communities, there may be particular responsibilities for prayer or ritual that the man will carry within the time that birth is taking place.[30] This may be easier to enact within the home setting, as Sered's study identified.[68] Men may not be allowed to be present, and it will be important for the midwife to understand the cultural principles and religious rules associated with birth by which the family live.

There have been few investigations of the spiritual effect of other children being present at the birth. It is evident that children are able to have a simple acceptance of life, and this seems to enable their acceptance of birth as a normal, natural process. There seems no reason to exclude children if the parents wish them to be there.

The unborn child

It is a challenge to consider the spiritual nature of the unborn child.[29] A woman's personal views of the value of her unborn child will be influenced by her culture, religion and beliefs.[29] Some have suggested that certain dreams in pregnancy are evidence of the child's spiritual potential, in particular dreams of white birds or light.[76,99,100] However, it is also suggested that, for this to occur, the mother has to accord spiritual meanings to such dreams from within a spiritually aware frame of reference.[75]

There is evidence to suggest that the mother will make some form of connecting relationship with her unborn baby during the pregnancy.[57,58,99,101,102] However, those women whose pregnancies carry some uncertainty or who are thought to be at risk may try not to get too attached emotionally until the perceived threat to the pregnancy has passed.[103] This may even be avoided until the baby is successfully born and is perceived to be well. The boundaries between mother and baby are intertwined and fluid and, at times, it is hard to discern where each ends and begins. There is obviously a dependence of the child upon the mother during pregnancy, and for some time after the birth, but there is also the complex need for the mother to recognize the infant as a separate being. It is possible that the child can form a connecting relationship with the mother through dreams. This is obviously speculative.

The possibility that the child in utero has a spiritual capacity leads to a further supposition: it is possible that the child will encounter a spiritual experience by going through the birth. Bergenheim, a Swedish midwife, goes further by stating that some infants may experience a spiritual emergency following birth and require special care to deal with their distress.[104] She suggested that 'spiritual bonding' includes giving physical contact, eye contact and talking to the child. It is essential for the carers at the birth to treat the infant with love, respect, care and gentleness. There has been much made of the potential danger physically of normal birth to the infant and yet little made of the potential danger to the emotional and spiritual side of a child by being pulled out mechanically or being cut off from the mother too soon. It has been speculated that this has a detrimental effect on people later in life.[25,99]

Spiritual distress

It is important to raise issues of what occurs if a woman's spiritual integrity is impaired. A diagnosis of spiritual distress may be given on such occasions.[105] For example, if a woman who is spiritually aware is cared for within a rigid maternity system that does not recognize her needs, she may become spiritually distressed. The result will be that she will shut herself down emotionally and spiritually in order to protect herself from further hurt and damage. This may affect her ability to labour and give birth and may subsequently lead to difficulty in her relationship with the child. It may be that some postnatal depression is associated with these kinds of unmet expectations.[106–108] It appears that transpersonal events and out-of-body experiences during labour may not be unusual.[95,109] Such dissociation events could be evidence of this kind of distress, or it could be a cultural, spiritual response.

Smucker suggested that the experience of spiritual distress may bring a person into deeper relationship with God.[105] In Shamanic practice, value is given to a time of spiritual conflict to allow a point of growth to be reached.[25] There is also a significant body of literature about the ultimate spiritual value of 'the dark night of the soul'. A negative experience of pregnancy or birth may allow this opportunity for a woman.[110] There is much work to be done to establish which women will find the experience of spiritual distress a time of growth or of devastation.

Midwives and spiritual issues

Earlier in the chapter, it was indicated that there is a place for investigating spiritual matters within midwifery care simply because international philosophies of practice for midwives require it to be explored. However, it is also clear from the issues outlined in relation to women's experiences that midwives should be aware of the role spirituality plays in normal birth. Box 3.2 indicates the elements of spiritual care identified from studies related to spirituality.[5] It is apparent that many of these could be qualities inherent within midwifery practice. However, over time, midwives have lost a lot of knowledge and skill through acquiescing in the overuse of technology in normal birth. A number of questions arise. What aspect of skills and knowledge makes midwifery care different or spiritual? What is it that is different about some midwives that results in the care they give being regarded as special or 'better', despite the fact that they are undertaking the same actions or procedures as others?[5] Is it possible that this is a spiritual link? Is it possible that midwives have lost the skills of the art of midwifery and no longer believe that women's

bodies are made to give birth? Research is currently under way, relating to what midwives view the art of midwifery practice to be, and how this links with holistic approaches (personal communication).

Intuition

It is suggested there is a type of 'tacit knowledge' which 'lies beyond rational understanding of patient situations' and that 'experienced nurses who are asked to explain their decisions about patient care often cannot articulate the reasons satisfactorily or scientifically'.[111] This kind of knowledge may be intrinsic within some midwives, even if they are not aware of it, and it is a skill recognized within those providing 'expert' care in labour.[112] However, the chances are that someone possessing these characteristics could be suppressed within the current fragmented and highly technological nature of many maternity services. In addition, the potential of students qualifying without seeing many truly physiological births means that they may lose such intuitive skills very early on, or even have missed the chance to develop them. In the absence of technological aids to diagnosis, midwives rely more heavily upon their senses to recognize and understand the process of normal birth.[113] They also rely more on their ability to use intuition as a tool for recognizing subtle changes within the process. The skill of intuition has been derided in an age of scientific knowledge; yet it has also been viewed as a major part of giving spiritual care.[36,43,56] In order for intuitive care to occur, it may be necessary for a relationship to have been formed. The midwife needs to be aware of her own self and limitations and to be able to trust her instincts and those of the women she is caring for. Clarke & Wheeler also suggest that a carer should feel confident in the knowledge that she is being cared for herself,[114] which indicates a certain level of security in herself and her relationships.[5] Such skills may be inherent but may also develop over time with experience. It is suggested that such skills may be enhanced or encouraged through education.[3,115] It is apparent that women recognize when midwives are practising intuitively, and that these skills are important to them.[112,116,117] Women's confidence appears to be reduced where there is a perceived lack of intuitive care.[117]

Support

There has been a great deal of research carried out in relation to the provision of support to women during labour. The evidence demonstrates the benefit of continuous support in labour,[116,118] and this benefit may be enhanced if a relationship has been formed during the antenatal period.[119] This relationship gives an opportunity for 'connecting' qualities to develop. Women have specified that their preference is to be cared for by someone with whom they have been able to develop a relationship of trust and care.[116,118–120] The relationship is one of 'professional intimacy', where a woman is allowed 'space' to be herself and yet also allows for 'connection'.[116] The ability to form this type of relationship may affect the midwife as well. Schemes offering continuity of carer show the importance to midwives, as well as women, and gave satisfaction through the development of a trusting one-to-one meaningful relationship.[121] However, it is also noteworthy that the provision of a one-to-one relationship is of no worth if the midwife is also 'distant' from the woman. It appears to be significant that there is a quality of 'presence' within a powerful caring relationship.

Osterman & Schwartz-Barcott established four images of 'presence' from the nursing literature. The first image is that of the nurse being physically in the room with the patient but totally self-absorbed and, therefore, not connected.[122] In the second, there is a partial presence, when the nurse is physically present but is intent on putting all her energy on a task instead of the other person. In the third, full presence is described: the nurse is physically and psychologically present and each patient interaction is 'personalized'. The final image is of transcendent presence, which is described as 'spiritual' presence. This is said to come from a 'spiritual source initiated by centring'. In this last case, the presence of the carer is felt as peaceful, comforting and harmonious. The ability to care appears to be boundless and she is able to recognize a 'oneness' or unity with the person being cared for.

Others have seen a spiritually healing power within the concept of presence.[109] Burkhardt described a need for the carer consciously to let go of the anxieties of the person she has left in order to be fully aware and present for the person that she next encounters.[123] Burkhardt & Nagai-Jacobson highlighted that the skills of being 'present' can and should be developed, and indicated how carers can enhance these skills.[8] Within midwifery, the concept of presence carries considerable meaning and significance, as it has been shown how valuable the supportive presence of a midwife is to women, and how it may benefit their future role as mothers.[71,112,119,124] It has been argued that qualities such as authenticity of being, conscience, commitment, presence, compassion, empathy and empowerment are needed if the relationship between midwife and woman is to have a beneficial and healing effect.[125]

Such concepts of relationships that border on being loving in their intensity may be regarded as spiritual in nature. However, there are complex issues to be addressed regarding the ability to develop such powerful relationships. The midwife obviously has her own life experiences and these will have an impact on how able she is to respond to others. She may feel the need to protect her own personal boundaries within a situation in a way that will subsequently affect her ability to be 'present'. She may also feel unable to give the kind of care she wishes to within an institution that suppresses spirituality. In order to give out to others, she will need to feel personal safety and trust within the situation. If, for any reason, she feels fearful or vulnerable, it will affect her ability to care and respond appropriately. As stated above, midwives as women in society may already be living in a framework of fear and this may produce an intolerance of risk that could conflict with that of the mother. Factors such as lack of experience or support, bullying, her own birth experiences, the threat of litigation, previous difficult births she has attended or a lack of trust in women's bodies may lead to high levels of midwifery fear.

Those midwives who fear the power of labour, or the openness of women, may be challenged by women who wish to 'let go' of themselves to give birth. These midwives may want to suppress the labour as a consequence. There needs to be open recognition of the impact that the threat of litigation has on midwives' practice, and on the boundaries set up by rigid protocols. In order to reduce the fear experienced by midwives, we may need to change the culture in which we practise. For example, we need to ensure that students' training is appropriate and that both students and newly qualified midwives are adequately supported. Where midwives are lacking experience in normal birth, this should be recognized and the opportunity provided for 'shadowing'. There should be the facilities for debriefing both previous birth experiences and midwifery experiences. There must be recognition of the potential for a blame culture to exist within maternity units and measures should be taken to eradicate this.

There should also be recognition of potential difficulties in situations where midwives are spiritually aware and are caring for women who are also spiritually aware but hold different views. The potential may be for conflict or for growth. It may also be appropriate for care to be handed to someone else if the relationship is proving detrimental. Alternatively, if a spiritually aware midwife cares for a mother, there is the possibility that she will enable or facilitate a woman to the extent of bringing her into a place of spiritual awareness.

Practical considerations

Midwives are in a powerful position to enhance the spiritual quality of birth. Place of birth is relevant. There is a contrast between the cold, clinical, bright hospital environment and the warmth and comfortable atmosphere created within most homes. There has been much effort in recent years to 'soften' hospitals, providing curtains and soft furnishings, televisions and music, and, in some places, water-birthing facilities. This is superficial and ineffective without an accompanying change in philosophy and attitude. There are also situations where women giving birth at home have experienced midwives trying to convert their home into a hospital room. It is clear there is more to birth than just the place.[126] The aim should be to facilitate an atmosphere of calm and serenity. Certain environmental props may be helpful: softer lighting, quiet or chosen music seem to be appropriate for some women. Some women appreciate the use of candles, but these may be impractical in a hospital setting because of the perceived risk of fire. Some women also welcome the aroma of particular substances to enhance their spiritual receptivity. Outside the therapeutic use of aromas, some women may use a particular scent or flowers or incense within their homes during labour. Others may participate in ritual, either of an orthodox religious nature or in some other way; some may use chanting, singing or prayer as a way to cope through the pain of labour. In a woman's home, the midwife is a guest, and unless some obvious harm is being done to the mother or baby, there should be no question of interference with such practices. The key fact is to respect the individual beliefs and values of the woman and her partner.[30] Caregivers should never impose their own beliefs.

Conclusions

The aim of this chapter has been to raise issues of spirituality in childbirth, to provide a basis for reflection about ways in which women's experiences might be affected and to suggest ways in which midwives might introduce spiritual awareness into their care. A holistic approach is fundamental, both towards the childbearing woman and her family, and in the way in which midwives' practice is configured within the broader social context of healthcare provision. However, spirituality cannot be forced. Inauthentic spirituality is a contradiction in terms. As Quinn has pointed out, there is no point in tagging on such practices to a system that is inherently flawed.[127] Furedi noted: 'A journey that is self-consciously about safety is very different to one that is about exploration and discovery. A safe journey attempts to avoid the unexpected – since the unexpected is more than likely to be dangerous'.[54] Worldwide, societies are moving towards a belief that birth is dangerous, and systems and individuals attempt to avoid the unexpected at all costs. A radical change of philosophy of maternity care provision is needed, away from one that is exclusively grounded in safety, and towards one which acknowledges the value of giving birth without excessive precaution and intervention, where mother and baby are well and healthy. This will have implications for training and practice, both of which will need to give greater priority to self-awareness. Midwives should start to take note of what they do and how they are when caring for women in labour, to identify places in themselves where they are not at peace, or fearful, and to find ways to deal with themselves first. Karll wrote: '… creating a birth of love and trust could influence an entire lifetime. Every birth contains the potential to make a difference. As midwives, this can be our highest offering'.[128] Midwives have the power to make a difference for birthing women, and one aspect of this has to be through recognizing the spirit.

References

1. Koenig H G, McCullough M E, Larson D B 2001 Handbook of religion and health. Oxford University Press, New York

2. Swinton J 2001 Spirituality and mental health care: rediscovering a forgotten dimension. Jessica Kingsley, London

3. Chamberlain T J, Hall C A 2000 Realized religion: research on the relationship between religion and health. Templeton Foundation, Radnor, PA

4. McSherry W 2006 Making sense of spirituality in nursing and health care practice: an interactive approach. Churchill Livingstone, Oxford

5. Hall J 2001 Midwifery mind and spirit: emerging issues of care. Books for Midwives, Oxford

6. Klassen P E 2001 Blessed events: religion and home birth in America. Princeton University Press, Princeton, NJ

7. Orchard H (ed.) 2001 Spirituality in health care contexts. Jessica Kingsley, London

8. Burkhardt M A, Nagai-Jacobson M G 2002 Spirituality: living our connectedness. Delmar, Albany, NY

9. Robinson S, Kendrick K, Brown A 2003 Spirituality and the practice of health care. Palgrave Macmillan, London

10. White G 2006 Talking about spirituality in health care practice: a resource for health professionals working in multidisciplinary teams. Jessica Kingsley, London

11. Wright S 2005 Reflections on spirituality and health. Whurr, London

12. Greenstreet W 2006 Integrating spirituality in health and social care: perspectives and practical approaches. Radcliffe, London

13. Labun E 1988 Spiritual care: an element in nursing care planning. J Adv Nurs 13:314–320

14. Price J L, Stevens H O, LaBarre M C 1995 Spiritual caregiving in nursing practice. J Psychosoc Nurs 33:5–9

15. Goddard N C 1995 'Spirituality as integrative energy': a philosophical analysis as requisite precursor to holistic nursing practice. J Adv Nurs 22:808–815

16. Davis-Floyd R 2001 The technocratic, humanistic and holistic paradigms of childbirth. Int J Gynecol Obstet 75:S5–S23

17. International Confederation of Midwives 2007 Philosophy and model of midwifery care. Online. Available: http://www.internationalmidwives.org/index.php?module=Con tentExpress&func=display&ceid=59&bid=22&btitle=IC M%20Documents&meid=52 (accessed 30 August 2007)

18. Hall J 2002 Spiritual care for childbirth: is this the weakest link? Sacred Space J 3:37–40

19. Stoll R I 1979 Guidelines for spiritual assessment. Am J Nurs 79:1579–1587

20. Koenig H G 2002 Spirituality in patient care: why, how, when, and what. Templeton Foundation, Radnor, PA

21. McSherry W, Ross L 2002 Dilemmas of spiritual assessment: considerations for nursing practice. J Adv Nurs 38:479–488

22. Clarke J 2006 Religion and spirituality: a discussion paper about negativity, reductionism and differentiation in nursing texts. Int J Nurs Stud 43:775–785

23. Swinton J 2006 Identity and resistance: why spiritual care needs 'enemies'. J Clin Nurs 15:918–928

24. Totton N 1999 Not just a job; psychotherapy as a spiritual and political practice. In: House R, Totton N (eds) Implausible professions: arguments for pluralism and autonomy in psychotherapy and counselling. PCCS Books, Ross on Wye, p 129–140

25. Grof S, Grof C (eds) 1989 Spiritual emergency: when personal transformation becomes a crisis – New Consciousness Reader. Warner, London

26. Watson K W 1994 Spiritual emergency: concepts and implications for psychotherapy. J Humanist Psychol 34:22–45

27. Ankrah L 2002 Spiritual emergency and counselling: an exploratory study. Counselling and Psychotherapy Research 2:55–60

28. Dombeck M B 1996 Chaos and self-organization as a consequence of spiritual disequilibrium. Clin Nurse Spec 10:69–73

29. Hall J 2006 Spirituality at the beginning of life. J Clin Nurs 15:804–810

30. Schott J, Henley A 1996 Culture, religion and childbearing in a multiracial society. Books for Midwives, Oxford

31. Cawley N 1997 An exploration of the concept of spirituality. Int J Palliat Nurs 3:31–36

32. Heath C D 2006 A womanist approach to understanding and assessing the relationship between spirituality and mental health. Mental Health, Religion and Culture 9:155–170

33. Chan C L W, Ng S M, Ho R T H 2006 East meets West: applying Eastern spirituality in clinical practice. J Clin Nurs 15:822–832

34. WHOQOL SRPB group 2006 A cross-cultural study of spirituality, religion and personal beliefs as components of quality of life. Soc Sci Med 62:1486–1497

35. Tanyi R A 2002 Towards clarification of the meaning of spirituality. J Adv Nurs 39:500–509

36. Waugh L A 1992 Spiritual aspects of nursing: a descriptive study of nurses' perceptions. PhD Thesis, Queen Margaret College, Edinburgh

37. Dobbie B J 1991 Women's mid-life experience: an evolving consciousness of self and children. J Adv Nurs 16:825–831

38. Karis S 2002 Theobiology and gendered spirituality. Am Behav Sci 45:1866–1874

39. Hunt M E 1995 Psychological implications of women's spiritual health. Women Ther 16:21–32

40. Tucakovic M 1994 Spiritual aesthetics in nursing. Aust J Holist Nurs 1:16–27

41. King U 1993 Women and spirituality, 2nd edn. Macmillan, London

42. Burkhardt M A 1994 Becoming and connecting: elements of spirituality for women. Holist Nurs Pract 8:12–21

43. Davis D 1995 Ways of knowing in midwifery. Aust Coll Midwives Inc J 8:30–32

44. Davis-Floyd R E, Davis E 1997 Intuition as authoritative knowledge in midwifery and home birth. In: Davis-Floyd R E, Sargent C F (eds) Childbirth and authoritative knowledge: cross-cultural perspectives. University of California Press, Berkeley, CA, p 315–349

45. Annandale E, Clark J 1996 What is gender? Feminist theory and the sociology of human reproduction. Sociol Health Illness 18:17–44

46. Mitchell E D 2002 Holistic midwifery: the reality. RCM News Appoint Dec:4

47. Kitzinger S 2000 Rediscovering birth. Little, Brown, London

48. McCool W F, McCool S J 1989 Feminism and nurse-midwifery: historical overview and current issues. J Nurs Midwif 34:323–334

49. Achterberg J 1990 Woman as healer. Rider, London

50. Wickham S 2004 Feminism and ways of knowing. In: Stewart M (ed.) Pregnancy, birth and maternity care: feminist perspectives. Books for Midwives, London

51. LoCicero A K 1993 Explaining excessive rates of caesarean section and other childbirth interventions: contribution from contemporary theories of gender and psychosocial developments. Soc Sci Med 37:1261–1269

52. Page L 2001 The humanization of birth. Int J Gynecol Obstet 75:S55–S58

53. Raphael-Leff J 1991 Psychological processes of childbearing. Chapman & Hall, London

54. Furedi F 1997 Culture of fear: risk taking and the morality of low expectation. Cassell, London

55. Richards H 1992 Cultural messages of childbirth: the perpetration of fear. Int J Childbirth Educ 7:27–29

56. Gaskin I M 2002 Spiritual midwifery. Summertown, Cambridge

57. LaChance C W 2002 The way of the mother: the lost journey of the feminine. Vega, London

58. Hebblethwaite M 1984 Motherhood and God. Geoffrey Chapman, London

59. Rubin R 1984 Maternal identity and maternal experience. Springer, New York

60. Bergum V 1989 Woman to mother: a transformation. Bergin & Garvey, Granby, UK

61. Rich A 1992 Of woman born: motherhood as experience and institution, 2nd edn. Virago, London

62. Hampton M R 1995 Searching for their roots in birth. Midwif Today 33:14–15, 40

63. Nichols F H 1996 The meaning of the childbirth experience: a review of the literature. J Perinat Educ 5:71–77

64. O'Shea M 1998 An exploratory study of women's experience of childbirth specifically identifying the spiritual dimension. BSc Midwifery Studies, The Nightingale Institute, King's College London, London

65. Taylor M 2002 Labour and spirituality. Practis Midwife 5:10–13

66. Baumiller R 2002 Spiritual development during a first pregnancy. Int J Childbirth Educ 17:7

67. Balin J 1988 The sacred dimensions of pregnancy and birth. Qualit Sociol 11:275–301

68. Sered S S 1991 Childbirth as a religious experience? Voices from an Israeli hospital. J Feminist Stud Relig 7:7–18

69. Kitzinger S 2000 Some cultural perspectives of birth. Br J Midwif 8:746–750

70. Leap N 2000 Pain in labour: towards a midwifery perspective. MIDIRS Midwif Digest 10:49–53

71. Lundgren I 2004 Releasing and relieving encounters: experiences of pregnancy and childbirth. Scand J Caring Sci 18:368–375

72. Odent M 2001 The scientification of love, 2nd edn. Free Association, London

73. Hall S M, Holloway I M 1998 Staying in control: women's experiences of labour in water. Midwifery 14:30–36

74. Stone J 1993 Whose pregnancy is it anyway? Health Matters 16:12–13

75. Kahn R P 1995 Bearing meaning: the language of birth. University of Illinois Press, Champaign, IL

76. Stockley S 1986 Psychic and spiritual aspects of pregnancy, birth and life. In: Claxton R (ed.) Birth matters. Unwin, London, p 75–98

77. Belbin A 1996 Power and choice in birthgiving: a case study. Br J Midwif 4:264–267

78. Weaver J 2000 Talking about caesarean section. MIDIRS Midwif Digest 10:487–490

79. Viisainen K 2001 Negotiating control and meaning: homebirth as a self-constructed choice in Finland. Soc Sci Med 52:1109–1121

80. Hofberg K, Ward M R 2004 Fear of childbirth, tocophobia and mental health in mothers: the obstetric–psychiatric interface. Clin Obstet Gynecol 47:527–534

81. Walsh D 2002 Fear of labour and birth. Br J Midwif 10:78

82. Bewley S, Cockburn J 2002 Responding to fear of childbirth. Lancet 359:9324, 2128–2129

83. Waldenström U I, Hildingsson I, Ryding E L 2006 Antenatal fear of childbirth and its association with subsequent caesarean section and experience of childbirth. BJOG 113:638–646

84. Nerum H, Halvorsen L, Sorlie T et al 2006 Maternal request for cesarean section due to fear of birth: can it be changed through crisis-oriented counseling? Birth 33:221–228

85. Lowe N K 1996 The pain and discomfort of labor and birth. J Obstet Gynaecol Neonat Nurs 25:82–92

86. Sjorgen B 1997 Reasons for anxiety about childbirth in 100 pregnant women. J Psychosom Gynecol Obstet 18:266–272

87. Saisto T, Kaaja R, Ylikorkala O et al 1999 Factors associated with fear of delivery in second pregnancies. Obstet Gynecol 94:679–682

88. Alehagen S, Mijma K, Wijma B 2001 Fear during labor. Acta Obstet Gynecol Scand 80:315–320

89. Saisto T, Kaaja R, Ylikorkala O et al 2001 Reduced pain tolerance during and after pregnancy in women suffering from fear of labor. Pain 93:123–127

90. Melender H-L 2002 Experiences of fears associated with pregnancy and childbirth: a study of 329 pregnant women. Birth 29:101–111

91. England P, Horowitz R 1998 Birthing from within. Partera Press, Albuquerque, NM

92. Hall J 2002 Finding the spiritual side of birth. Practis Midwife 5:4–5

93. Booth C L, Meltzoff A N 1984 Expected and actual experience in labour and delivery and their relationship to maternal atachment. J Reprod Infant Psychol 2:79–91

94. Lahood G 2007 Rumour of angels and heavenly midwives: anthropology of transpersonal events and childbirth. Women Birth 20:3–10

95. Price J 1999 Motherhood: what it does to your mind. Pandora, London

96. Belenky M, Clinchy B, Goldberger M 1996 Women's ways of knowing: the development of self, voice and mind, 10th anniversary edn. Basic Books, New York

97. Parvati Baker J 1993 Wombside earthside. Compleat Mother, Fall:18–19

98. Rawlings L 1995 Re-imagining birth. Birth Gazette 11:14–17

99. Verny T, Kelly J 1982 The secret life of the unborn child. Sphere, London

100. Salter J 1987 The incarnating child. Hawthorn Press, Stroud

101. Reading A E, Cox D N 1982 The effect of ultrasound examination on maternal anxiety levels. J Behav Med 5:237–247

102. Schwartz L 1991 Bonding before birth. Sigo Press, Boston, MA

103. McGeary K 1994 The influence of guarding on the developing mother–unborn child relationship. In: Field P A, Marck P B (eds) Uncertain motherhood: negotiating the risks of the childbearing years. Sage, London, p 139–162

104. Bergenheim A 1995 Spiritual emergency of the newborn. Birth Gazette 11:14–15

105. Smucker C 1996 A phenomenological description of the experience of spiritual distress. Nurs Diagn 7:81–91

106. Axe S 2000 Labour debriefing is crucial for good psychological care. Br J Midwif 8:626–628, 630–631

107. Saisto T, Salmela-Aro K, Nurmi J E et al 2000 Psychosocial predictors of disappointment with delivery and puerperal depression: a longitudinal study. Acta Obstet Gynecol Scand 80:39–45

108. Ayers S, Pickering A D 2001 Do women get posttraumatic stress disorder as a result of childbirth? A prospective study of incidence. Birth 28:111–118

109. Kennedy H P 2002 Altered consciousness during childbirth: potential clues to post traumatic stress disorder? J Midwif Womans Health 47:380–382

110. Brown Y 1993 Perinatal loss: a framework for practice. Health Care Women Int 14:469–479

111. Carlsson G, Drew N, Dahlberg K et al 2002 Uncovering tacit caring knowledge. Nurs Philos 3:144–151

112. Downe S, Simpson L, Trafford K 2006 Expert intrapartum maternity care: a metasynthesis. J Adv Nurs 57:127–140

113. Hall J 2001 Sense and sensibility in midwifery. Midwif Today 60:60

114. Clarke J B, Wheeler S J 1992 A view of the phenomenon of caring in nursing practice. J Adv Nurs 17:1283–1290

115. Rew L 1989 Intuition: nursing knowledge and the spiritual dimension of persons. Holist Nurs Pract 3:56–68

116. Halldorsdottir S, Karlsdottir S I 1996 Empowerment or discouragement: women's experience of caring and uncaring encounters during childbirth. Health Care Women Int 17:361–379

117. Berg M, Lundgren I, Hermansson E 1996 Women's experience of the encounter with the midwife during childbirth. Midwifery 12:11–15

118. Hodnett E D, Gates S, Hofmeyr G J 2003 Continuous support for women during childbirth. Cochrane Database Syst Rev, Issue 3. Art. No.: CD003766. DOI: 10.1002/14651858.CD003766.pub2

119. Flint C, Poulengeris P 1987 The 'know your midwife' report from Peckarmans Wood. 49 Peckarmans Wood, London

120. Bluff R, Holloway I 1994 'They know best': women's perceptions of midwifery care during labour and childbirth. Midwifery 10:157–164

121. Sandall J 1997 Midwives' burnout and continuity of care. Br J Midwif 5:106–111

122. Osterman P, Schwartz-Barcott D 1996 Presence: four ways of being there. Nurs Forum 31:23–30

123. Burkhardt M A 1998 Reintegrating spirituality into healthcare. Altern Ther Health Med 4:127, 128

124. Oakley A 1992 Social support and motherhood. Blackwell, Oxford

125. Siddiqui J 1999 The therapeutic relationship in midwifery. Br J Midwif 7:111–114

126. Page L 2002 Building for a better birth. Br J Midwif 10:536, 538

127. Quinn J F 2000 The self as healer: reflections from a nurse's journey. AACN Clin Issues: Adv Pract Acute Crit Care 11:17–26

128. Karll S 2001 Making a difference: a blueprint for harmony. Midwif Today 58:22–23

Section **Two**

Aspects of normality

CHAPTERS

4

Normal birth: women's stories

Beverley A. Lawrence Beech and Belinda Phipps

Chapter contents

Introduction

This chapter is a collaboration between the UK National Childbirth Trust (NCT) and the Association for Improvements in the Maternity Services (AIMS). Box 4.1 sets out a brief history of both organizations. These organizations, and others such as the Maternity Alliance, have had a major impact on change in maternity care in the UK since the 1960s. Pubic shaving, routine episiotomy and routine electronic fetal monitoring were all first challenged by women's childbirth organizations. They are no longer accepted as appropriate routine interventions. Rooming in, the presence of fathers at birth, protection of the right to home birth, parents' rights and woman-centred care all owe a major debt to consumer pressure. Our message in this chapter is that the way birth happens matters to women, babies and society. We want to emphasize not only how disempowering a bad birth experience is but also the positive and long-lasting benefits of a good birth. Throughout the chapter, we have used quotes from women who responded to an electronic discussion on the nature of birth and of normal birth. The discussion was conducted among members of the NCT. While it is acknowledged that members of any organization may have a different view from the population as a whole, we also use comments from women who have contacted AIMS over the years to discuss their birth experiences. These women made contact for support, not because they belonged to the organization. The NCT and AIMS stories do not differ in their underlying message. This suggests that, for some women at least, the accounts are typical. The names of the respondents have been changed to preserve anonymity.

The importance of birth

There are very few events in the life of a woman that compare to the birth of a child. Women themselves know this and, among themselves, may talk of it. If asked (and unfortunately they rarely are), most

Box 4.1

Childbirth campaigning influence of the main organizations

The National Childbirth Trust charity was launched in 1957. The original aims of the charity included a desire that women should be humanely treated during labour and never hurried, bullied or ridiculed. They also stated: 'the idea fostered by many medical people today that natural childbirth includes routine internal examinations, routine administration of analgesia, routine episiotomy should be dispelled'.

AIMS focus has always been to address the shortcomings in maternity care by helping women to get the care they feel is appropriate for them, and to assist those who wish to complain about the care they have had.

Both organizations have long recognized the importance of the woman's perspective in decisions about birth and the way it should be conducted. The Association for Improvements in the Maternity Services' focus has always been on women who have had unsatisfactory experiences or who want to ensure they have a satisfactory experience. The National Childbirth Trust has focused on supporting, informing and empowering all parents to enable them to have a life-enhancing experience of pregnancy, birth and early parenthood.

women would compare the importance of the birth of their child to their own wedding or the death of a close relative.

I would liken it (birth) to a major life experience such as losing your virginity, etc. It's a rite of passage. (Nina)

Relative to marriage or first time sex, I would put my birth experiences way beyond these … they strike at the very heart and soul of you, they touch new emotions not experienced before and bring a whole new perspective to life. (Rona)

Nothing can compare to the experience of giving birth and holding your child for the first time. It definitely altered my relationship with my partner, but for the better. (Kristine)

Birth memories are long-lasting and imprinted onto a woman's mind until her death. Try asking an elderly woman about the birth of one of her children and she will be able to tell you in great detail about the experience. Many women want to talk about their births and their accounts are almost invariably being relived as the woman talks. She is remembering the birth as it happened at the time, fully associating with the experience, seeing it again from her own viewpoint. Birth is rarely recalled dispassionately.

This (home birth) was a hugely empowering experience and after the birth I simply felt wonderful (apart from the usual sore bits!) – my self-esteem was restored and since then I have noticed a huge improvement in my general wellbeing, my relationship with my husband and I have been careful to take care of myself. I realised that I had been depressed ever since my first birth experience but this was now gone. I once again enjoy sex and have lost 3 stone in weight – all as a result of regaining my confidence in myself. For me my first birth experience in hospital with every intervention was something I wanted to forget but my second birth experience, my homebirth, was the most significant, empowering and important experience of my life. The way a woman gives birth can affect the whole of the rest of her life – how can that not matter unless the woman herself doesn't matter? (Hannah)

I can't tell you how different the two birth experiences were. During the home birth I felt relaxed, in control, unpressured. I could eat and drink. I could move about easily and adopt any position I wanted. I could use my own bathroom and get into my own bed afterwards. After the birth my husband did not have to leave me unsupported at a time when my need was greatest. He felt much more involved in the birth. (Lisa)

To me a vaginal birth mattered very much. Physically I was not prepared for how I would feel after the caesarean section, I was not back to normal for weeks. From what I have read I also understand that a vaginal birth is better for the baby. Mentally too I found a caesarean section much harder than a vaginal birth although perhaps if the caesarean section is planned this is less of a problem. (Diane)

To me having a vaginal birth mattered immensely. I would have been devastated to have had to undergo a c-section. Again it's all about it being a rite of passage. I didn't feel comfortable with the idea of my baby's first moments being in an operating room, being pulled from my womb by hands unrelated to it, then being whisked away. (Nina)

Our society fails to acknowledge the importance of the birth experience. It is generally expected that the woman should be satisfied with the birth of a live baby, irrespective of the way the birth happened. The failure to acknowledge and address the mother's experiences leaves too many women with traumatizing memories, rather than positive and empowering ones. Often this is because we have allowed systems to develop that interfere with the birth process.

My life was devastated by my experience and it has made me a worse mother – a barely functioning suicidal mother at times, who was deeply wounded by the careless expression of 'never mind at least you have a healthy baby' – of course I mind! Having a baby is an important rite of passage, which I have been robbed of. Of course I am delighted to have a healthy baby but my feelings matter too. (Sarah)

Birth experiences, however the woman perceives them, are critical events in women's lives. They have an impact on how well she makes the transition to motherhood, on her self-esteem, on her physical and mental health, on her relationships with the child, on the well-being of the child and on the family which is created. When the memory is traumatic, disempowering and negative, this can have long-term adverse effects.

The worst adverse effect is maternal suicide. The most recent data on maternal mortality indicated that suicide is currently the leading cause of maternal deaths in the UK, exceeding rates of deaths from hypertensive disease, yet it receives far less attention. The latest Confidential Enquiry now investigates and highlights this problem,[1] but it only records maternal deaths as those occurring within one year of the birth of a baby. This may exclude the deaths of some women who, for the sake of their children, live with a depth of misery that others would have found intolerable. Their suicides may not occur until much later.

In a Swedish study,[2] women who had post-traumatic stress reactions after emergency caesarean were reported to be 'twice as likely to feel wronged by delivery staff as those who did not feel traumatized'. Mothers can feel particularly bitter towards midwives who stood by and did nothing while a doctor they knew to be unsatisfactory traumatized them.[3]

Definitions of normal birth

As discussed in Chapter 1, carrying out research into the effects of normal birth, and even counting the number of normal births, is made difficult by hazy definitions as to what constitutes normality and even what terminology to use. Much of the research that purports to be about normal birth is, in fact, about highly managed obstetric deliveries. Soo Downe and her colleagues have noted that 'within the maternity services abnormality is becoming more often defined as a deviation from the average, rather than as a pathological entity in its own right'.[4] In this section, we set out a number of definitions that have been suggested, and we propose a terminology which we believe will be most understandable for women.

The designation *normal* to describe labour and childbirth has been in use for centuries.[5] The current UK *Midwives Rules and Standards* talk about a 'deviation from the norm' when referring to areas outside the midwives' competence.[6] It is commonly taken to mean a physiological labour and a vaginal birth with little or no external intervention.[7]

At the beginning of its thorough document on care in normal labour, the World Health Organization defined normal birth as 'spontaneous in onset, low-risk at the start of labour and remaining so throughout labour and delivery. The infant is born spontaneously in the vertex position between 37 and 42 completed weeks of pregnancy. After birth mother and infant are in good condition'.[8] As the labours and births of many women with so-called high-risk pregnancies have a normal course, a number of the recommendations in this paper also apply to the care of these women.

The UK Royal College of Midwives has described the elements in and outside of normal birth (Table 4.1) and has also proposed a definition.[9] In this

Table 4.1	UK Royal College of Midwives' description of normal birth[9]
Normality includes	**Normality excludes**
Spontaneous onset of labour	Induced and augmented labour
Labour is considered as a continuum	Timing of labour
Holistic, alternative methods of pain relief, water, ambulation	Medical methods of pain relief
Permit food and fluids	Withholding food and fluid in labour
Spontaneous physiological rupture of membranes	Artificial rupture of the membranes
Encourage mobility	Restricted mobility
Calm, gentle and non-threatening environment, auscultation	Clinical environment – institutionalization of birth
Intermittent fetal monitoring	Continuous fetal monitoring
Specific indications only, preference for abdominal examinations	Routine vaginal examinations
Judicious use of episiotomy	Routine episiotomy

case, there is acknowledgement of the symbiosis between mother and infant, and of the transforming possibilities of childbirth. The elements in this version are shown in Box 4.2. There is debate about what terminology to use. Normal has the disadvantage of often meaning usual or most common. Marianne Mead

Box 4.2

UK Royal College of Midwives: components of normal birth

- Birth is a unique dynamic process
- Fetal and maternal physiologies interact symbiotically
- [Birth] occurs within 24 hours of commencement of labour
- Minimum trauma occurs to either mother or baby
- Spontaneous onset is between 37 and 42 weeks
- It follows an uncomplicated pregnancy

explores this concept of normality in Chapter 5. Normal may also imply that any other sort of birth is abnormal, and this can be guilt inducing for some women and healthcare professionals. An alternative possible term is physiological birth; however, this would have little meaning for the average parent. The Association for Improvements in the Maternity Services has proposed that birth should be divided into three categories:[10]

1. Operative delivery or instrumental (i.e. caesarean section, ventouse or forceps).
2. Obstetric delivery (i.e. a vaginal delivery preceded by a variety of interventions such as artificial rupture of membranes, prostaglandin pessary, induction or acceleration, epidural anaesthesia and episiotomy.
3. Normal birth.

In this paper, Beech noted that:[10]

When parents talk about 'normal birth' or 'normal delivery' they mean a physiological birth where the baby is delivered vaginally following a labour which has not been altered by technological interventions. It does not, therefore, refer to a vaginal birth where the mothers have had artificial rupture of membranes, induction or acceleration by drugs, an intravenous glucose drip, epidural anaesthesia or episiotomies.

The NCT uses the term 'straightforward vaginal birth' to mean a birth that starts, progresses and concludes spontaneously, without major interventions such as a caesarean, an instrumental delivery or a series of other medical procedures.

Building on the work of Beech[10] and Downe et al,[4] the Web-based organization BirthChoiceUK attempted to construct normal birth rates for every unit in England and Scotland.[11] However, this work was hampered by the fact that records were not complete, and that data were not collected at the national level for many technological interventions. The definition finally used for this work, and later adopted into government statistics, was a birth without caesarean, assisted delivery, induction of labour or regional anaesthesia. Historical statistics are available for England and are cited on the Web site. They show a dramatic decline in normal birth

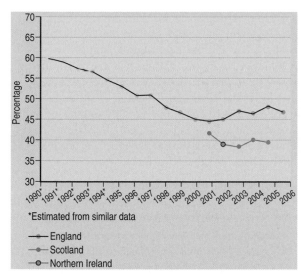

Fig 4.1 • Normal birth rates in England (from BirthChoiceUK). Normal birth is defined as birth without caesarian section, assisted delivery, induction or regional anaesthetic.[12]

rates since the early 1990s, as demonstrated in Figure 4.1. In 1992, an estimated 57.2% of births were categorized as normal using this definition; by 2001 that had fallen to 44.4%. Medical intervention has often been justified on the grounds that it saves lives; yet, during this rapid increase in obstetric delivery, there has been no corresponding fall in maternal or neonatal deaths. For more statistical data on normal birth rates, see the BirthChoiceUK Web site.[11]

Although there is no single universal definition of normal birth, the existing definitions cover similar aspects. The concept of unique normality that was discussed in Chapter 1 may provide a more fruitful direction than the proliferation of more definitions. Wherever the debate takes us, it is time for normality to be reclaimed and seen as different from that which is commonly happening in many maternity units across the world.

Normal birth experiences

As the majority of research is carried out in hospitals, there is little relevant valid research on births without intervention. However, a body of information does exist in the form of birth stories. These are a vital source of information in this area.

My second birth was … weaved into the fabric of everyday life … we approached it as a 'birth' day for my 2-year-old daughter's sake … she helped put up streamers and balloons whilst I was 'niggling' and we had a birthday cake. She'd had a bath in the pool with me as a rehearsal and knew 'her' baby would be born in it. She slept upstairs whilst I laboured and came down to meet her new brother when she stirred and best of all she joined me and Sam in bed that night. All in my own home, no white walls, no bright lights, no distracting noises, just me, Pete and the 2 midwives with me ALL of the time … is this normal? Sadly no, I'm viewed as 'brave' and a minority. But I wouldn't swap it for anything in the world. Birth matters. (Rose)

Having 'breathed out O's head', his body followed almost immediately with a slither and a gush. It was 2.26 a.m. Lorna passed him through my legs to the front where I held his lovely, slippery, warm body. I shan't forget that moment. Just to feel him and hold him when he was wet and new. What a contrast to C's delivery when I only got to hold a cleaned and wrapped up bundle, a good hour after he was born. When the midwives had gone, we dressed O, Guy made some tea and toast, and by 6.00 a.m. we all three were in bed asleep! It seemed so right for us all to be together at home. A hospital delivery could never compare to the calm, relaxing and safe atmosphere of our bedroom that night. (Lisa)

The moment when each of my babies was put into my arms is burned clearly into my mind. The fact that I was surrounded by people who cared about me and the fact that inside of my head a voice was singing 'I did it!' made the first moments of being that child's mother confident. I gave birth to 3 of my 4 children at home. (Celia)

The subtle, long-term effects of childbirth experiences have yet to be properly evaluated or recognized. In 1998, a woman contacted AIMS because she was very concerned about her daughter, Elizabeth, who was 9 years old and was constantly seeking attention from anyone who visited the home. Throughout her childhood, Elizabeth would be the first of Jenny's children to climb on the lap of any visitor and the last to break away. Now that Elizabeth was approaching puberty, Jenny was becoming increasingly worried by her behaviour. She was also unhappy about her own attitude towards her daughter and commented that Elizabeth was beginning to make critical comments about her failure to cuddle or touch her. Jenny had two other children but she did not feel this way about them. She described the birth of Elizabeth as different from the birth of the other children. She had gone into hospital early and ended up with a standard 'medicalized' birth experience: artificial rupture of membranes, continuous electronic fetal monitoring, a painful oxytocin-driven labour and, eventually, a vaginal birth with a routine episiotomy. Elizabeth had been removed immediately and only given back some time later. This caused Jenny to have an unfounded anxiety that there might have been a problem with her baby. Her wish to hold and examine her baby immediately was ignored. She described how she had been left alone for most of the labour and how worried both she and her husband had felt. This was their first child, and they were not sure what would happen. After the birth, she felt exhausted and was unable to breastfeed successfully. However, during the labours of her other two children, she managed to avoid most of the routine interventions she had suffered during the first birth and felt much more attached to these children. Jenny recognized that her behaviour towards her daughter was probably the reason for her daughter's behaviour and she felt guilty that she acted in this way.

Jenny's experience was mirrored by that of Sharon. She described how, although she loved both her sons equally, she did not have the same response to the eldest child as she did the youngest. When Peter, the eldest, fell over and ran to her crying, she would cuddle him, because that was what mothers did, but she would also urge him as soon as possible not to be such a big baby and stop crying and go off and play. When her second son arrived, having experienced a normal, physiological birth without any need for pain relief, and well supported by the midwives, she found that when he fell over and hurt himself, her heart gave a lurch and she would rush to comfort him. Realizing the different attitudes to these two children, she deliberately worked hard to treat them similarly. It was not until a family crisis occurred, when her eldest son was 9 years old and his despair at his father's departure threw them together in joint distress, that she noticed feelings emerging for her elder son as she comforted him that she had had for her youngest son.

Neither Jenny nor Sharon felt that the midwives who attended them were unkind, unsympathetic or cruel. Their descriptions of their birth experiences were similar to hundreds and thousands of other women who have experienced medicalized births. How many of these commonly occurring traumatizing births have adversely affected the mother-child relationship? We do not know because this research has not been done.

My first child was born in hospital. I was induced when she was 11 days late. However, the induction, which took place at midnight (my husband was not allowed to stay with me), sent me into immediate and very scary labour, with labour pains very close together from the start. My husband was called back at 5 a.m. when my waters had broken and I was unable to walk by myself to the delivery suite. The baby became distressed, I was given a painful episiotomy and she was taken out with a Ventouse. I then went into shock, did not care whether the baby was OK (for which I still feel guilt to this day). I was then in so much pain after being badly stitched up, that everything was too much effort. I enjoyed breast feeding her, she fed well and I loved her immediately, but the trauma of the birth, followed by a very painful internal infection, remnants of the placenta being left in my womb and subsequently becoming infected took a very long time for me to recover. My daughter has never slept well, is not a relaxed child, suffers from eczema and has had osteopathy and chiropractic treatments to help her. I love her completely, but sometimes I have to work hard at it.

My second child was born at home. Midwife led care, labour started naturally and I walked around my garden throughout. I went into my bedroom at 4.45 and she was born at 5.05. She was put onto my stomach immediately and fed straight away. She was contented, fed immediately and has always slept well, she has none of her sister's allergies and my maternal bond with her was instant and still requires no effort. (The writer asked to remain anonymous.)

History of childbirth intervention

At this point, we want to revisit briefly the fairly well-known recent history of childbirth intervention. Because of its importance in the life of a woman and of her society, birth is associated with many rituals and practices. These vary, depending on the time in history and the culture in which the birth is occurring. For most of history and for much of the world, this has been an overwhelmingly female concern. Women supported women in labour, with the male influence absent or as an observer. In recent times, however, and especially in the Western world, there has been a trend to increasing involvement of men in birth. In the UK, this trend began during the Middle Ages, when the church sought to register 'good women'. In parallel with this, the development of childbirth technologies, and specifically the Chamberlen forceps, meant that men could further justify their involvement by having secret means to assist obstructed labour. In time, childbirth became a lucrative source of income, and midwife involvement was relegated to those in the population who could not afford to pay. As time progressed and lying-in hospitals were established, these units offered the medical men a captive audience upon whom they could practise and research. This did not occur without protest from some midwives.

Donnison[13] has noted that, in 1760, Elizabeth Nihell published her 400 page polemic against male practice under the title *A Treatise on the Art of Midwifery*. She was unusual in that she had obtained the privilege, rare for a foreigner, of training at the Hotel-Dieu (a renowned French maternity unit). There the midwives worked without male supervision or interventions, and from her observation of their successful practice she had concluded that instruments were seldom, if ever, necessary. Worse still, complained Nihell, the male practitioner, adding insult to injury, was so adept at concealing his errors with 'a cloud of hard words and scientific jargon', that the injured patient herself was convinced that she could not thank him enough for the mischief he had done.

Such sentiments have a modern echo when we hear from women who have traumatic birth experiences that investigation reveals involved a variety of unnecessary procedures, which led to major emergency action. Those women often acknowledge how 'lucky' they were to have been in hospital, unaware that, had they had their babies at home, they would not have had the procedures in the first place and, therefore, there would have been no need for emergency action.

Little research has been undertaken on the differences in attitudes between male and female practitioners towards the use of interventions in vaginal births, although a recent study in the USA has found that male obstetricians in training used forceps in 12.4% of vaginal births compared with 9.9% for births attended by their female colleagues.[14]

This disparity raises the question: 'Why?'. An insight was revealed through an interview with Professor Marsden Wagner, a respected paediatrician and epidemiologist, for APERIO, a Czech childbirth group. He was asked why the social model of birth has little appeal for obstetricians. He replied:[15]

The first time I attended a birth outside hospital, yes, I was invited by a midwife to a homebirth, I was shocked. I had already practiced medicine for years but this was the first time I witnessed the full power of a woman in control of her own body. Believe me, it's a most scary experience for a man. It took me a long time to figure out the truth: men are afraid of women, afraid of unleashed nature, afraid of childbirth. We've all heard about 'penis envy' but here's 'womb envy', an abiding sense of male inadequacy in the face of women's unique childbearing gift. You know, men are outsiders at birth, always have been, always will be. But watch out. Hell hath no fury like a man devalued. When men are afraid and angry at being afraid, they cope through denial of their fear and through controlling whatever they're afraid of. So the male dominated obstetric profession tries to control birth, an impossible task unless you find a way to stop the process.

The increasing involvement of men and the increasing use of technology have both been justified in the name of safety. Concepts of risk and safety are discussed further in Chapter 7. The rise of faith in science and technology has led to women and their caregivers trusting the machine rather than women's reported experience of their own observations. So, for example, if a woman states that she is progressing rapidly, midwives often do not believe her until they have done a vaginal examination to prove this fact for themselves.

When I was in labour the midwives arrived and examined me to find I was 'only' 3 cms dilated. This was at half-past midnight. I told them that my previous labour had been fast and furious and I had delivered my previous baby within two hours of the initial examination. However, after a further 45 minutes had passed – and I was labouring very intensely – the midwives still wouldn't let me get into the birthing pool because their protocol said I had to be 4 cms dilated as it could 'slow things down'. By this time even a steam roller wouldn't have slowed things down. I refused to be examined again because the first time had been so painful so I told the midwives I was going to get into the water regardless but I did concede that if anything appeared to be 'slowing down' I would get out again in order to let them reassess the situation. They didn't argue with that and I got into the water and my daughter was born at 2.25 a.m. – exactly 1 hour and 55 minutes after the initial examination. (Hazel)

The catalogue of medical and midwifery interventions and drugs used in labour that are not supported by good-quality research is substantial. Discussion of the differential implementation of evidence arising from studies of electronic fetal heart monitoring and of caesarean section for breech presentation were explored in detail in Chapter 1. In the next section, we highlight some of the research around three other interventions. The first two, routine perineal shaving and routine use of episiotomy, are now rare in UK practice, not least because of the vigorous challenge made to them by organizations such as the NCT and AIMS. However, they are still prevalent in some European countries, and in tertiary referral centres across the world. The third one, routine ultrasound in pregnancy, is still in evidence in many maternity services across the world, with little research to evaluate its long-term effects.

Pubic shaving

As early as 1922, researchers demonstrated that pubic shaving did not prevent infections.[16] Little changed until the 1980s, when this research was repeated and organizations campaigning for more humane birth, such as AIMS and the NCT, gave women information on the results of the research and helped to challenge the need for this procedure. Over the next few decades, practice began to change as midwives themselves began to question the practice and enact change.

Episiotomy

Unlike the situation in the USA, the liberal use of episiotomy did not occur in the UK until the 1960s. The Association for Improvements in the Maternity Services received a constant stream of letters and phone calls from women with post-episiotomy problems, and even one report from a woman who was given an episiotomy after the baby's head was born because the midwife did not want to be criticized for failing to abide by the hospital's policy of a 100% episiotomy rate.

The Association for Improvements in the Maternity Services challenged the medical profession to provide the evidence that episiotomy was of benefit. In the early 1980s, Sheila Kitzinger produced her survey of women's experiences of episiotomy for the NCT.[17] In 1984, Jennifer Sleep and colleagues revealed the results of their trial of 1000 women, which found that episiotomy did not prevent tears and that women who had an episiotomy resumed their sexual lives later than those who suffered a tear.[18] Over the next few years, midwives joined in the criticisms. Routine episiotomy is rarely performed in the UK today.

Ultrasound examination in pregnancy

One of the promises held out by antenatal scanning is that technologists will be able to identify the baby with problems and do something to help it. However, a large German study found that, in 2378 pregnant women undergoing ultrasound, only 58 of 183 growth-retarded babies were diagnosed before birth.[19] Forty-five were wrongly diagnosed as being growth retarded when they were not. Only 28 of the 82 severely growth-retarded babies were detected before birth, despite the mothers having an average of 4.7 scans.

Women can also be told that the scan has found that they have placenta praevia (a condition where the placenta is very low and can prevent the baby birthing vaginally). A large randomized controlled trial of 9310 women in Finland revealed that 250 of the 4691 women screened by ultrasound at 16–20 weeks were diagnosed as having placenta praevia.[20] By the time the women reached the full term of their pregnancies, only 4 still had the condition; they were compared with 4619 women who did not have ultrasound and, ironically, 4 of them were also found at term to have placenta praevia. All 8 women had caesarean sections and there was no difference in the health of the women and their babies. In addition, there were 20 miscarriages after 16–20 weeks in the screened group and none in the controls.

In a later study in London,[21] researchers randomized 2475 women to either routine Doppler ultrasound examination of the umbilical and uterine arteries at 19–22 weeks and 32 weeks or standard care without Doppler ultrasound. There were 16 perinatal deaths of normally formed infants in the Doppler group compared with 4 in the standard care group.

The significance of these results appears to have been ignored by practitioners, despite attempts by AIMS to draw attention to the inconvenient appearance of adverse effects from an intervention introduced without adequate evidence of safety and benefit. The most recent review we found on the use of routine ultrasound in pregnancy for all women was published in 2000.[21] This looked at three areas: routine ultrasound in early pregnancy (9 trials); routine late pregnancy ultrasound (7 trials); and routine Doppler ultrasound in pregnancy (5 trials). Though the associated Cochrane review has recently been withdrawn for reasons of datedness, we have not located any more recent trials in this area. The authors of the review concluded: 'Routine ultrasound in early pregnancy appears to enable better gestational age assessment, earlier detection of multiple pregnancies and earlier detection of clinically unsuspected fetal malformation at a time when termination of pregnancy is possible. However, the benefits for other substantive outcomes [such as outcomes of diagnosed multiple pregnancies and

ultimate fetal outcome] are less clear'; and 'Based on existing evidence, routine late pregnancy ultrasound in low risk or unselected populations does not confer benefit on mother or baby'; and finally 'routine Doppler ultrasound in pregnancy … has not been shown to be of benefit and may even increase the risk of adverse outcome'.[22]

The widespread use of ultrasound has been justified on the grounds that women want it. This is not surprising, given that few women are told of any possible risks of the process, and that it promises the opportunity to visualize their baby while it is still in utero. It has been claimed that this process can be a major factor in helping the mother to bond with the baby. This ignores the fact that the mother is already experiencing hormonal and sensual cues that are likely to be building that bond from the very early stages of pregnancy. Claims have also been made that, if they are present for the scan, fathers, and even grandparents, can increase their connection with the baby. There is no formal evidence to substantiate these claims.

The majority of ultrasound research focuses on what ultrasound can reveal and little or none considers the effects of the process on the mother and baby beyond the first postnatal year. Long-term research is necessary on potential clinical, emotional and psychological consequences of false-negative or false-positive screening via ultrasound.

The pioneer of ultrasound examination in pregnancy, Donald, warned that 'the possibility of hazard should be kept under constant review'.[23] Those words of caution appear to have been largely ignored. Indeed, some practitioners explicitly dismiss any suggestion that routine ultrasound examination of the fetus may cause harm:

A great deal of research has been done over the past 30 years to investigate if foetal ultrasound has any effect on the baby and there is no evidence whatsoever of harm.

(The Sunday Times, 12 September, 2004)

The Association for Improvements in the Maternity Services wrote to Professor Stuart Campbell, the author of this quote, asking him to explain his claim in light of the adverse effects reported by the Davies[21] and the Saari-Kemppainen[20] studies. Unfortunately, he did not reply.

Mother versus baby

One impact of the developing capacity to visualize and treat the baby separately from the mother has been an increasing focus on the importance of the baby relative to the woman. Women who complain about traumatic births and long-term damage to their bodies are often told that they should be grateful that they have a live baby. Paediatricians are now claiming to represent the interests of the baby to justify some of the interventions in labour and birth, as described by Ann McCabe:[24]

I gave birth to triplets in March 1999 by planned caesarean section. The birth was clinically straightforward and the children were fine weighing in at 6lb 12ozs, 4lb 9ozs and 4lb 1oz. I had reached 36 weeks' gestation with ease and, whilst not 100 per cent happy to deliver so early, I decided to trust the medical advice.

Trauma for me was largely caused by staff thoughtlessness and my own passivity induced by diamorphine – given without my knowledge. Both meant I was barely involved in the birth, not even as a spectator. It was further exacerbated later when I read the relevant research. It shows the caesarean to have introduced significant risk to my babies and to me contrary to the advice of the obstetric staff. I had always wanted to deliver vaginally and changed my decision on safety grounds.

My exclusion from the birth and separation from the babies within 30 minutes of their birth gave me a sense of overwhelming loss. Four days after the birth I became very distressed and sought help from the obstetrician whom I had seen throughout my pregnancy and who performed the caesarean. His response, sadly, was unsupportive and defensive. So, instead of starting to heal, the pain worsened. Over the subsequent eight weeks or so I learned about the diamorphine and the very personal procedures carried out without my knowledge on the other side of the screen. The screen itself had been erected despite agreement weeks beforehand that it wouldn't be. The resulting sense of being manipulated and demeaned brought emotional pain, shock, and anger that I struggled to deal with.

As well as feeling traumatized, I felt guilty. I had three healthy babies, there were no physically horrendous aspects of the birth to describe. I was fine, so how could I complain? This was clearly the view of the medical staff and showed in their comments and behaviour towards me. Their reaction to my distress exacerbated it.

Paediatricians also appear to have been selective in their concern for the fetus. They have vigorously expressed their anxiety about water birth, and the possible risk to the fetus of a raised core temperature because of the mother's immersion in a water birth pool that had a temperature higher than recommended. Water birth services were suspended in many hospitals in the UK as a result of this suggestion. There is no evidence at all for this hypothesis, but there is evidence of fever in women who have had an epidural in place for more than six hours.[25] In the UK, not a single paediatrician has raised public concerns about the possible effects of this in the fetus. To our knowledge, no epidural services have been suspended for this reason.

Women's views of interventions

One of the few pieces of work that reflects women's views of which interventions are most likely to cause distress is that of Clement and colleagues.[26] They developed an intrapartum intervention score to quantify the degree of intervention in childbirth. Women found a series of what are often considered by professionals to be minor interventions, such as artificial rupture of membranes, episiotomy, urinary catheterization and electronic fetal monitoring, to be equally disturbing as one large intervention, such as use of forceps. The authors noted that scores from the many respondents may well differ markedly from the perceptions obstetricians and midwives have of the effect of interventions on a woman. The following quotes from the respondents to the NCT debate on intervention and normal birth illustrate this point.

I then went into labour at about 11.00 p.m. on 15th April and after an hour or so we went to the hospital as they would go ahead with the c-section anyway. I knew from class that I would be examined internally to see how dilated I was, but what I didn't know was how painful that would be when the midwife did it, and also how much more painful it would be when the doctor repeated the examination a short time later! (Kirsten)

I … had a natural 3rd stage this time which resulted in heavy bleeding for 2 days and a cessation of lochia by day 10 as well as a 5 day period of enforced rest due to heavy blood loss directly after the birth. With syntometrine I bled sluggishly for 6 weeks. I know which I preferred and it wasn't the artificial method. I also have tried both stitches and natural healing. I have been left with a large patch of unnecessary scar tissue from an overeager amount of stitching first time round, which resulted in 9 months of discomfort and a nosedive in libido. This time healing took 10 weeks (probably being over cautious) and I've not had a twinge since. (Clare)

The result of these interventions is that, for some women, the experience of birth is damaging, with little improvement to her well-being or that of her baby. The irony is that, while there are a minority of babies and mothers who need medical intervention, it is the majority who are unnecessarily subjected to them. It is vital that those mothers and babies with problems are identified and receive the medical care they need. However, the process of optimizing systems to uncover and treat pathologies should not exclude recognition of the birth experience. After over 40 years of campaigning about medicalized birth, women are still subjected to intervention without good evidence of efficacy. The women who challenge the advice they are given are often labelled as 'difficult patients' and are required to justify their failure to comply. Kitzinger wrote:[27]

When interns in a Boston hospital were asked to define a 'good patient', one reply was, 'She does what I say, hears what I say, believes what I say …'. A good patient is compliant. Not only does she conform, but she thanks the professionals because they 'save' her baby. She is grateful regardless of what they do to her. Women who fail to conform in this way are seen as 'difficult patients'.

Many women know, intuitively, what is best for them and their babies. The needs of those who are happy with technical oversight can be met in most maternity units, assuming that the support they are given is also respectful and caring. However, in the current climate of centralized obstetric care, it is often extremely difficult for women who want minimum technical input to negotiate the kind of care they want.

Being critical of the evidence

The evidence used to promote both technical and 'natural' process for birth can be suspect. In addition, the way this evidence is promoted in the media provides interesting insights into the predominant concerns of society. We illustrate these claims next.

The first example is a questionnaire sent to a selective group of 75 female obstetricians in London. The authors concluded that 31% of the respondents would choose an elective caesarean section.[28] This selective research received considerable publicity. At the same time, a survey of midwives found that almost all of them (129 out of 135) would not choose an elective caesarean.[29] A Scottish survey of female obstetricians also found that 77% would not choose an elective caesarean.[30] Neither of these latter surveys attracted media attention.

In terms of asking women their views, care needs to be taken to understand the multilayered and complex context that informs women's responses. If, as frequently happens, women are asked to respond to simple linear questions without context, there is a risk of drawing simplistic or even erroneous conclusions. An example illustrating this is a survey seeking women's views that was published in 1999 by a former Assistant Master of the National Maternity Hospital in Dublin.[31] A questionnaire was handed out to 400 women on their first visit to the hospital antenatal clinic. Almost half the women were expecting their first child. They were given seven statements, with which they could agree, disagree or say they did not care or did not know:

1. I don't want my waters to be broken.
2. I want a quick labour.
3. I want my labour to be as free of pain as possible.

4. I want to avoid a labour that lasts more than 12 hours.
5. I want to avoid a caesarean in labour.
6. I want to avoid a forceps or vacuum delivery.
7. I want an epidural.

From the responses to these questions, the author concluded that 'Many women want a quick and painless labour and do not object to the interventions that help achieve this'. There are a number of issues with this conclusion, but the primary one is that a large percentage of the respondents were having their first baby, and all the respondents were asked for their views in the first trimester of pregnancy. The conclusions, therefore, can only relate to women's views at that stage. In addition, women were not given information about the implications of the choices they made in response to the questions.

Criticism of much of the research in this area can be extended to include the topics chosen for that research. For example, while research has been undertaken into 'alternative' settings for birth (see Ch. 3), it appears, surprisingly, that no investigation has been undertaken into the effects on labour of transporting a woman from her home tens of miles to a centralized, unfamiliar obstetric unit. From the perspective of evidence-based practice, this raises serious concerns about the whole project of hospitalization for birth.

Conclusion

Over the last 50 years of medicalized, centralized birth, women's hopes and desires have been remarkably consistent. They want to come through the experience physically and mentally whole and in a fit state to start life as a parent with a live and healthy baby. Parents who will not benefit from medical intervention have been misled into believing that the best way to achieve their hopes for the birth is by an operative or obstetric delivery. As a result, the medical resources of the health service are spread thinly across too many births and poor care may be provided both for those who only need non-medical support to have a normal birth and for the minority who need medical intervention to preserve the life or well-being of mother or baby. Parallel issues are explored in the context of birth in Egypt in Chapter 7.

For many years, the evidence on the importance of birth, and particularly normal birth, has been there in women's stories and in qualitative research, but professionals have largely ignored this source. At last, an interest is beginning to be taken in the effect of the birth experience on the psychosocial well-being of the mother, baby and family. There are indications that normal birth, in the widest sense of a spontaneous physiological, straightforward birth that occurs in the context of supportive, caring, respectful professional care, may enhance the woman's self-esteem, and her physical and mental health. It may also impact upon her relationship with the child and offer a good foundation for future family well-being. If more women, and especially marginalized women, could give accounts of their births, such as the one below, the childbirth organizations in the UK would feel that they had succeeded in their mission.

The whole experience was truly amazing. It was so calm and soothing, I hardly felt like I had given birth at all. N came into the world so peacefully, we couldn't have asked for a better birth experience. I suffered no ill effects, lost no blood, needed no stitches, and was out and about within a day or two. (Sue)

References

1. CEMACH 2004 Why mothers die 2000–2002. Sixth report of the Confidential Enquiries into Maternal Deaths in the United Kingdom. RCOG Press, London

2. Ryding E L, Mijma K, Wijma B et al 1998 Fear of childbirth during pregnancy may increase the risk of emergency caesarean section. Acta Obstet Gynecol Scand 77:542–547

3. Robinson J 1998 Suicide: a major cause of maternal deaths. Br J Midwif 6:767

4. Downe S, McCormick C, Beech B L 2001 Labour interventions associated with normal birth. Br J Midwif 9:602–606

5. Towler J, Bramall J 1986 Midwives in history and society. Croom Helm, London

6. Nursing and Midwifery Council 2004 Midwives rules and standards. NMC, London

7. Lee B 1999 Royal Society of Medicine forum: what is normal birth? RCM Midwives Journal 2:386–387

8. World Health Organization 1999 Care in normal birth: a practical guide. Report of a technical working group. WHO, Geneva

9. Bates C 1997 Debating midwifery: normality in midwifery. Royal College of Midwives, London

10. Beech B A L 1997 Normal birth: does it exist? AIMS Journal 9:4–8

11. BirthChoiceUK 2005 Normal birth rate 1990–2005. Online. Available: http://www.birthchoiceuk.com/Professionals/ NormalBirthHistory.htm (accessed 30 October 2007)

12. BirthChoiceUK. Data taken, with permission, from http://www.birthchoiceuk.com/Professionals/ BirthChoiceUKFrame.htm? http://www.birthchoiceuk. com/Professionals/NormalBirth.htm

13. Donnison J 1988 Midwives and medical men: a history of the struggle for the control of childbirth. Historical Publications, London

14. Bonar K, Kaunitz A M, Sanchez-Ramos L 2000 The effect of obstetric resident gender on forceps delivery rate. Am J Obstet Gynecol 182:1950–1951

15. Labusoua E 2003 An interview with Marsden Wagner. AIMS Journal 15:5–8

16. Johnston R A, Sidall R S 1922 Is the usual method of preparing patients for delivery beneficial or necessary? Am J Obstet Gynecol 4:645–650

17. Kitzinger S 1981 Some women's experiences of episiotomy. National Childbirth Trust, London

18. Sleep J, Grant A, Garcia J et al 1984 West Berkshire perineal management trial. Br Med J 289:587–590

19. Jahn A, Razum O, Berle P 1998 Routine screening for intrauterine growth retardation in Germany; low sensitivity and questionable benefit for diagnosed cases. Acta Obstet Gynecol Scand 77:643–689

20. Saari-Kemppainen A, Karjalainen O, Ylostalo P et al 1990 Ultrasound screening and prenatal mortality; controlled trial of systematic one-stage screening in pregnancy. Lancet 339:387–391

21. Davies J A, Gullivan S, Spencer J A D 1992 Randomised controlled Doppler ultrasound screening of placental perfusion during pregnancy. Lancet ii:1299–1303

22. Bricker L, Garcia J, Henderson J et al 2000 Ultrasound screening in pregnancy: a systematic review of the clinical effectiveness, cost-effectiveness and women's views. Health Technol Assess 4(16):i–vi, 1–193

23. Donald I 1980 Sonar: its present status in medicine. In: Kurjak A (ed.) Progress in medical ultrasound, vol 1. Excerpta Medica, Amsterdam, p 1–4

24. McCabe A 2002 My experience of post childbirth trauma. AIMS Journal 14:15–16

25. Fusi L, Steer P J, Maresh M J A et al 1989 Maternal pyrexia associated with the use of epidural analgesia in labour. Lancet 69:634–638

26. Clement S, Wilson J, Sikorski J 1999 The development of an intrapartum intervention score based on women's experiences. J Reprod Infant Psychol 17:53–61

27. Kitzinger S 2000 Rediscovering birth. Little, Brown, London

28. Al-Mufti R, McCarthy A, Fisk N M 1997 Survey of obstetricians' personal preference and discretionary practice. Eur J Obstet Gynaecol Reprod Biol 73:1–4

29. Dickson M J, Wilett M 1999 Midwives would prefer a vaginal delivery. Br Med J 319:1008

30. MacDonald C, Pinion S B, MacLeod U M 2002 Scottish female obstetricians' views on elective caesarean section and personal choice for delivery. J Obstet Gynaecol 22:586–589

31. Impey I 1999 Maternal attitudes to amniotomy and labor duration: a survey in early pregnancy. Birth 26:211–217

5

Midwives' practices in 11 UK maternity units

Marianne Mead

Introduction

Numerous studies have demonstrated variations in intrapartum care. Some have dealt with overall care;[1-4] others have dealt with more specific aspects such as nutrition,[5] pain relief[6] or the use of guidelines.[7] The variation in caesarean sections between systems of care and across countries has perhaps been subjected to the greatest amount of investigation. Studies have compared national[8-20] and international rates.[21-24] Some have suggested explanations for these variations, including maternal characteristics,[25] fear of litigation,[26] previous obstetric history,[27] intrapartum events,[28,29] maternal choice[30-33] and medical control.[34]

The amount of information available on alternatives for optimum intrapartum care demonstrates the complexity of the issue. It is, therefore, not surprising that there is an element of confusion among practitioners, obstetricians, midwives and childbearing women.

Most, if not all, midwives would claim that they are the specialists in normal pregnancy, and the official worldwide definition of the midwife[35] supports that claim. But the question arises as to how midwives demonstrate that they are indeed specialists in this area. Given the physiological nature of pregnancy, there ought to be consistent similarities between the role of the midwife wherever it is examined. Unfortunately 'normal midwifery care' or 'normality' is a complex concept that has not been described accurately or definitely. This is particularly true for labour and delivery[36,37] and begs a number of questions. What are the criteria that define 'normal' labour or 'normal' delivery? Is a delivery 'normal' or 'spontaneous' if intrapartum interventions have been used, such as induction of labour, artificial rupture of membranes (ARM), augmentation of labour with oxytocics, use of epidural analgesia and of episiotomy? This chapter sets out to provide some answers to these questions, from the perspective of midwives working in the UK, Belgium and France.

Research

Aims and methods

The research presented in this chapter follows an earlier feasibility study that demonstrated that the use of the data from several UK units using the same computerized maternity records enabled the systematic exclusion of women who were not suitable for midwifery-led care. This initial study also demonstrated that neighbouring UK units had significantly different intrapartum practices, despite the fact that they provided clinical experience to student midwives from a single university and that their midwives primarily used the same institution for most of their continuing education.[3]

These findings led to an initial question of whether UK midwives' perception of intrapartum risk might be affected by their units' level of intrapartum intervention. A further study tested the hypothesis that midwives working in units with higher rates of intrapartum intervention would have a different perception of intrapartum risk than midwives working in units with lower rates of intervention. Four specific objectives were identified for this initial study:

1. To examine the policies of these 11 units for the care of women suitable for midwifery-led care on admission and during the first stage of labour.
2. To survey midwives to describe the care they and their colleagues would adopt on admission and in the first stage of labour.
3. To compare the intrapartum intervention rates of women suitable for midwifery-led care in these 11 units.
4. To survey midwives' perceptions of the labour and birth risks for women suitable for midwifery-led care, and to compare this across units classified as having higher or lower rates of intervention.

Following the publication of the results of the UK study, the phase of work dealing with midwives' reported personal practice and perception of risk was extended to Belgium (Flanders) and France (Alsace and Lorraine regions).

In the UK, 11 maternity units, all using the St Mary's Maternity Information System (SMMIS) were used. The SMMIS data contained information on 35 367 labours and births for the year 1998. A series of data reduction steps was used to exclude women deemed unsuitable for midwifery-led care.[38] The proportion of non-Caucasian women varied considerably in these units and the decision was taken to only include Caucasian women in the analysis. About one-third of the women were excluded on the basis of ethnic background and another third because of other factors, including previous medical history (hypertension, diabetes, epilepsy, haemoglobinopathies), previous obstetric history (caesarean section, perinatal mortality) or present pregnancy abnormalities or situations which would mean that the women were not suitable for exclusive midwifery care (prematurity, postmaturity, multiple pregnancies, pregnancy-induced hypertension, induction of labour, elective caesarean sections). Nearly 10 000 women (9887) who could be considered suitable for midwifery-led care, including 4090 nulliparous women, remained in the analysis at the end of the data reduction. The remaining women accounted for about 50% of the Caucasian women who were initially considered.

All midwives (828) who had undertaken births in the previous year were sent a questionnaire via the delivery suite and 249 (30%) were returned. The return rate was low and could be explained by several reasons, including insufficient funds to send the questionnaires directly to the midwives' home address or include a stamped self-addressed envelope for the return of the questionnaires, and the length and complexity of the questionnaire. The latter issue was probably compounded by the attempt to identify risk probabilities, an approach that many midwives are not familiar with. The questionnaires were collected from the 11 units after a given deadline. Despite the low rate of return, the number of respondents did allow useful statistical analysis.

In Belgium, an invitation to attend the Flemish midwives' 2004 annual conference provided the opportunity to replicate the study. All 845 midwives and 143 student midwife members of the Flemish Midwives Association (Vlaamse Organisatie van Vroedvrouwen – VLOV) were sent a questionnaire with their invitation to take part in the annual conference. Funding was limited to the translation and printing of the questionnaires that could only be returned at the conference. Two hundred and seventy-five midwives and 107 students attended the conference, and returned 128 questionnaires: 99 midwives (36% of the attendees), 26 students (24% of attendees) and 3 unidentified respondents. This convenience sample represents 12% of all midwives and 18% of all students in the Belgian Flanders at that time.

In France, a similar opportunity presented itself when an invitation was made to attend the French midwives annual meeting held in Strasbourg in 2005. A similar funding issue limited the study to the two local regions of Alsace and Lorraine. The questionnaire was translated (MM), and the two schools organized the printing, distribution and return of the questionnaires to all 750 midwives involved in intrapartum care in their region: 270 (36%) midwives returned their questionnaire.

Design

The first part of the survey to midwives dealt with their practice on admission of a woman in spontaneous labour and during the first stage of labour. A standardized scenario was used.

The mother was presented as a 24-year-old primigravida, with no previous medical history, a normal singleton pregnancy, in spontaneous labour at 39+ weeks' gestation who presents herself at the delivery suite. Her contractions started three hours earlier, are now regular and moderately strong at a rate of two or three per ten minutes. She has had a show and her membranes are intact.

In the UK, three versions of this scenario, randomly distributed to the midwives, were designed to mirror choices of care that women might opt for:

- *Janet Jones* – does not have a birth plan and wishes to rely on the midwives' best judgement.
- *Brigit Smith* – has a birth plan and wishes to have the very barest minimum of intervention.
- *Lynn Brown* – has a birth plan and wishes to have 'high-tech' care and supervision.

This initial study demonstrated that the different scenarios were only associated with an increased use of electronic fetal monitoring and epidural for 'Lynn Brown'. The decision was therefore made to use only the first scenario in Belgium and France.

Respondents were asked to identify the care that they would provide on admission and during the first stage of labour. Respondents in the UK were asked what they thought their colleagues might do, because it was felt that midwives might be more likely to describe the practice they may ideally wish to adopt, but might better identify actual practice through the description of their colleagues' options.

The following observations or actions were investigated: on admission – temperature, pulse, blood pressure, urinalysis, abdominal palpation to assess contractions, presentation and descent of the fetus, type of fetal auscultation or monitoring and notification of admission to the medical staff. Midwives were asked similar questions on the care they would provide during the first stage of labour, including vaginal examinations, ARM, pain relief and, more specifically, epidural analgesia, nutrition in labour and fetal monitoring.

The standardized scenario presented the description of a mother suitable for a home birth. Midwives assisting women at home normally carry out observations of both mother and baby, but do not have recourse to the technology often used in hospital practice. The practice used in the context of home birth could therefore be judged as the standard for normal practice.

Results

To reduce costs to a minimum, questionnaires were distributed in delivery suites in the UK and France and with their organization magazine in Belgium, where the collection of the questionnaire was only available at the annual conference. This will have influenced the return rates. The response rates identified were calculated on the basis of the questionnaire sent or distributed, and may therefore be artificially low. This may raise some concerns about representation, but the numbers were sufficient to describe practice and risk perception and establish interesting comparisons between the three countries. In the UK and France, the questionnaires were sent to midwives working in the delivery suites, whether exclusively or not;

all hospitals were public NHS hospitals in the UK but, in France, respondents worked either in public (72% of the respondents), or private (21%), or both public and private (7%) maternity units. In Belgium, 8 respondents (8%) were midwife teachers and 7 (7%) worked exclusively in the antenatal/postnatal areas; the other 74 (75%) worked in the delivery suite, and 7 of them worked there exclusively.

A total of 828, 850 and 750 questionnaires were sent out to UK, Belgian and French midwives respectively, with a response rate of 249/828 (30%) in the UK, 99/277 (36%) midwives and 26/107 (24%) student midwives attending their annual conference in Belgium, or a 12% and 18% overall population response rate, and 270/750 (36%) midwives in France.

Admission

The majority of respondents undertook admission observations such as temperature, pulse, blood pressure, urinalysis and abdominal palpation, but respondents were less likely to do so in Belgium than in the other two countries (Table 5.1). The overwhelming majority of Belgian respondents would notify a medical practitioner, compared to 19% in France and 4% in the UK. These findings are in line with previous information gathered on midwifery practice in the EU.[39]

The majority of respondents in the UK (73%) and Belgium (89%), and practically all respondents in France (99%), reported using admission cardiotocography (CTG).

Care during the first stage of labour

Midwives were first asked if they would undertake a range of maternal observations: temperature (with intact membranes, spontaneous or artificial rupture), pulse, blood pressure and urinalysis. They were also asked to identify the frequency of vaginal examinations, the preferred method of fetal heart monitoring and the type of nutrition they would recommend. Marked variations were observed between the three countries (Table 5.2). Respondents in the UK were more likely to undertake routine observations, and this was particularly so when compared to their Belgian colleagues. Respondents were less likely to take a woman's temperature if her membranes were intact, but UK respondents generally took a woman's temperature if her membranes were ruptured, irrespective of whether this was a spontaneous or artificial rupture, whereas in Belgium and France, the respondents were more likely to take a woman's temperature during labour where the membranes had been ruptured spontaneously than artificially. Belgian respondents were less likely to check the pulse and only about 60% checked a woman's blood pressure during labour, whereas more than 90% of their British and French colleagues did so. Urinalysis was hardly undertaken in Belgium and France, but ketonuria was checked for by about 74% in the UK, compared to 2 or 3% in the other two countries. The rate of vaginal examination varied between the countries too. In Belgium and France, 87% and 96% of the respondents reported that women had a

Table 5.1 Admission observations (%)

Observations	UK (N = 249)	Belgium (N = 125)	France (N = 270)
Temperature	96	51	3
Pulse	100	59	94
Blood pressure	100	98	100
Proteinuria	90	52	83
Glycosuria	81	34	77
Ketonuria	74	13	49
Electronic fetal monitoring	73	89	99
Inform a doctor	4	80	19

Table 5.2 Intrapartum observations and care (%)

	UK (N = 249)	Belgium (N = 125)	France (N = 270)
T° – intact membranes	75	6	29
T° – spontaneous rupture of membranes	95	51	71
T° – artificial rupture of membranes	94	45	51
Pulse	97	19	81
Blood pressure	97	59	91
Proteinuria	64	3	6
Glycosuria	56	2	4
Ketonuria	74	2	3
Vaginal examinations	(4 h) 90	(1&2 h) 87	(1&2 h) 96
Fetal monitoring			
Fetal stethoscope	40	2	–
Intermittent CTG	57	76	44
Continuous CTG	3	22	56
Nutrition			
Nil by mouth or water only	6	40	84
Any solid food	81	38	5

vaginal examination hourly or two hourly, whereas 90% of British respondents reported a four-hourly rate. Methods of observing the fetal heart during labour also varied markedly: 0–2% of respondents reported the use of the Pinard's stethoscope in France, compared to 40% in the UK. Only 3% of UK respondents reported using continuous monitoring, compared to 22% in Belgium and 56% in France. Nutrition followed a similar pattern: extremely restricted in France where 84% of the respondents opted for a 'nil by mouth' or water only policy, but only 40% in Belgium and 6% in the UK; 81% of the UK respondents identified that any solid food would be acceptable, compared to 38% in Belgium and only 5% in France.

Intrapartum risk perception

The second part of the questionnaire asked midwives to identify the risks that they associated with specific outcomes, on admission and during labour, given specific levels of interventions, for 100 women similar to Janet Jones, and therefore suitable for midwifery-led care. The initial comparison of 11 maternity units allowed the categorization of intrapartum intervention rates; the results of the UK respondents are therefore given here according to the type of maternity units they worked in.

At the point of admission, the respondents were asked to identify the likelihood of various outcomes: fetal presentation, engagement of the fetal head, birth weight and fetal oxygenation. The birth weight options selected by respondents matched the distribution of birth weight in the UK, but the other items demonstrated a greater rate of pessimism than expected for healthy women at term and in spontaneous labour. The likelihood of a breech presentation at term in the SMMIS database was 2–3%, yet this was identified as 5–8% in the three countries. Similarly the likelihood of normal fetal oxygenation in labour was only set at 79–83%, thereby suggesting that 17–21% of babies would be likely to have an abnormal fetal heart rate/pattern. Although actual figures could not be found for comparison, this rate of abnormality seems unduly high for babies of healthy women at term of a normal pregnancy, and in spontaneous labour. Although the admission risks identified might be greater than reality, the differences in respondents' perception varied little between the

Table 5.3 Risk perception on admission				
	UK (N = 249)		Belgium (N = 125)	France (N = 270)
	Intervention −	Intervention +		
Cephalic presentation	94	93	90	93
Breech presentation	5	5	8	6
Head engaged	82	80	69	29
Birth weight 3–4 kg	75	75	71	72
CTG normal	83	82	79	82
CTG slightly abnormal	13	13	17	13
CTG pathological	4	5	5	5

three countries. However, where the engagement of the head was concerned, there was a marked difference, with French respondents identifying that in only 29% of cases the head would be engaged, compared to 69% in Belgium and at least 80% in the UK (Table 5.3).

The perception of risk during the first stage of labour was divided into three distinct scenarios: the woman has no intervention, has an artificial rupture of membranes (ARM) or an epidural. Midwives were asked what they thought the likelihood of the following outcomes might be for each of the three situations: birth within 12 hours, use of continuous electronic fetal monitoring, adequacy of fetal oxygenation, maternal request for an epidural (for the first two options) and type of birth. The perceived risk of mild and severe fetal hypoxia increased slightly between 'no intervention' and the other scenarios, but were very similar between the three countries. There were, however, some marked differences: the Belgian and French respondents were more likely to think that women would give birth within 12 hours and would have a spontaneous vaginal birth, irrespective of the care options. However, they were more likely to think that the mothers would request an epidural. The French respondents thought unanimously that women would have continuous electronic fetal heart rate monitoring (EFM) by the time of birth, irrespective of the level of intrapartum intervention. They also believed that their colleagues would note a high level of EFM use for women who had an epidural (Table 5.4).

Whatever the level of intervention, the Belgian and French respondents reported a risk perception for caesarean section that was very low – a maximum of 7–8% with the epidural scenario, compared to 14–15% in the UK. The previous study on risk perception in the UK had already identified that the risk perception was over-pessimistic for healthy nulliparous women in spontaneous labour at term, when compared to reality.[38] The overall caesarean section rate is lower in Belgium (18% in 2005)[40] and France (20% in 2003)[41] than in the UK (22% in 2004),[41] but the epidural rates are higher (Belgium 65%,[40] France 63% in 2003[42] compared to 31% for epidural and spinal analgesia in the UK).[43] Previous randomized controlled studies have not identified any statistically significant links between epidurals and caesarean sections, but did show an increased rate of operative vaginal deliveries and therefore a corresponding reduction in spontaneous vaginal delivery rate.[44]

A previous retrospective study of women suitable for midwifery-led care demonstrated a statistically significant link between epidural and caesarean section, but this may not have controlled adequately for associated variables such as prolonged labour and birth weight.[45]

These results from Belgium and France call into question the findings of the initial UK study where respondents were shown to be over-pessimistic for the risks of healthy women in spontaneous labour at term and progressing without intervention, or just an ARM, and over-optimistic for the outcome of labour of similar women where labour had progressed with an epidural. The over-optimism is much greater for

Table 5.4 Intrapartum risk perception by level of intervention

Outcome	England (N = 249)		Belgium (N = 125)	France (N = 270)
	Units with low rates of intervention	Units with high rates of intervention		
No intervention				
Delivery <12h	66	63	77	85
Continuous CTG	56	60	53	100
Mild/severe hypoxia	18	17	17	19
Requesting epidural	46	61	63	75
Spontaneous vaginal delivery	72	66	81	80
Forceps/ventouse	16	22	14	13
Emergency caesarean	12	12	5	7
ARM				
Delivery <12h	76	68	83	91
Continuous CTG	53	60	56	100
Mild/severe hypoxia	22	21	21	21
Requesting epidural	50	65	69	77
Spontaneous vaginal delivery	71	64	78	79
Forceps/ventouse	17	23	16	14
Emergency caesarean	12	13	6	7
Epidural				
Delivery <12h	59	54	83	90
Continuous CTG	91	82	90	100
Mild/severe hypoxia	22	23	25	22
Spontaneous vaginal delivery	57	51	69	75
Forceps/ventouse	29	34	23	18
Emergency caesarean	14	15	8	7

the epidural scenario in Belgium and France, but this may be linked to the much higher rate of use and the fact that, despite this much higher rate, the overall caesarean section rates remain lower than in the UK in these two countries. The explanation of these differences would require further research, but might include obvious differences in the approach to health care: a greater number of obstetricians and a much greater use of private care, greater patient autonomy and choice, but a much lower rate of midwives too.[41] Possible hypotheses may include the suggestion that the longer lasting relationship that women and gynaecologists establish over a period of many years in the private sector may play a role in trust that both the physicians and the women have in the ability to give birth normally. It is also possible that physicians who provide continuity of care may feel more responsible for ensuring that the women they know and will most probably continue to care for over many years, and possibly further pregnancies, will have as normal pregnancies and deliveries as it is possible to ensure.

Normal or the norm

The scenario presented a woman suitable for midwifery-led care, and therefore suitable for home birth, but identified as delivering in hospital. The rate of home birth is low in all three countries, but more actively discouraged in Belgium and France than in the UK. The UK study had three versions of the same scenario, and it is conceivable that 'Lynn Brown' would not have opted for a home birth, even if it had been offered to her, since she wanted to avail herself of the medical technology only available in a hospital context. However, only the use of electronic fetal monitoring and epidural analgesia demonstrated notable differences between the three scenarios. The simplification of the study to only one scenario was therefore justified, as the purpose was to identify the type of care that midwives would recommend and their perception of risk.

Several questions arise from this study in terms of how midwives construct normality and, as the study was extended to other countries, how this may vary according to different midwifery or obstetric 'cultures'. What is normal midwifery practice for women suitable for midwifery-led care? The answer to the question would really depend on how the word 'normal' is interpreted. The analysis of the 1998 data, of the care provided to 9887 healthy UK women in spontaneous labour at term of a healthy singleton pregnancy, allowed the identification of some common UK practices. If normal equals the norm, as might be understood from a statistical point of view, then clearly hospital care is normal because the great majority of UK women (96.7%) selected this option. The same can be said of the other two countries where the proportion of home births is lower than in the UK. The proportion of UK women who opt for home delivery was low (3.3% – varying between 0.2% and 9.0%), demonstrating perhaps a difference in the perception of what midwives, rather than women, view as acceptable.

Similarly, the use of electronic fetal monitoring must be seen as normal, since 60–100% of the respondents reported that they would use either intermittent or continuous electronic fetal monitoring at some point during labour. Bearing in mind that fetal monitoring is a screening rather than a diagnostic test,[46] that women who opt for a home birth do not have access to such technology, yet that home birth is at least as safe as hospital birth,[47,48] it is worrying to note that 17–25% of the respondents believed that these healthy women would have an abnormal tracing on admission in spontaneous labour and during labour. Although this was not specifically explored with the Belgian and French respondents, the comparison of the 11 UK maternity units confirmed that the interpretation of CTGs is far from consistent and there is no reason to believe that this might be systematically different in the other two countries. The risk perception rates for an abnormal fetal heart trace on admission or in labour were very similar in the three countries, and this suggests that better training and regular updates in this area may be a widespread need.[49] Given the potentially very low predictive value of an abnormal fetal heart tracing, one must question the value of using CTGs in a healthy population in the first instance. Indeed the inherited guidelines from the Royal College of Obstetricians and Gynaecologists (RCOG)[50] adopted by the National Institute for Health and Clinical Excellence (NICE) recommend intermittent auscultation with a Pinard's stethoscope or a hand-held Doppler for the healthy mother with an otherwise uncomplicated pregnancy.[51]

The contrast between normal practice (the most likely practice to be adopted) and recommended practice demonstrates that the norm is not necessarily practice based on evidence. This suggests that the adoption of best practice might present difficulties for midwives who might find themselves at odds with the general practice adopted in their unit, whether consciously and explicitly or not.[52] This may be more marked in the UK where health care is more centralized, where private obstetric practice is less common and where evidence-based practice and guidelines have been established for a longer period.

Figure 5.1 clearly demonstrates the close correlation that existed between the perception of respondents regarding their own practice and that of their colleagues, and the recommendations made by unit policies.[45]

The responses of respondents regarding nutrition during labour demonstrated wide variations from available evidence.[53] The UK study had suggested that the unit philosophy or ethos had an influence in the care women received, but the comparison of the three countries suggests more important cultural influences, particularly in the case of the French respondents. Very similar conclusions can be drawn for the practice of fetal monitoring on admission and during labour (Fig. 5.2).

The discrepancies illustrated in Figure 5.1 suggest that UK respondents who work in a context that they perceive as being at odds with their own

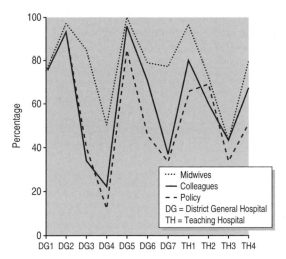

Fig 5.1 • Support for solid food for women in labour.

philosophy may be confronted with decisions that set them apart from their colleagues or their unit policy. Respondents were systematically more likely to allow solid food in labour or to use intermittent auscultation than they felt their colleagues would. Where respondents identified that their unit policy was particularly restrictive (e.g. DG4 for nutrition during labour or DG3 for intermittent auscultation), the differences between respondents' practice and routine practice or policy were more obvious. In DG4, only 10% of respondents thought the policy would allow solid food during labour, yet they perceived that just over 20% of their colleagues

would allow it and 50% of the respondents would do so themselves. Similarly in DG3, no respondents thought that intermittent auscultation was unit policy, yet they thought that it would be the practice for just under 10% of their colleagues; 50% of the respondents would adopt the practice themselves. This aspect might be worthy of examination in Belgium where respondents reported a relatively lower level of medicalization, but perhaps not so useful in France where respondents reported a very high and very systematic level; this was particularly so for their approach to nutrition and electronic fetal monitoring during the first stage of labour.

The respondents' answers to what they would adopt as personal practice in the standardized scenario were at odds with reality. This confirms a previous study,[54] but also raises important questions about what respondents consider normal practice and how the environment in which they practise may encourage them away from normality and into a model of intrapartum intervention rather than watchful observation, which may reveal a degree of mistrust rather than trust in the physiology of labour. The comparison of the three countries raises further questions about the usual assumption that more intervention is associated with worse outcomes. Clearly the example of France negates this assertion as the level of intervention is much higher, and yet the caesarean section rate is substantially lower than in the UK, and midwives' perception of risk in this study was more optimistic than in the UK.

Towards normal labour

It might be useful to think of normal labour as a concept situated somewhere between two distinct perspectives: the physiological approach on one end of the spectrum and the technological approach on the other. This view might allow an approach which would address the problem from two distinct standpoints: encouraging an uncritical emphasis on a physiological approach to pregnancy, labour and birth on the one hand, even where this is not optimal, and challenging the use of inappropriate technology or interventions on the other.

If physiological processes are to be supported, all stakeholders, including women, partners, midwives,

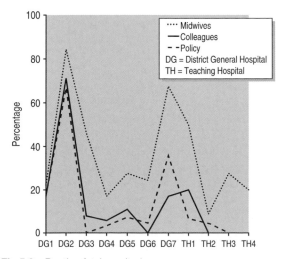

Fig 5.2 • Routine fetal monitoring.

general practitioners, obstetricians, anaesthetists and policy makers, will have to engage in very meaningful dialogues and research to establish how best to encourage and nurture the spontaneous process of labour. The situation we are experiencing today is primarily the result of good intentions, namely the desire to reduce maternal and perinatal mortality and morbidity. However, in the absence of sound programmes of research, these good intentions have contributed to an increase in maternal morbidity, particularly an increase in intervention in pregnancy and childbirth, and a disproportionate rise in caesarean sections, without a corresponding improvement in neonatal outcome.[55]

If normal labour is to be encouraged for healthy women presenting at term with an otherwise normal pregnancy, it may be useful to look critically at the present situation in Europe. The overwhelming majority of births take place in hospital. Routine intrapartum care includes practices that are not necessarily beneficial to either mother or fetus.[56] Electronic fetal monitoring is widely used[3,57,58] despite awareness of disadvantages such as high false-positive rates and increased intrapartum interventions and caesarean sections,[59-61] and recommendations on limiting their use.[50,51,62] Artificial rupture of membranes is also widely performed, and, more worryingly, is often perceived not to be a form of augmentation of labour, despite available information as to the potential negative consequences.[63-65] The rate of epidural analgesia is growing despite awareness of its potential consequences[66-68] and recommendations on its use.[62]

Midwives and obstetricians are extremely familiar with these practices and may find it difficult to return to a more physiological approach. Indeed the de-skilling of midwives is now a concern for those who wish to see a less interventionist maternity service.[69] It is also important to be aware that fear of the perceived risk of litigation may have contributed to the present situation.[26,70-72] This may be of some importance if one considers that there is also increased evidence that the wishes of women are not necessarily acceded to.[73]

But the picture is not altogether negative. A substantial body of knowledge exists on the aspects of care that are known to be helpful and positive. It has already been established that the option of home birth is safe for healthy women. The same has generally been said for birth centres,[74-80] although a randomized controlled trial conducted in Sweden has raised a question mark on a possible increase in perinatal mortality for nulliparous women in integrated birth centres.[79,80] Social support has also been shown to be useful at all stages of pregnancy,[80] and so has continuity of care.[81-83] The different healthcare systems of the three countries may exert an influence on the way that evidence is used in maternity services. The UK has a very small level of private obstetric practice, but this is much more important and influential in Belgium and France. This may have an influence on the relationship between women and their main care provider – the midwife in the UK and the obstetrician in Belgium and France. There is evidence, particularly in the UK, that women wish to be involved in the decisions regarding their care during pregnancy and labour,[73,84,85] but effective partnership between midwives and women needs to develop further.[52,86] It may be more difficult for women's involvement in the care decisions to take place in the context of private practice. Although this may at first seem paradoxical, there is some evidence that obstetricians are generally more reluctant to abandon the 'safety' of obstetric technology.[87-90] The woman may be looked after by a midwife, but still rely heavily on the information provided by her obstetrician; this may prevent the woman from accepting a philosophy of care that is at odds with what she may have become familiar with during her pregnancy.

Evidence-based information is also widely available on the optimum intrapartum care for healthy women. The main principle is simple: 'In normal birth there should be a valid reason to interfere with the natural process'.[62] This may be the mid-point at which the physiological process may meet the medical model, the point at which practitioners wishing to support the physiological process need to demonstrate how their care will ensure the optimum safety both of mothers and babies, and that at which practitioners who are inclined to practise along a more medicalized model need to justify every intervention which can be seen to interfere with the physiological process of labour and delivery. In the language of the English court, each healthy woman suitable for midwifery-led care should be seen as 'innocent until proved guilty'.

There is little doubt that the UK maternity services have been run along a medical regimen rather than a woman-centred approach and that this approach has been encouraged by the recommendations of successive reports.[91] This was eventually challenged, however, first in the 1980s[92] and then finally in the 1990s when the Department of Health endorsed the Expert Maternity Group report *Changing Childbirth*.[93] Despite initial reticence,[50] there is evidence that the stance taken by many obstetricians and, indeed, by their Royal College has changed and is opting for more evidence-based practice.[51,94,95] It is possible that the development of the movement for evidence-based medicine may have encouraged this process.

However, obstetricians cannot change the way maternity services are delivered on their own. Information on pregnancy and labour available to the general public tends to reinforce the stereotype of the medical model or portray obstetrics and perinatal medicine as everyday heroic or extraordinary activities, either saving women from the jaws of certain death or providing them with medical miracles. There is evidence that the levels of risk perceived by women influences their choices during pregnancy and labour,[96,97] and it follows that accurate information would have to be provided to enable women to understand the potential benefits of a physiological approach to labour.

Risk assessment tools could be used, but these have been shown to be of doubtful value,[98] so in the absence of known or recognized health issues, women may benefit from referral to the primary healthcare team, and in particular midwives, unless or until abnormalities which require referral to specialist services are demonstrated. This is relatively easy in countries that have a national form of health care, as in the UK, but more challenging where private practice has a much greater profile and where women therefore go to where their private obstetricians have access. Although obstetricians working in tertiary referral centres tend to be employees, this is not the case for those who have access contracts with maternity units situated in secondary level hospital care. It is unusual for these obstetricians to provide care in the primary sector.

It is unlikely that the trend towards hospital delivery would decrease dramatically in the next few years,[99] and it follows therefore that midwives and obstetricians working in hospital will have a major role to play in achieving a more physiological approach to intrapartum care and delivery in the context of a secondary care setting.[100]

The benefit of some aspects of care is no longer in doubt. Physical, emotional and psychological support together with continuity of carer are known to be beneficial,[53] for example in reducing the use of analgesia.[80] Women ought therefore to be able to expect that maternity services will be structured in such a way that these forms of support will be available. Some other aspects are promising, though their advantages have not yet been identified through randomized controlled trials. This includes the freedom to move during labour and the use of touch and massage to relieve pain.[53] Midwives, where appropriate in collaboration with private obstetricians, must ensure that they facilitate and indeed encourage women to move during labour; they must also become skilled at the art of touch and massage.

If normal labour can be interpreted as a concept situated somewhere on the continuum between the physiological and the medical approach, it is helpful to look at useful medical interventions as well as interventions which have been shown to have a potentially negative effect on the normal development of labour. Perhaps the most widely accepted form of intervention in the UK is the active management of the third stage of labour that is associated with a lower rate of postpartum haemorrhage (PPH).[53] However, it is not routine practice in Sweden where there is a greater stress on the physiological aspects of labour,[101] and it is worth noting that the administration of oxytocin is commonly associated with side effects such as nausea, vomiting and headaches, and very rarely with severe maternal cardiac or pulmonary complications and even death.[102] Midwives must therefore, in conjunction with the mother, develop decision strategies that take into consideration the advantages and the disadvantages of the active management of the third stage of labour, as well as the risks associated with particular intrapartum circumstances.

Recent publications, and in particular the guidelines developed by RCOG[50] and adopted by NICE,[51] have reviewed the evidence to date on fetal monitoring, and recommend the use of intermittent auscultation for women suitable for midwifery-led care. It is to be hoped that midwives and obstetricians will perceive that the level of authority of both the RCOG and NICE will strongly support midwives and obstetricians who wish to implement a reduction in the use of continuous electronic fetal monitoring for those women for whom it has not been shown to be advantageous. A similar approach to the development of evidence-based guidelines for care is being developed in France through the auspices of the 'Haute Autorité de Santé' (http://www.has-sante.fr/), but nothing of that magnitude is presently being developed in Belgium.

The association between epidural analgesia and caesarean sections is more controversial. A number of studies have been undertaken, but with conflicting results. Some studies support the hypothesis that epidural analgesia is not associated with an increase in caesarean section rate,[103–105] whereas others report opposing findings.[106–108] Other retrospective studies have examined different aspects, particularly in nulliparous women and, irrespective of the pre-labour plans of women, those who opted for an epidural generally had a longer labour and were more likely to have their labour augmented, both before and after the insertion of the epidural.[103] A systematic review undertaken by Lieberman & O'Donoghue has explored the many aspects of the question,[109] and in particular the potential effects of trial sizes and non-compliance with treatment allocation on the findings following analysis according to intention to treat. They conclude that there is now little doubt that the rate of normal vaginal delivery is lower for women who opt for an epidural and the rate of caesarean section is also increased, and this is particularly so for nulliparous women.

Conclusion

There is now little doubt that a pattern of care which resembles that available in the home setting would have benefits for healthy mothers and babies. But this will need a shift in the perception of midwives, obstetricians, general practitioners, women and maternity care commissioners. Instead of approaching labour from a perspective of a catastrophe waiting to happen, it is time that professionals regain their trust in the physiology which enables healthy women to labour and deliver, mostly without interference. Pregnancy and labour should be seen as normal until proven otherwise. A programme of research to complement the study reported in this chapter is currently underway with midwives in five Nordic countries (Denmark, Finland, Iceland, Norway and Sweden), as well as Germany and Luxembourg, and will be extended to obstetricians in collaboration with the European Board and College of Obstetricians and Gynaecologists (EBCOG). It is hoped that this research will enable comparison between countries, but also between obstetricians and midwives of individual countries. At a later stage, the project intends to introduce support systems that may encourage midwives and obstetricians to adopt more physiological evidence-based approaches to intrapartum care. Research should then be advocated to examine the influence of a shift in philosophy on the practice of midwives and obstetricians, and on the outcomes of labour, including the well-being of mothers, babies and families.

References

1. Garcia J, Garforth S 1989 Labour and delivery routines in English consultant maternity units. Midwifery 5:155–162

2. Kaczorowski J, Levitt C, Hanvey L et al 1998 A national survey of use of obstetric procedures and technologies in Canadian hospitals: routine or based on existing evidence. Birth 25:11–18

3. Mead M, O'Connor R, Kornbrot D 2000 A comparison of intrapartum care in four maternity units. Br J Midwif 8:709–715

4. Mead M, Bogaerts A, Reyns M et al 2006 Midwives' perception of intrapartum risk in England, Belgium and France. Eur Clin Obstet Gynaecol 2:1–8

5. CNM Data Group 1999 Oral intake in labour. Trends in midwifery practice. The CNM Data Group, 1996. J Nurse Midwifery 44:135–138

6. CNM Data Group 1998 Midwifery management of pain in labor. The CNM Data Group, 1996. J Nurse Midwifery 43:77–82

7. Alfirevic Z, Edwards G, Platt M J 2004 The impact of delivery suite guidelines on intrapartum care in 'standard primigravida'. Eur J Obstet Gynecol Reprod Biol 115:28–31

8. Guihart P, Blondel B 2001 Trends for risk factors for caesarean section in France between 1981 and 1995: lessons for reducing the rates in the future. Br J Obstet Gynaecol 108:48–55

9. Leung G M, Lam T H, Thach T Q et al 2001 Rates of cesarean births in Hong Kong: 1987–1999. Birth 28:166–172

10. Thomas J, Paranjothi S 2001 National Sentinel Caesarean Section Audit Report. RCOG, London

11. Koroukian S, Rimm A 2000 Declining trends in cesarean deliveries, Ohio 1989–1996: an analysis by indications. Birth 27:12–18

12. Belizan J M, Althabe F, Barros F C et al 1999 Rates and implications of caesarean sections in Latin America: ecological study. BMJ 319:1397–1400

13. Zanetta G, Tampieri A, Currado I et al 1999 Changes in cesarean delivery in an Italian university hospital, 1982–1996: a comparison with the national trend. Birth 26:144–148

14. Rabilloud M, Ecochard R, Guilhot J et al 1998 Study of the variations of the cesarean sections rate in the Rhône-Alpes region (France): effect of women and maternity service characteristics. Eur J Obstet Gynecol Reprod Biol 78:11–17

15. Guillemette J, Fraser W 1992 Differences between obstetricians in caesarean section rates and the management of labour. Br J Obstet Gynaecol 99:105–108

16. Anderson G, Lomas J 1989 Recent trends in cesarean section rates in Ontario. Can Med Assoc J 141:1049–1053

17. Lomas J, Enkin M 1989 Variations in operative delivery rates. In: Chalmers I, Enkin M, Keirse M (eds) Effective care in pregnancy and childbirth. Oxford University Press, Oxford, p 1182–1195

18. Hager R, Oian P, Nilsen S T et al 2006 [The breakthrough series on Cesarean section]. Tidsskr Nor Laegeforen 126:173–175

19. Paranjothy S, Frost C, Thomas J 2005 How much variation in CS rates can be explained by case mix differences? BJOG 112:658–666

20. Liu S, Rusen I D, Joseph K S et al 2004 Recent trends in caesarean delivery rates and indications for caesarean delivery in Canada. J Obstet Gynaecol Can 26:735–742

21. Walker R, Turnbull D, Wilkinson C 2002 Strategies to address global cesarean section rates: a review of the evidence. Birth 29:28–39

22. Flamm B L 2000 Cesarean section: a worldwide epidemic? Birth 27:139–140

23. Notzon F, Cnattingius S, Bergsjo P et al 1994 Cesarean section delivery in the 1980s: international comparison by indication. Am J Obstet Gynecol 170:495–504

24. Notzon F 1990 International differences in the use of obstetric interventions. JAMA 263:3286–3291

25. Bell J S, Campbell D M, Graham W J et al 2001 Do obstetric complications explain high caesarean section rates among women over 30? A retrospective analysis. BMJ 322:894–895

26. Dubay L, Kaestner R, Waidmann T 1999 The impact of malpractice fears on cesarean section rates. J Health Econ 18:491–522

27. Enkin M 1989 Labour and delivery following previous caesarean section. In: Chalmers I, Enkin M, Keirse M (eds) Effective care in pregnancy and childbirth. Oxford University Press, Oxford, p 1196–1215

28. Seyb S, Berka R, Socol M et al 1999 Risk of cesarean delivery with elective induction of labor at term in nulliparous women. Obstet Gynecol 94:600–607

29. Macara L, Murphy K 1994 The contribution of dystocia to the caesarean section rate. Am J Obstet Gynecol 171:71–77

30. Lee B 2000 Too posh to push: the issue of caesarean section on demand. Midwives 3:52–53

31. Mould T, Chong S, Spencer J et al 1996 Women's involvement with the decision preceding their caesarean section and their degree of satisfaction. Br J Obstet Gynaecol 103:vii–viii

32. Paterson-Brown S, Fisk N 1999 Caesarean section: every woman's right to choose. Curr Opin Obstet Gynecol 9:351–355

33. Turnbull D, Wilkinson C, Yaser A et al 1999 Women's role and satisfaction in the decision to have a caesarean section. Med J Aust 170:580–583

34. Castro A 1999 Commentary: increase in caesarean section may reflect medical control, not women's choice. BMJ 319:1401–1402

35. ICM, WHO, FIGO 2005 Definition of the midwife. ICM, London

36. Downe S, McCormick C, Beech B 2001 Labour interventions associated with normal birth. Br J Midwif 9:602–606

37. Thomson A M 1993 Pushing techniques in the second stage of labour. J Adv Nurs 18:171–177

38. Mead M M, Kornbrot D 2004 An intrapartum intervention scoring system for the comparison of maternity units' intrapartum care of nulliparous women suitable for midwifery-led care. Midwifery 20:15–26

39. European Midwives Liaison Committee (EMLC) 1996 Activities, responsibilities and independence of midwives within the European Union, 1st edn. EMLC, Northampton

40. Cammu H, Martens G, De Coen K et al 2006 Perinatale activiteiten in Vlaanderen 2005. Studiecentrum voor Perinatale Epidemiologie, Brussels

41. World Health Organization Europe 2004 European health for all database. WHO, Copenhagen

42. Vilain A, De Peretti C, Herbet J-B et al 2005 La situation périnatale en France en 2003 – Premiers résultats de l'Enquâte nationale périnatale. Etudes et Résultats

43. Richardson A, Mmata C 2007 NHS maternity statistics, England: 2005–06. National Statistics, London

44. Anim-Somuah M, Smyth R, Howell C 2005 Epidural versus non-epidural or no analgesia in labour. Cochrane Database Syst Rev, Issue 4. Art. No.: CD000331. DOI: 10.1002/14651858.CD000331.pub2

45. Mead M M, Kornbrot D 2004 The influence of maternity units' intrapartum intervention rates and midwives' risk perception for women suitable for midwifery-led care. Midwifery 20:61–71

46. Grant A 1989 Monitoring the fetus during labour. In: Chalmers I, Enkin M, Keirse M (eds) Effective care in pregnancy and childbirth. Oxford University Press, Oxford, p 846–882

47. Ackermann-Liebrich U, Voegeli T, Gunter-Witt K et al 1996 Home versus hospital deliveries: follow up study of matched pairs for procedures and outcome. Zurich Study Team. BMJ 313:1313–1318

48. Johnson K C, Daviss B-A 2005 Outcomes of planned home births with certified professional midwives: large prospective study in North America. BMJ 330:1416

49. Young P, Hamilton R, Hodgett S et al 2001 Reducing risk by improving standards of intrapartum fetal care. J R Soc Med 94:226–231

50. Royal College of Obstetricians and Gynaecologists Clinical Effectiveness Support Unit 2001 The use of electronic fetal monitoring. RCOG, London

51. National Institute for Health and Clinical Excellence 2007 Intrapartum care: care of healthy women and their babies during childbirth. NICE, London

52. Kirkham M, Stapleton H 2000 Midwives' support needs as childbirth changes. J Adv Nurs 32:465–472

53. Enkin M, Keirse M, Renfrew M et al (eds) 2000 A guide to effective care in pregnancy and childbirth, 2nd edn. Oxford University Press, Oxford

54. Dover S, Gauge S 1995 Fetal monitoring – midwifery attitudes. Midwifery 11:18–27

55. Tew M 1995 Safer childbirth? A critical history of maternity care, 2nd edn. Chapman & Hall, London

56. Williams F L, Florey C V, Ogston S A et al 1998 UK study of intrapartum care for low risk primigravidas: a survey of interventions. J Epidemiol Community Health 52:494–500

57. Martin C 1998 Electronic fetal monitoring: a brief summary of its development, problems and prospects. Eur J Obstet Gynecol Reprod Biol 78:133–140

58. Mead M 2001 Decision making by midwives involved in the intrapartum care of women suitable for full midwifery care. Fifth World Congress of Perinatal Medicine, 26 September. World Association of Perinatal Medicine, Barcelona

59. Goddard R 2001 Electronic fetal monitoring. Is not necessary for low risk labours. BMJ 322:1436–1437

60. Mires G, Williams F, Howie P 2001 Randomised controlled trial of cardiotocography versus Doppler auscultation of fetal heart at admission in labour in low risk obstetric population. BMJ 322:457–462

61. Alfirevic Z, Devane D, Gyte G M L 2006 Continuous cardiotocography (CTG) as a form of electronic fetal monitoring (EFM) for fetal assessment during labour. Cochrane Database Syst Rev, Issue 3. Art. No.: CD006066. DOI: 10.1002/14651858.CD006066

62. World Health Organization 1996 Care in normal birth: a practical guide. WHO, Geneva

63. Brisson-Carroll G, Fraser W, Breart G et al 1996 The effect of routine early amniotomy on spontaneous labor: a meta-analysis. Obstet Gynecol 87:891–896

64. Cammu H, Van Eeckhout E 1996 A randomised controlled trial of early versus delayed use of amniotomy and oxytocin infusion in nulliparous labour. Br J Obstet Gynaecol 103:313–318

65. Johnson N, Lilford R, Guthrie K et al 1997 Randomised trial comparing a policy of early with selective amniotomy in uncomplicated labour at term. Br J Obstet Gynaecol 104:340–346

66. Lieberman E, Lang J M, Frigoletto F et al 1999 Epidurals and cesareans: the jury is still out. Birth 26:196–198

67. Rogers R, Gilson G, Kammerer-Doak D 1999 Epidural analgesia and active management of labor: effects on length of labor and mode of delivery. Obstet Gynecol 93:995–998

68. Leong E W, Sivanesaratnam V, Oh L L et al 2000 Epidural analgesia in primigravidae in spontaneous labour at term: a prospective study. J Obstet Gynaecol Res 26:271–275

69. Akbar A 2002 Rise in caesareans is harming midwifery. The Independent, 19th August, Sect. 6

70. Clements R, Huntingford P 1994 Introduction. In: Clements R (ed.) Safe practice in obstetrics and gynaecology: a medico-legal handbook, 1st edn. Churchill Livingstone, London, p1–4

71. Symon A 2000 Litigation and defensive clinical practice: quantifying the problem. Midwifery 16:8–14

72. Symon A 2000 Litigation and changes in professional behaviour: a qualitative appraisal. Midwifery 16:15–21

73. O'Cathain A, Thomas K, Walters S J et al 2002 Women's perceptions of informed choice in maternity care. Midwifery 18:136–144

74. Dickinson C, Jackson D, Swartz W 1994 Making the alternative the mainstream. Maintaining a family-centered focus in a large freestanding birth center for low-income women. J Nurse Midwifery 39:112–118

75. Rowley M, Kostrzewa C 1994 A descriptive study of community input into the evolution of John Hunter Hospital Birth Centre: results of 'open entry' criteria. Aust N Z J Obstet Gynaecol 34:31–34

76. Garite T, Snell B, Walker D et al 1995 Development and experience of a university-based, freestanding birthing center. Obstet Gynecol 86:411–416

77. Spitzer M 1995 Birth centers. Economy, safety, and empowerment. J Nurse Midwifery 40:371–375

78. Waldenström U, Nilsson C 1997 A randomized controlled study of birth center care versus standard maternity care: effects on women's health. Birth 24:17–26

79. Waldenström U, Nilsson C, Winbladh B 1997 The Stockholm birth centre trial: maternal and infant outcome. Br J Obstet Gynaecol 104:410–418

80. Hodnett E D, Downe S, Edwards N et al 2005 Home-like versus conventional institutional settings for birth. Cochrane Database Syst Rev, Issue 1. Art. No.: CD000012. DOI: 10.1002/14651858.CD000012.pub2

81. Page L, McCourt C, Beake S et al 1999 Clinical interventions and outcomes of one-to-one midwifery practice. J Public Health Med 21:243–248

82. Hodnett E D, Gates S, Hofmeyr G J et al 2003 Continuous support for women during childbirth. Cochrane Database Syst Rev, Issue 3. Art. No.: CD003766. DOI: 10.1002/14651858.CD003766.pub2

83. Farquhar M, Camilleri-Ferrante C, Todd C 2000 Continuity of care in maternity services: women's views of one team midwifery scheme. Midwifery 16:35–47

84. Gibbins J, Thomson A M 2001 Women's expectations and experiences of childbirth. Midwifery 17:302–313

85. Chalmers B 2002 How often must we ask for sensitive care before we get it? Birth 29:79–82

86. Fleming V E 1998 Women and midwives in partnership: a problematic relationship? J Adv Nurs 27:8–14

87. Schimmel L, Schimmel L, DeJoseph J 1997 Toward lower cesarean birth rates and effective care: five years' outcomes of joint private obstetric practice. Birth 24:181–187

88. Oakley D, Murray M, Murtland T et al 1996 Comparisons of outcomes of maternity care by obstetricians and certified nurse-midwives. Obstet Gynecol 88:823–829

89. Davis L, Riedmann G, Sapiro M et al 1994 Cesarean section rates in low-risk private patients managed by certified nurse-midwives and obstetricians. J Nurse Midwifery 39:91–97

90. Blanchette H 1995 Comparison of obstetric outcome of a primary-care access clinic staffed by certified nurse-midwives and a private practice group of obstetricians in the same community. Am J Obstet Gynecol 172:1864–1868

91. Standing Maternity and Midwifery Advisory Committee CJP 1970 Domiciliary midwifery and maternity bed needs. HMSO, London

92. Maternity Services Advisory Committee 1984 Maternity care in action, Part II – Care during childbirth. HMSO, London

93. Department of Health 1993 Changing childbirth: report of the Expert Maternity Group. HMSO, London

94. Tindall V C (ed.) 1995 Women in normal labour: report of a CSAG committee on women in normal labour, 1st edn. HMSO, London

95. National Institute for Health and Clinical Excellence 2003 Antenatal care – routine care for the healthy pregnant woman. NICE, London

96. Callister L 1995 Beliefs and perceptions of childbearing women choosing different primary health care providers. Clin Nurs Res 4:168–180

97. Marteau T M, Kidd J, Cook R et al 1991 Perceived risk not actual risk predicts uptake of amniocentesis. Br J Obstet Gynaecol 98:282–286

98. Alexander S, Keirse M J N C 1989 Formal risk scoring during pregnancy. In: Chalmers I, Enkin M, Keirse M (eds) Effective care in pregnancy and childbirth. Oxford University Press, Oxford, p 345–364

99. Chamberlain G, Wraight A, Crowley P 1999 Birth at home. Pract Midwife 2:35–39

100. Vandenbussche F P, De Jong-Potjer L C, Stiggelbout A M et al 1999 Differences in the valuation of birth outcomes among pregnant women, mothers, and obstetricians. Birth 26:178–183

101. Righard L 2001 Making childbirth a normal process. Birth 28:1–4

102. Prendiville W, Elbourne D 1989 Care during the third stage of labour. In: Chalmers I, Enkin M, Keirse M (eds) Effective care in pregnancy and childbirth. Oxford University Press, Oxford, p 1145–1169

103. Dickinson J E, Godfrey M, Evans S F et al 1997 Factors influencing the selection of analgesia in spontaneously labouring nulliparous women at term. Aust N Z J Obstet Gynaecol 37:289–293

104. Cammu H, Martens G, Van Maele G 1998 Epidural analgesia for low risk labour determines the rate of instrumental deliveries but not that of caesarean sections. J Obstet Gynecol 18:25–29

105. Anim-Somuah M, Smyth R, Howell C 2005 Epidural versus non-epidural analgesia for pain relief in labour. Cochrane Database Syst Rev, Issue 4. Art. No.: CD000331. DOI: 10.1002/14651858.CD000331.pub2

106. Thorp J, Parisi V, Boylan P et al 1989 The effect of continuous epidural analgesia on cesarean section for dystocia in nulliparous women. Am J Obstet Gynecol 161:670–675

107. Thorp J A, Hu D H, Albin R M et al 1993 The effect of intrapartum epidural analgesia on nulliparous labor: a randomized, controlled, prospective trial. Am J Obstet Gynecol 169:851–858

108. Dickinson J E, Paech M J, McDonald S J et al 2002 The impact of intrapartum analgesia on labour and delivery outcomes in nulliparous women. Aust N Z J Obstet Gynaecol 42:59–66

109. Lieberman E, O'Donoghue C 2002 Unintended effects of epidural analgesia during labor. A systematic review. Am J Obstet Gynecol 186:S31–S68

Midwives constructing 'normal birth'

Sue Crabtree

Introduction

Reflecting an international trend, New Zealand women and midwives continue to work in an environment of increasing intervention during childbirth. The midwifery role in promoting and defining 'normal birth' is widely discussed at midwifery conferences and in midwifery publications.[1-4] These accounts emphasize the need to develop and support skills in maximizing physiological birth as one strategy to decrease unnecessary intervention, questioning the practices and definitions that are ever present.

Sociological, anthropological and gender studies and midwifery literature contain a number of examinations of so-called 'medicalization' or technological hegemony in midwifery and obstetric practice and, as a consequence, in women's childbirth experiences.[5-16]

This chapter discusses some issues of contemporary medicalization in primary midwifery practice (lead maternity care) in New Zealand and some of the approaches midwives have adopted while working to promote the normalcy of birth in the context of a medically dominant environment. The work presented is one section of a study that examined constructions of normal birth held by a particular group of lead maternity care midwives in New Zealand.[17] All quotations in this paper arise from midwives in the study and pseudonyms are used to ensure anonymity. Having introduced the New Zealand maternity system, I then briefly describe how the research was carried out and present a summary of the research findings. This is followed by a discussion of some midwives' construction of normal birth within the current New Zealand context.

New Zealand maternity system

This research was carried out in New Zealand during 2000. At this time, midwives were the lead maternity carer for 71% of childbearing women.[18] Under a government-funded maternity service, women choose a lead maternity carer for primary maternity care. The lead maternity carer can be a midwife, a general practitioner or an obstetrician. The New Zealand College of Midwives claims that 'continuity of midwifery care enhances and protects the normal process of childbirth'.[19] The lead maternity carer is responsible for assessment of the woman's needs, for planning care and for ensuring provision of maternity services during pregnancy, labour, birth and until six weeks after birth.[20] This is in line with the International Confederation of Midwives (ICM) definition of the role of the midwife, to provide full care in partnership with the woman.[21] Likewise, the New Zealand government expectation is that all maternity care is planned with the woman and her family, and is based on partnership, information and choice.[20]

Midwives can choose to work as lead maternity caregivers, either employed by a hospital service or in self-employed practice. Midwives also provide a 'core' midwifery service, providing midwifery care in antenatal clinics and wards, 24-hour inpatient care and labour care for women requiring secondary and tertiary obstetric services; and for those women who choose to have a medical practitioner as their lead maternity carer. New Zealand has an annual birth rate of approximately 57 000 and a midwifery workforce of approximately 2000 midwives, 93% of whom work in direct clinical practice. Around half of these midwives work as lead maternity carers.

Overview of the study

The study on which this chapter is based was designed to explore the meaning of normal birth in lead maternity care midwifery practice in the early 21st century in New Zealand and to understand the complex influences surrounding midwives' construction of normal birth. A qualitative descriptive approach with feminist underpinnings was selected as the framework for the study.

Midwives were recruited to participate in the study via information sheets distributed by regional chairpersons of the New Zealand College of Midwives. Those who were interested made contact by telephone, and interviews were arranged if they met the criteria for inclusion. These criteria were that the midwife provided full lead maternity carer midwifery services throughout the pregnancy, labour and birth, and to six weeks postpartum (i.e. continuity of carer), and provided care for women planning either home or hospital birth.

Semi-structured interviews were undertaken at a location that was convenient for both the participant and interviewer. All the interviews took place in homes or practice rooms. Interviews were recorded on audiotape, transcribed and then returned to the midwives for accuracy checks and amendment. Transcripts were then analysed using thematic analysis.

Nine midwives participated in the study; they all identified as Pakeha (New Zealanders who are not Maori) and were aged between 43 and 55 years. They had all completed a registered nurse to registered midwife education programme. Five respondents had been in self-employed (independent) practice for over 15 years, three for between 5 and 7 years, and one for 18 months.

The midwives all had a caseload of between 30 and 60 women per year, in line with the New Zealand College of Midwives' guidelines. Between them, they were based in urban, semi-urban and rural locations. They worked across a variety of settings, including homes, birthing centres, small community-based units and secondary and tertiary city hospitals. However, the majority of births they attended took place in a hospital environment.

Throughout the research process, I continued to work as an independent/home-birth midwife, and reflected on my own practice and how my interpretations of the data 'fitted' into my day-to-day practice reality. Practising midwifery alongside undertaking midwifery research gave me a unique perspective and balance between what I was reading in the literature and the data, and the 'real world' of midwifery practice. At the completion of the research, I was more acutely aware of the multiple and competing influences on midwifery decision making. My own conviction of the normality of birth was solidified.

Summary of findings

As stated above, the initial focus for this study was on midwives' construction of normal birth. However, as the study progressed, I found that it was not possible to focus on normal birth without looking at the wider context within which birth takes place. During the interviews with the midwives, it was quickly confirmed that there are multiple and competing influences on midwifery practice and a woman's birthing course. Data analysis revealed that these experiences occur in a contested context that remains firmly entrenched in a medically dominant model of care. The themes and codes identified from the data are given in Box 6.1.

The main finding from this study was the midwives' awareness of the contested and medicalized nature of their working environment, and the lack of consensus and clarity around their constructs of normal birth. Within this context, the midwives had a strong commitment to supporting women. They found ways to adapt to the environment in order to promote healthy birthing experiences. This finding has been confirmed by Earl & Hunter in their study of the work of 'core' midwives in tertiary hospitals.[22]

Box 6.1

Themes arising from the data

1. Birthing in a contested context
   The nature of normal birth
   The place of birth
   Acceptance and expectation of intervention
   Fear present in the birthing context
   Midwifery referral and its pitfalls
   Agreeing/acquiescing
2. Adapting to the environment
   Supporting women's choices
   Protecting women: being a buffer
   'Shutting the door'
   'Keeping women away from medicalization'
   Making definitions fluid
   Returning birth to normality
   Keeping birth as normal as possible

Theme one: birthing in a contested context

Defining normal birth

Data published by the Ministry of Health (MOH)[23–25] reflect an increasing trend to intervention. In 2000, 68.7% of births were reported under the heading 'normal delivery'; however, at that time, the MOH provided no definition for what 'normal delivery' actually meant. The only births that were excluded from the 'normal delivery' category were the 31.4% of births that occurred by caesarean section (20.4%) or operative (forceps or ventouse) delivery (11%).

More recently, the MOH defined a normal birth as 'the birth of a baby without obstetric operative intervention' (p 107).[25] However, the category of 'normal delivery/birth' continues to include other obstetric interventions such as epidural anaesthesia, induction of labour, augmentation of labour, episiotomy, active management of the third stage, artificial rupture of membranes and continuous electronic fetal monitoring (cardiotocography (CTG)).

Many of the midwives in the study had experienced the impact of increasing interventions in practice. For example, as Liz and Mary said:

What worries me is that, I saw [a midwife] talking, 'I had a nice normal birth,' but I know that I watched that midwife arrive, the client wasn't there. The IV [intravenous] trolley and the epidural trolley were outside the room, the woman walked in smiling, 'Gidday', and no obvious contractions, from coming in the door to the room, which would have taken two minutes. Looking very unstressed. I saw the anaesthetist go in within half an hour, but [the midwife says] she had a lovely normal birth. That was a second baby, I didn't want to ask the circumstances. So that would be client choice. (Liz, p 11)

And certainly the practitioners that we see from say [other practice], will proudly say they have had a lot of normal births and you know, we've got something like a 90% epidural rate for primips amongst the practitioners. And they will say that's a normal birth. A normal birth has now become a spontaneous vaginal birth, you know with epidural and syntocinon. And ARM [artificial rupture of membranes], scalp clip, fetal blood sampling and continuous fetal monitoring. (Mary, p 12)

Enabling a woman to labour undisturbed can be seen as part of a midwife's effort to act as a guardian to normal birth. The midwifery model in this way 'normalizes' individual women's labour processes, recognizing 'the individuality of each woman's pregnancy and childbirth experience'.[19] In contrast, those who take a medicalized approach attempt to 'pathologize' women's uniqueness as deviance or abnormality, and to correct the deviance with interventions. Midwifery, as constructed by Liz and Mary, defines 'normal' on a one-to-one basis with each woman:

I think that I can last a lot longer [than other midwives] because I have seen so many people achieve, with time. I don't think that there is a rush in labour. I don't have a Friedman's curve timeline in my practice. (Liz, p 9)

We don't have routines. We don't routinely do anything to anybody. Every woman starts her labour at this point and goes to that point and there are things that we may or may not use along the way. We don't really have standard expectations or interventions. (Mary, p 10)

This view is further supported by Banks: 'In the depth and breadth of women's experiences of childbirth defining normality is not just problematic – it is impossible. Just as the meaning of midwife (with woman) is defined in the singular, practice of the midwife's art and science must be tailored to the individual woman.' (p 35).[26] Sue discusses the individuality of the process:

It [natural birth] needs to be re-framed, so that people understand what natural is … It's not a rigidly determined thing. It's something that involves judgement, it involves process. It's processing with women and that is a really vague thing to transmit to people. (Sue, p 17)

Medical definitions do not allow for women's individual experiences of labour and birth. Rather, they introduce rigid boundaries and expectations that mean many women will 'fail'. In the midwifery model propounded by the midwives in this study, more appropriate fluid definitions of birth allow for the uniqueness of individual women's expression and experiences, with room for birth as complex and multilayered. Even when birth is defined as abnormal by medical parameters, midwives have a vital role to play. This includes women experiencing vaginal birth after caesarean section (VBAC), 'post dates' or 'prolonged' labours.

Many factors impact on a woman's labour and birth and on midwifery practice, with the use of intervention not easily explained. The midwives discussed the context of birth from their practice perspective and a number of interrelated aspects emerged. These were: the place of birth; acceptance and expectation of intervention; fear of the birthing process; midwifery referral; and midwifery agreement or acquiescing to intervention. From the respondents' narratives, all of these seemed to have an influence on whether a birth could be considered normal or not.

Place of birth

As discussed in Chapter 3, place of birth has the potential to shape the woman's experience, determining who is in control and what interventions are available. The majority of women in New Zealand give birth in institutions controlled by obstetricians and obstetric policies and protocols, with only an estimated 5–7% giving birth at home.[23-25] Imogene said:

The place of birth is crucial to the way that I practise and how I feel about working really. It makes a big difference as to how I practise as a midwife. (Imogene, p 13)

In the hospital environment, midwives are more aware of the expectations of the institution and it is more likely that medicalization will frame a woman's birthing experience. In such settings, Banks argues: 'While the woman may be free from unnecessary intervention, it will only be within the framework of the policies and protocols of the hospital. Should her situation transgress the rigid rules, she will inevitably be subject to medicalised childbirth' (p 5).[6]

At a home birth, the attendants are visitors in the cultural context of the family, whereas in hospital, it is the woman (and midwife) who must adapt to the hospital context. Judy and Liz demonstrate the hidden or implicit ways that the hospital setting directs their practice.

I alter my practice when I'm doing hospital births. I think that we all do to a certain extent. But I'm very aware that they're [health professionals who work from a medicalized framework] watching me and they are auditing notes ... they are not supportive of midwifery, of midwives who practise in the midwifery model. They like midwives to practise according to the medical model and the way they relate to midwifery practice. [Asked in what ways do they change your practice?] They make me a little bit more conservative when I practise in hospital ... They tie you down; the protocols; tie you down too tight. (Judy, p 4)

I know that when I arrive in there [in hospital] and the room has been prepared for me by the hospital staff, there is a [CTG] monitor by the bed, there's a thermometer on the locker, and the bed is in the middle of the room. And there is an expectation that the woman will come in and lie down and be monitored ... It's amazing what this platform is like when you walk in there. It dominates the whole room; and that's what birth is? Lying on the bed? (Liz, p 15)

Walsh argued that research in the UK showed consultant-led hospitals to be associated with more birth interventions, more maternal morbidity, less 'normal birth', more low Apgar scores, more birth asphyxia and more birth trauma.[27] He continues this argument in Chapter 7. Further, such sites are more expensive to run than smaller locations, and women are less satisfied. In conclusion, Walsh stated that midwives have an ethical obligation to inform women about the possibility of adverse effects in many hospitals.[27] Nevertheless, the need for medical surveillance and objective confirmation of normality is well entrenched in most Western societies, and in those that have adopted Western ways of birthing, as illustrated in Chapter 7. Many women continue to believe hospital to be more appropriate and the 'safest' place to give birth to their babies, unaware of the dangers inherent in medically managed birthing.

Acceptance and expectation of intervention

Technology and intervention have become an accepted and expected part of having a baby. Banks stated: 'The philosophy and practice of manipulating and controlling labour are so firmly entrenched that they have changed our societal view of birth' (p 106).[6] Many people now have expectations about things that are known to happen and women expect them to happen in the course of their labour and birth. One such example is that of women labouring while lying on a bed. Liz, one of the contributing midwives, said:

Women in a semi-reclining position or flat on their back in lithotomy is common. I don't know whether there are many midwives who encourage their women to not be on the bed. (Liz, p 16)

Other examples include artificial rupture of membranes and CTG:

[Midwives] do the blood pressure and the pulse because that's the hospital guidelines, and temperature. A [CTG] monitoring for 20-minutes early in labour, and actually some of them come in so early in labour that that's not an issue. But if you've got someone in really pounding labour it's ridiculous to strap them on ... Rupturing the membranes is common, epidural is common, active management of third stage is common. (Liz, p 15)

Invasive interventions such as induction of labour and epidural anaesthesia are also expected and acceptable to some women:

One was a social induction ... you have this family who want this baby to be born and you think, now, do I want to be part of this? So you call an obstetrician and the obstetrician says, 'yeap sure, which day do you want to do it?' So you go along with this thinking, well I don't really think I want to be here, but what can I do? I can't really just leave them. I can't just disappear. (Lynley, p 15)

In researching American women's experiences of childbirth, Davis-Floyd found that a significant number of women actually welcomed the medical intervention and technology.[28] It made them feel powerful and that they were full participants in their cultural construction of childbirth. Judy discusses women's expectations in relation to epidural pain relief:

That's their perception of normal birth, isn't it? … Some women, in fact I had one woman having her third baby and she'd had two without any pain relief and she insisted on having an epidural for her third. She had the epidural and about half an hour later she delivered. She waited for that epidural to go in before she actually delivered. Now she said that that was a great birth and who am I to say that it's not? But is it normal? No, it's not. But for her it was fine. (Judy, p 8)

These midwives' accounts reinforce the hypothesis that many people have lost touch with the 'normalcy' of birth, as part of the process of life, and that many women have lost faith in their inherent ability to give birth to their babies. Further, Jo Murphy-Lawless writes:[29]

… real care can so easily be dismantled by a different take on birth, promoted especially by entrenched and complex medical interests … the moment of birth is devalued so that women emerge from a deeply medicalized birth … asking no further questions and seeing birth in that mode as acceptable, appropriate and even desirable'. (p 443)

Fear of the birthing process

The midwives discussed the background of fear, which they felt informed much of the birthing context. Sadly, fear is a deep part of pregnancy for some midwives and women, as Jennifer Hall explored in Chapter 3: fear that something can or will go wrong; that the woman cannot do this; fear of pain; fear of litigation; fear of exposure, public shame and censure; fear of something 'wrong' with the baby; fear that it will be damaged or not 'normal'.[30] Maureen and Mary both acknowledge the fear present in practice:

And the fear thing is there: the atmosphere of fear through litigation and through, you know, the odd person who has had a hard thing to deal with. (Maureen, p 6)

I guess, the degree of fear that we operate under now, because of things like [the] Health and Disability Commissioner … A lot of midwives do have this element of fear creeping into their practice about litigation. So sadly, on occasions, and probably increasingly, your practice is bound by defensive practice really. (Mary, p 9)

Pearse identified fear as a major hurdle that the New Zealand midwifery profession is facing.[31] She believes that it is a hurdle that potentially carries considerable risk to the care which women receive from midwives:[31]

Fear is a very negative and potentially damaging way to live, as it has the capacity to paralyse us. It robs us of our joy; it takes away our trust of women; it alienates us from our colleagues both medical and midwifery; it makes us defensive and compliant and unchallenging. It also means that we start doing things for the wrong reasons and that can result in harm. (p 10)

Liz explained the relationship between medicalization and defensive practice:

Sometimes I'm a defensive practitioner, because if I'm not seen to be safe by the medical model (sic) and I then have to refer women, especially in management of third stage. If I know that I'm going to have to consult I do … I may modify how often I do things. (Liz, p 6)

Holland also argued that, in the New Zealand context, 'we live in litigious times' (p 17),[32] and midwives are especially aware of this. She believed that high-profile cases reported in the media, along with an increased number of cases being referred for consideration of disciplinary action, have made 'us all a bit nervous' (p 17).[32] Sue explained what she thinks stops midwives remaining true to midwifery ideals:

Fear mainly and things like that midwife appearing in the media … I think has been a major thing, so that's reinforced the fear and it is very hard to pick actual things out because we are living in an historical moment, which is a fearful moment about birth. It's really hard to say what exactly it is because it's actually the culture that we are in. Which is fearful and we can't actually stand outside of that. (Sue, p 17)

Cartwright & Thomas described the context of obstetric care in the USA as a complicated environment that included 'biomedical technologies, corporate interests and an amalgamation of fears and feelings of vulnerability among both "patients" (sic) and practitioners' (p 220).[33] They argued that the most common response to this environment is to create protocols and rituals that are designed to reduce risk, 'even in the absence of data supporting their routine use' (p 220).[33] These protocols and rituals have increased intervention in healthy birthing women, simply because of the belief that 'without a certain kind of care it [birth] becomes more risky' (p 443).[29] More and more women are having labours and births that are coached, controlled and managed. The more that women and society see intervention, the more we accept it and the less we know about the physiological processes of an 'unmanaged' birth. While it is obstetricians who carry out the actual procedures, it is midwives who initiate the referral for the 70% of women for whom they are the lead maternity carer. It is, therefore, appropriate for New Zealand midwives to examine their role in initiating referral.

Midwifery referral and its pitfalls

The majority of pregnant women in New Zealand receive an obstetric referral at some stage during their maternity experience. This is, in part, a result of the 'Referral guidelines' issued by the Ministry of Health and now included in the Maternity Services Notice Pursuant to Section 88 of the New Zealand Public Health and Disability Act 2000.[20] The referral guidelines identify a broad range of clinical scenarios that warrant a consultation with a specialist. Guilliland considered that the 'requirement' of referral has the effect of 'heavily medicalising childbirth despite midwives being Lead Maternity Carers' (p 12).[34] The majority of midwives in the current study stated that they 'follow the guidelines' and use them to frame their practice. As Imogene and Maureen said:

I'll offer women referrals as per the guidelines, and sometimes they will choose not to have the referral, but I usually offer it to them and most women take it up. (Imogene, p 9)

I do refer ... appropriately but I would talk to the women about it and then someone said, well I don't want to go. And I go, well look ... this is recommended for these reasons and if you absolutely won't go I need to document that you're not going for these reasons ... No one is going to force you. He's not going to come round and force you up there. But I do work closely with the obstetricians here, because it's a small place. (Maureen, p 12)

Maureen does recognize that obstetric referral can alter a woman's course. She said:

It stops being a normal birth the minute you involve an obstetrician, in my book. Often way back at the referral process too. (p 15)

Reflecting on the referral process, Diane said:

Yes, and hindsight is an awful thing. If only, we do tend to maybe do too much, too much intervention. And as soon as they are into that referral, you know that that particular mum is probably going to be induced or maybe offered a Caesar, when you wouldn't be talking about it until the labour when you see how things went. (Diane, p 10)

When midwifery care conforms to medical parameters and is framed by medicalization, then a woman will experience a medically managed labour and birth, regardless of whom she has chosen as her lead maternity carer. Kaufman argued that midwifery care that follows medical protocols and concepts is not the same as midwifery care that focuses on individual women's uniqueness and trust in the social, sexual and physiological processes of birth.[35] Midwifery care can and does reflect and mimic medical care, when the care midwives give is based on following medical protocols, parameters and research.

Midwives are working within a medically dominated environment and at times follow medical parameters and protocols, because they agree with them or because they can see no other way forward and so comply and support the medicalization of labour and birth in well, healthy birthing women. In this way, the midwives are acting as agents for medicalization.

Agreeing/acquiescing

Choi suggested that people decide and act in a given situation based on a model of thinking identified as appropriate for that situation.[36] Further, he said that without a model there will be no decision and no action. A situation is uncertain if one cannot identify an appropriate model to associate with it. To make a decision is to resolve uncertainty. Uncertainty is an integral part of women's birthing processes. We all make decisions and take actions when practising midwifery. The medicalized way of practising is readily accessible, clearly defined and generally accepted, and, as Sue said:

I think it depends where you practise, how you practise as to where your definition starts, the boundaries start moving into things, like epidural. I think a lot of midwives would consider epidural, so long as the birth was vaginal, that it was normal. (Sue, p 5)

Enkin, Keirse & Chalmers proposed the existence of collective uncertainty 'among those who provide care about the effectiveness and safety of many of the elements of care given during pregnancy and childbirth' (p 2).[37] In spite of this, midwives will feel the pressure to conform to medical expectations and parameters or the 'cultural consensus'.[38] In discussing medical practice, Enkin said: 'clinicians often fail to practise what they know to be the most effective form of care, because of the many other factors that tend to motivate and determine their behaviour' (p 13).[39] I believe this comment also applies to midwives, even if they have a strong belief in a midwifery model. The midwifery model of practice has no power in mainstream obstetrics. Hillier concluded: 'Traditional midwives' knowledge is not power, midwifery knowledge is not power, women's knowledge is not power because their knowledge has little status within the dominant scientific system' (p 146).[40] For example, Judy strongly felt the pressure to conform to medical protocols because of the power that she perceived the institution (hospital) held over her:

It's very frustrating because you know what you would like to be doing, but you go in there and you have to practise according to the hospital [protocols] because otherwise they will remove your access contract and I can't afford for that to happen. (Judy, p 4)

Maureen also recognized the way that the medical culture impacts on her midwifery practice:

I know that I am influenced by the medical model, I really am. Because of where I work mostly and the people that I associate with. (Maureen, p 19)

Imogene and Liz showed the strong familiarity that midwives have with medical expectations and parameters in the following comments:

For instance, having an active management of third stage I am much more likely to do in a hospital setting than I would in a home birth setting. Because I know that the protocol says that they recommend strongly that all women have an active management of third stage. (Imogene, p 13)

The obstetric model is so hard sometimes to ignore and the doctors say that this is my time frame, and I must do it by this time, I must do it by that [time]. (Liz, p 8)

Davis-Floyd & Davis found that the home-birth midwives they interviewed had 'in-group jargon filled with technomedical terms, their midwifery bags bulge with technologies and their home birth charts look quite hospital-like, with maternal temperature and blood pressure and fetal heart tones duly recorded at proper intervals' (p 326).[38] All the midwives interviewed for this study demonstrated an awareness of, and a pressure to conform to, the cultural consensus around birth. They must constantly weigh their trust in the process of birth with the consequences of straying too far outside the medical parameters, which are the measures used by many forums in society.

I can see the boundaries of my practice, of what's normal. There's the boundary in me that says if the mother's all right and the baby's all right then you can go for as long as you like. There is also the boundary that says that if you are standing up in court because this baby has died or something has happened to the mother, what's going to be seen as being too far to go. So I have these blue prints of how things will look from the outside and how they look from the inside. And I keep working those two boundaries so I actually work out what's logically safe to do and what seems like it's going too far. So that I can actually be rational about and can defend what I've done and what I've supported. And where I don't think that's defensible, I'll tell the parents that. So it's [my practice decisions] not a fixed thing, it's movable, but it has to be rational. (Sue, p 8)

The current birthing environment is a contested context in which medicalization remains the dominant construction of birth, as indicated in the foregoing discussion. There is increasing intervention in the birthing process and increasing normalization of intervention despite midwives' efforts to protect normal birth. The next section addresses these efforts and assesses their place in the midwives' struggle to manage the contested issue of normal birth.

Theme two: adaptation to the environment

The midwives in this study reported a number of ways in which they adapted to the medicalized environment. They saw themselves as using these techniques to support women and to promote healthy and fulfilling birth experiences. They supported women to remain outside the system by promoting planned home birth and by supporting their refusal to use technology. Within the system, midwives provided a 'buffer', using strategies such as shutting the door and keeping women away from medicalization. Midwives also created a new paradigm for normality, using strategies of 'fluid definitions', 'returning birth to normal' and keeping birth 'as normal as possible'.

Supporting women's choices

The midwives supported women in choices that didn't always conform to the 'expected' management, as Judy and Imogene explain:

I love the women who don't want to use the sonic aid, they don't want to have the scanning. All that sort of thing, because these women have

just incredible faith in their ability to grow this baby well and to birth and the confidence in their body. (Judy, p 11)

I had to make that decision whether I'd transfer her or not, but she was so determined that she wanted to stay there and she was making [very slow] progress, and she did achieve that birth. I suppose it's the women really that determine it. And making women strong, and I don't know what is going to make women strong sometimes. (Imogene, p 7)

Many women who have constructed their concept of birth based on the dominant cultural construct value the choice of hospital birth. However, all midwives in the current study also supported women who wished to give birth at home. In New Zealand, this is a minority of women. The midwives recognized that home as the planned place of birth is perhaps the only place where both the woman and the midwife can retain their autonomy and the only place that one may see 'normal' physiology and 'normal' emotional, sexual, spiritual and social responses to labour.[41]

Childbirth just shouldn't be in hospital unless people are very sick. I don't think it should be in hospital. It just wastes too much money, there is way too much money spent and I'm very one eyed about that. I think it's really really silly that we've got hospital births for normal birth. (Sue, p 13)

I'd love to just do home birth, but you have to convince them to have home birth and we're not really in an environment that you can do that. (Lynley, p 16)

I love nothing more than to be at a normal birth with a woman at home. I want more of those and I'm getting more each year. And I'm converting a few women. Those are the victories. (Mary, p 17)

It is interesting to note that in the last two quotes, women's choice is conflated somewhat with the midwives' desires to undertake birth at home. Judy has a slightly different take on this:

I would like to do more home births, but there are a lot of midwives now that are doing home birth and I think that that's just kind of diluted it down. And I don't try and insist on them [home birth], I don't. I will very rarely visit a multip in her home if she is in labour. Because if she has expressed a desire to have her baby in hospital I think that I should honor that and I will meet her at the hospital. (Judy, p 5)

Davis-Floyd & Davis explained that women choosing to birth at home are placing 'themselves quite consciously as far out of the reach of the technocratic model as they can get, choosing to give birth in the sanctity and safety of their own homes' (p 316).[38]

Women's choice is a cornerstone of maternity care in New Zealand. The midwifery model of care and the participants in the current study are grounded in supporting women's choice. The very concept of choice, however, has its own problems, as choice itself can be a 'slippery' and contested concept. What choices are really available to women in labour and birth, when, as Benoit argued, 'society and culture shape birthing women's desires about what they want and the maternity care they receive' (p 201).[42] Further, maternity services have been described as suffering from 'cultural inertia', where health professionals steer women towards making decisions that reinforce the status quo,[43,44] as Imogene has experienced:

Once they [the women] see an obstetrician, usually they are not given a choice. Unless they are very strong and highly motivated and really sure about what they want to do. (Imogene, p 12)

In the light of these comments, it is also important for midwives to consider how far their personal beliefs about birth may act as a subtle directive for women's choices in labour.

Protecting women: becoming a buffer

The ways that the midwives identified to support women in their choice of hospital birth, while promoting 'normal birth', are now considered. Mary explained:

If ... that [spontaneous normal birth] is her goal, that's where she wants to be, that is her choice, and she's well informed. Then that's where she

is going to be and that's okay. Yes, you can have spontaneous normal birth in hospital, but she has to be guarded and protected by her caregivers to allow that to happen.

Yes

And she has to be strong, as I say if you can, get into your room and shut your door. (Mary, p 13)

All participants agreed with Mary that it is possible for women to birth in hospital without intervention, despite the difficulties previously discussed. When I asked Diane if women could experience 'normal birth' in hospital, she answered:

Absolutely, yes and that's yeah I sort of feel like I've done my job then. (Diane, p 13)

The attitude and belief system of the midwife are crucial and can be more important than the place of birth. In researching home-like versus conventional institutional settings for birth, Hodnett et al concluded: 'there is much stronger evidence to support the need for changes in caregivers' behaviour than there is to support the need for structural changes to labour wards' (p 7).[45] This was also a finding in the Ontario Women's Health Council Report, which stated that the attitude of caregivers is a critical factor for attaining and maintaining a low caesarean section rate.[46] Diane and Sue both recognized this:

I think, because I really do believe in normal, I go in there thinking this woman will go well. I don't actually go in there thinking what's going to go wrong. The majority of the time, that's fine. (Diane, p 6)

[Despite] being in a hospital room I still think that they can do it, because they've decided that they are going to shrink themselves into that space and they do. And the women have babies normally and they breastfeed them and go home. I mean I can't say that that's not a normal birth. But you see we've got very good rooms in the hospital where you take them and you can shut the door and we're pretty much on our own. And you have to be able to do that for it to be anything like normal. Shut out the rest of the world and that becomes your home ... And that's an attitude that you have yourself that you take with you.

That this is a sacred space and it is what you are going to do in this space. (Sue, p 13)

The majority of midwives interviewed commented on two specific actions for supporting women in a hospital setting: shutting the door and keeping the woman away from medicalization.

Shutting the door

Shutting the door was seen as a way of protecting women in order that they could achieve normal birth. Shutting the door was an actual physical action, but it was also symbolic. This was seen as creating privacy, safety and a way to enable the woman to make the hospital room 'her own space/ place'. Diane and Judy provided good examples of comments made by the majority of participants:

For a lot of the births that I do [at the hospital] it is just the woman and I anyway. We close that door and I just try and think that, well this is your space. I don't do a lot different. I mean it's nicer at home, but I actually do, I try and keep it low key. (Diane, p 12)

Ah privacy, so that I expect that when I go into the hospital I shut the door and I don't expect anybody to open it unless they knock first and are invited in ... It is important to establish an environment in which the woman feels really relaxed and comfortable and that sometimes takes a lot. Takes a long time of being in the hospital. I try and take out all of the things that I think are not conducive, like the CTG machine, not always, but sometimes. I try and be as unobtrusive as possible myself, unless I'm needed to do back rubbing and things like that. I try and get members of her family or support people to do that sort of thing ... I guess I just try and find, try and get an atmosphere in which the woman feels comfortable and confident for the birth. (Judy, p 2)

Keeping women away from medicalization

A second action that the midwives undertook was to keep women away from medicalization. This was again a physical action of keeping the women away

from the hospital by visiting at home in early labour and delaying transfer to the hospital.

I mainly care for my clients in their home until such time as they are getting to the last third of their labour and we come into hospital then. (Liz, p 14)

Bringing them [women] in as late as possible in their labour. It's really important not to get them there too early. To wait until they are really well established in their labour ... I think that certainly they can achieve a normal birth in hospital. (Imogene, p 11)

We have ... always based our care on keeping women at home as long as possible, even if they are birthing in the hospital. So we still do that, our policy is that when a woman goes into labour, we communicate with them frequently; we visit them at home as often as they require, just to confirm that they are doing okay. (Mary, p 11)

It could also mean keeping women away from obstetric management, if possible.

I guess what I try and do, as long as it's safe, I try to keep women away from having to refer, because I know that as soon as I have the obstetrician involved, her chance, the woman's chance of a normal birth are less, because they have their scope of practise and that's where they're operating. (Diane, p 16)

I think it's really nice that we've got that autonomy too, you know unless things are going really wrong. It's great that we can work through. Like yesterday's one, the woman got really tired and headachy and sort of got a little bit stuck. What will I do here? So I said that she ... needed to get up and have a good walk around and put some fluids up. And that got her over it. I didn't want to have to call in an obstetrician, I knew she could do it and she did ... So she ended up with a lovely birth. (Diane, p 13)

Liz explained how she uses the obstetric referral guidelines[20] in ways that support women. The woman declined obstetric referral during pregnancy and Liz explained how she would 'wear' it if necessary, in this way providing a buffer between the system and the woman's choice:

I also like my clients to be well informed before they go off [for obstetric referral] and they also have a choice to go. And I've had somebody who had had a previous Caesar who did not want to go because of very bad memories of the hospital. She has had a home birth the second time, which was great. She had had a posterior position the first time, so there was no contraindication pelvis wise, that I could see to her achieving a vaginal birth. So we knew, and I said [to the woman] that you just have to realise when we go in [to hospital], if we have to go in there, they're going to go, 'Oh, why didn't you come and see us?' You can just say that Liz must have forgotten to refer me. And I will wear it. (Liz, p 7)

In order to promote intervention-free birthing experiences, midwives used different ways and means to provide a buffer between the women and the medicalized environment present in the hospital setting. Anderson suggested that this may be the 'essence' of midwifery: 'doing nothing but guarding a protected space where a woman can labour undisturbed and offering one's watchful presence as an unobtrusive safety net' (p 209).[47] Liz put it another way:

And I think that's the job of the midwife: to keep that space around them so that they are in a safe bubble. (Liz, p 10)

Returning birth to 'normal'

Lynley hinted at the subtleties involved in keeping birth normal or returning birth to normal:

And I think that we have lost that patience too in that we've had so many times put on us, you know particularly that time around when women are starting to sense that something is different and it is changing, being patient then. Some women go to sleep then, they might curl up and have a sleep for a couple of hours, what's the matter with that. You know, there's nothing, there is no pressure coming on the baby. It's safe, it's inside its mother's body, so why, why push on it. (Lynley, p 10)

Midwives also discussed the importance of fluid time-frames for labour while ensuring the wellness of mother and baby. Sue described this fluidity:

A normal labour is, is an event that people just participate in themselves, you know the woman and the husband, or the partner, whatever. Or the friend, or whoever it is, works together and it takes as long as it takes. So long as it doesn't seem to be obstructed or there doesn't seem to be a major problem and the woman's physiologically okay and the baby's okay. I have to actually be responsible for making sure that the baby is okay and that the mother is okay. Which are simple things, simple enough things to do, and she delivers where she is comfortable and she doesn't bleed excessively. (Sue, p 7)

Davis-Floyd & Davis argued that medicalized care has deconstructed labour and then reconstructed it to fit narrow and concrete parameters.[38] In this way, medicine reshapes labour to 'fit', by using medical intervention. In contrast, Davis-Floyd & Davis found that the home-birth midwives they interviewed continually redrew the parameters of normal, expanding the definitions to allow for the wide range of experiences. In this way, labour is 'a meaningful expression of the birthing woman's uniqueness, to be understood on its own terms' (p 335).[38] They quoted Maggie, a home-birth midwife:

What I resolved for me is that where birth is not normal, part of a midwife's job is to return it to normal. For example, in the case of a VBAC, which is regarded medically as high risk and almost universally by midwives as not high risk, what we're doing in that case is returning birth to normal. And when we go four, five, six hours of pushing, we are also returning birth to normal, a normal that says if the woman pushes for three hours and she's exhausted, then she can take a rest, and maybe in a couple of hours, she'll get her strength up, and then she'll be able to push again – she will get her baby out. When we do things like that, we're returning birth to normal.

As normal as possible

Often in the current New Zealand maternity environment, birth does not proceed without alteration or intervention. The midwives participating in the study also discussed ways of making birth 'as normal as possible' for the women, in spite of the use of medical intervention. Mary described a woman's birth story with the outcome of what she identified as a 'normal' birth. This woman experienced multiple obstetric referrals in pregnancy and an induction of labour. Mary was pleased with the end result, for the woman, as she explains:

So I feel like I've actually worked well with her to achieve what she wanted to achieve. While it was potentially a high-risk situation ... [I] protected her to have a normal birth, even though it was induced. It could have been a lot worse for her. They would have had monitors and scalp clips and God knows what else. (Mary, p 16)

A number of the participants found it difficult to identify clear boundaries, discussing both epidural anaesthesia and induction of labour as clinical areas in which the boundaries become 'murky', where women can experience a 'normal' birth, but with some additional assistance during the labour. In these situations, Imogene and Maureen hinted at keeping birth as normal as possible, under the circumstances.

It's difficult. Because, who defines normal birth and is it a normal birth because they have had an epidural on board, plus syntocinon, but they have eventually pushed their baby out? [She was asked if she would consider that a normal birth.] Probably not, because it is an assisted birth. I probably wouldn't call it a normal birth. No, because it has been assisted and it has been interfered with. The actual passage of the baby is normal, but the labour is not normal. And that is where the dilemma comes of course. (Imogene, p 11)

Epidurals are sometimes great for women's pain [but] your body forgets about how to do what it is meant to do. Not totally, but often. Because if it's one with which the woman still has good mobility, like I've had people on their hands and knees with epidural, still having a normal vaginal birth. (Maureen, p 16)

Gould undertook a concept analysis of 'normal labour' which revealed that her midwifery colleagues were enmeshed within the medical model of childbirth.[48] She believed that it is the underlying medical culture which has led to a paradox where many midwives 'may believe natural childbirth to be normal but do not really believe that normal childbirth has to be natural' (p 420).[48] In discussion with her colleagues, Gould found they defined normal labour as a 'purely physiological event with no intervention'; they then went on to explain the many interventions used, but they did not necessarily believe that the intervention put the woman into the realms of 'abnormal labour'. Gould summarized with her belief that midwives have been 'coerced into accepting the medical profession's measurable parameters of normal labour as defining factors' (p 420).[48] Gould's findings have been confirmed in the present study. Liz provided a further example, stating:

Normal is unassisted by anything but the woman and the support she's got around. Yeah, that is my bottom line. (Liz, p 3)

However, she contradicted this definition later in the interview when she shared a birth story:

They [the family] didn't want to, but she went to all the specialists ... and we ended up having a lovely normal birth ... via an epidural. She'd been in labour; we induced her at 38 weeks for maternal distress. (Liz, p 10)

Mary also demonstrates the way that midwives have come to accept medical intervention as a 'normal' part of birth:

I guess we are just as guilty as anyone else of saying 'Hey I had a normal birth today' and she may well have been an induction of labour. So in my kind of heart, I know that normal birth is defined as physiological birth, where there is no intervention, there is no time pressures and the woman just gets on and does it ... When I look back over my last six months worth of statistics, I say I've had 85% normal births, when I look further down the line at my statistics, I've had 43% induction. (Mary, p 5)

Can something remain 'as normal as possible'? This statement either demonstrates a lack of clarity around the way intervention and medicalization alter the normal physiological processes of labour and birth or suggests a fluid understanding of 'normal birth'. I argue that there is a subtle difference between bringing birth 'back to normal', as outlined in the previous section, and seeing a birth 'as normal as possible', with the dangers of midwives internalizing and accepting medical intervention. This confirms Banks' argument[6] that we have a fallacy of normal birth in the New Zealand maternity system, or, as Mary said:

… that whole concept of what people perceive as being an acceptable birth and calling it a normal birth. (Mary, p 12)

Liz mused on our discussion at the end of her interview:

Yes, what's normal? I never challenge, challenged that. I mean even when I read your script I heard in my mind yes, normal birth I've got normal birth. But some of my normal births have not been a normal labour. They've been a spontaneous, a vaginal birth with assistance of some sort of thing, either an induction, and/or an epidural … umm, it makes you think. (Liz, p 17)

It is clear from the foregoing discussion that midwives in this study were unable to define normal birth and tended to differentiate between a labour that has had interventions and a normal birth where no interventions such as caesarean section, forceps or ventouse have been used. As birth is part of labour, is it reasonable to make such a distinction? If not, how many births in which midwives are the lead carers can truly be said to be normal births?

Discussion

This chapter has described a small qualitative study undertaken with nine midwives. As with all such work, no claim to be able to generalize from the results is being made. The process of undertaking this research, including the interviews with the midwives, a foray into the literature and reflection on my own midwifery practice, has generated and refined my thoughts and ideas. The following discussion is a reflection of my own journey into exploring how this group of midwives constructed normal birth.

I argue that the concept of normal birth is increasingly fragile and subject to formidable challenge. The study verified previous conclusions[49-51]

that there is no clear consensus on how midwives construct normal birth. In addition, sadly, normal birth has not been protected as a highly valued goal of maternity services. Rather than being the norm, it can be described as 'an added bonus' (Judy, p 9).

For my own midwifery practice, I can now see and feel more acutely the medical boundaries and expectations. They can be overwhelming, in all settings. Whether in a totally medical setting or in a woman's home, as a lead maternity care midwife I am constantly aware when I am supporting a woman to move to the edge or outside of those boundaries. It is difficult, on a daily basis, to be on what Davis-Floyd & Davis termed 'the ragged edge far outside of the safety net of cultural consensus' (p 336),[38] as 'midwifery of its very being fronts up against the medical model on a daily basis'.[52]

I argue that, despite midwives being the lead maternity carer for the majority of women, our cultural construction of labour and birth continues to remain deeply entrenched in a medicalized approach, which is being continually reconstructed by midwives and women as well as by medical practitioners. Medicalization is the default mode. It is always present and expected to happen unless it is actively contended. This is verified by the 'cultural fallacy' that exists around normal birthing. More and more women are experiencing medical procedures during their labour and birthing processes,[23-25] and it is not possible to identify if intervention-free births are actually happening in our current environment. The official figures do not record the women who have given birth without recourse to surgical, technological or pharmacological interventions. This silence in itself may send a message about what society values and what is held as important.

Claiming that midwifery practice and women's birthing is subjugated and constructed within the medical model of birth is by no means a new idea. The medical or technocratic model of medicine has been discussed in the childbirth literature extensively since the late 1970s.[5-7,9-11,13,14] Women and midwives have mounted serious challenges to the dominance of the scientific 'management' of pregnancy and birth, working to break down and challenge the existing paradigm and re-establish a strong and dynamic body of knowledge that is unique to the culture of midwifery. What is significant about this research is that I have attempted to explore the notion of normal birth in the one place where I would have most expected to find it alive and well. By interviewing this particular group of midwives, I have visited an area where it could be expected that the role of guardian of 'normal birth' would be very much in evidence. This was only partially true.

If we, as midwives, now support the view that 'normal' includes a wide range of medical intervention, then we have little hope of educating women and the community that normal does not include those things. As a profession, I believe we need to increase our vigilance and challenge ourselves, asking: 'from what basis am I making this decision or taking this action?'. Some midwives have an awareness of the contested context in which they operate and attempt to honour the woman's process and work with a midwifery model: to keep birth normal, to return birth to normal, or to 'as normal as possible' within the constraints. However, we also need a very real and acute awareness of when normal physiology is undermined and defined as problematic by medicalization and midwifery action, and we need an awareness of when unnecessary intervention is normalized by midwifery actions influenced by the dominant medical and technocratic culture.

Conclusion

In the process of presenting this work, I have not offered any simple solutions to the issues raised. I do not believe that there are any simple solutions. Rather, it is my intention to stimulate debate and contribute to the growing recognition that midwives, in a rejection of the 'prevailing hegemony of the technocratic model of childbirth ... are now seeking a deeper understanding of that elusive phenomenon: the normal birth process'.[47] The most important way forward is a change of consciousness about the problems that we face, including a willingness to see that nothing will alter fundamentally without our active acknowledgement that the medicalization of labour and birth is being continually recreated by midwives as well as by medical practitioners.

The midwives in this study were political, experienced and articulate midwives. They provided continuity of midwifery care and actively worked in a women-centred midwifery model. They all supported women to birth at home, if this was the woman's choice. Some had worked throughout the changes in the maternity services in New Zealand. They all participate in an annual Midwifery Standards Review process and are active members of the New Zealand College of Midwives. Even these strong, politically aware midwives experienced difficulties in standing outside of the powerful medicalized discourse evident in the current New Zealand context.

Data collection for this research project on normal birth was undertaken during 2000. Since then, there has been a steadily increasing understanding of the importance of discussing and defining normal birth among midwives and women. At the commencement of my data collection, many midwives could not fathom that a midwife would find it necessary to research what a normal birth actually was. It is exciting to now see the increase in workshops, research and publications, conference papers, debate and discussion regarding the midwifery view of normal birth.

For example, Gilkison and colleagues explored defining normal birth from a student perspective and concluded that, while more questions were uncovered than answers found, their study highlighted an awareness of issues around the concept of 'normality'.[53] Earl & Hunter explored how 'core' midwives employed in tertiary obstetric settings work to keep birth normal, and concluded that a strong midwifery philosophy and belief in normal birth existed, alongside complexity and the daily battle experienced by these midwives to keep birth normal.[22] Likewise, Skinner & Lennox reviewed interest in birth centres as a vehicle to reduce intervention during labour and birth. They concluded that 'there are three areas requiring attention: working for policy changes, involving the community and supporting midwives to use primary birthing facilities' (p 15).[54]

However, the steady trend towards surgical birth and vaginal birth with medical intervention continues. The normal vaginal birth rate continues its slow but steady overall decrease. The reported normal birth rate of 67.4% in 2003 in New Zealand includes 1 in 5 women who have an induction of labour and 1 in 4 who use epidural anaesthesia during labour and birth. Encouragingly, the Ministry of Health[25] data do show that women who choose a midwife as lead maternity carer have a slight increase in normal birth rates: 70.7% in 2002 and 72.6% in 2003. In addition, a further trend is the increase in women choosing a midwife as her lead caregiver: 70% in 2000 and, by 2003, 78% of women selected a midwife lead caregiver.[25,26]

Medicalization continues to remain an important and contemporary issue that we, as midwives and birthing women, must confront within the ordinary, everydayness of our midwifery practices and midwifery relationships. The texture and meaning of the 'normal', 'expected' and 'taken for granted' must be deconstructed and articulated in order for us to gain a deeper understanding of birth. At the same time, midwives must resist the desire or need to define normal birth with such concrete boundaries as those put forward by the medical profession. By being more acutely aware of the overt and subtle ways in which the medical ideology frames our practice and continues to operate, we can continue to seek ways in which to challenge, resist and reframe this practice.

References

1. Downe S 2002 Preston National Symposium on the evidence base for normal birth. Practis Midwife 5:10

2. Downe S 2002 The current evidence base for normal birth: report from the Preston National Symposium. Found Nurs Stud Newslett Summer:6–7

3. Downe S 2006 Engaging with the concept of unique normality in childbirth. BJM 14:352–356

4. Thomson A 2002 Normal birth. Midwifery 18:1–2

5. Arney W R 1982 Power and the profession of obstetrics. University of Chicago Press, Chicago, IL

6. Banks M 2000 Home birth bound: mending the broken weave. Birthspirit Books, Hamilton

7. Davis-Floyd R 1994 The technocratic body: American childbirth as cultural expression. Soc Sci Med 38: 1125–1140

8. Donley J 1986 Save the midwife. New Women's Press, Auckland

9. Ehrenreich B, English D 1973 Witches, midwives and nurses: a history of women healers. Feminist Press, New York

10. Katz Rothman B 1982 In labor: women and power in the birthplace. Norton, New York

11. Katz Rothman B 1990 Recreating motherhood: ideology and technology in a patriarchal society. Norton, New York

12. Oakley A 1984 The captured womb: a history of the medical care of pregnant women. Basil Blackwell, Martin Robertson, Oxford

13. Papps E, Olssen M 1997 Doctoring childbirth and regulating midwifery in New Zealand: a Foucauldian perspective. Dunmore Press, Palmerston North

14. Rooks J P 1999 The midwifery model of care. J Nurse Midwifery 44:370–374

15. Tew M 1990 Safer childbirth? A critical history of maternity care. Chapman & Hall, London

16. Towler J, Bramall J 1986 Midwives in history and society. Croom Helm, London

17. Crabtree S M 2002 Lead maternity carer midwives' construction of normal birth: a qualitative study. MA Midwifery Thesis, Massey University, Palmerston North

18. Ministry of Health 2001 Commonwealth nursing and midwifery action plan. New Zealand progress report to June 2001. Ministry of Health, Wellington

19. New Zealand College of Midwives 2002 Midwives handbook for practice, updated edn. New Zealand College of Midwives, Christchurch

20. Ministry of Health 2002 Maternity services notice pursuant to Section 88 of the New Zealand Public Health and Disability Act 2000. Ministry of Health, Hamilton

21. ICM, WHO, FIGO 2005 Definition of the midwife. ICM, London

22. Earl D, Hunter M 2006 Keeping birth normal: midwives experiences in a tertiary obstetric setting. NZ Coll Midwiv J 34:21–23

23. Ministry of Health 2001 Report on maternity 1999. Ministry of Health, Wellington. http://www.moh.govt.nz

24. Ministry of Health 2004 Report on maternity 2002. Ministry of Health, Wellington. http://www.moh.govt.nz

25. Ministry of Health 2006 Report on maternity 2003. Ministry of Health, Wellington. http://www.moh.govt.nz

26. Banks M 2001 But whose art frames the questions? Practis Midwife 4:34–35

27. Walsh D 2002 The impact of the birth environment. Research update: report from the Preston National Symposium on the current evidence base for normal birth. Preston, UK

28. Davis-Floyd R 1992 Birth as an American rite of passage. University of California Press, Berkeley, CA

29. Murphy-Lawless J 2006 Birth and mothering in today's social order: the challenge of new knowledges. MIDIRS Midwif Digest 16:439–444

30. Katz Rothman B 2001 Spoiling the pregnancy: prenatal diagnosis in the Netherlands. In: de Vries R, Benoit C, van Teijlingen E, Wrede S (eds) Birth by design: pregnancy, maternity care and midwifery in North America and Europe. Routledge, New York

31. Pearse J 2000 Legal advisors column: address at the New Zealand College of Midwives Biennial Conference. Reprinted in New Zealand College of Midwives: Midwifery News 19:10–11

32. Holland D 2001 Practice wisdom: mentoring: a personal analysis. N Z Coll Midwiv J 23:15–18

33. Cartwright E, Thomas J 2001 Constructing risk: maternity care, law and malpractice. In: de Vries R, Benoit C, van Teijlingen E, Wrede S (eds) Birth by design: pregnancy, maternity care and midwifery in North America and Europe. Routledge, New York

34. Guilliland K 2002 The New Zealand context: similarities and difference. N Z Coll Midwiv J 26:12

35. Kaufman L 2000 Have we yet learned about the effects of continuity of midwifery care? Birth 27:174–176

36. Choi Y B 1993 Paradigms and conventions: uncertainty, decision making and entrepreneurship. University of Michigan Press, Ann Arbor, MI

37. Enkin M, Keirse J N C, Chalmers I 1989 A guide to effective care in pregnancy and childbirth. Oxford Medical, Oxford

38. Davis-Floyd R E, Davis E 1997 Intuition as authoritative knowledge in midwifery and home birth. In: Davis-Floyd R E, Sargent C F (eds) Childbirth and authoritative knowledge: cross-cultural perspectives. University of California Press, Berkeley, CA, p 315–349

39. Enkin M 1994 Six myths that can lead us astray. N Z Coll Midwiv J 11:13–21

40. Hillier D 2003 Childbirth in the global village: implications for midwifery education and practice. Routledge, London

41. Banks M 1998 Breech birth woman wise. Birthspirit Books, Hamilton

42. Benoit C 2001 Introduction to Part III: society, technology and practice. In: de Vries R, Benoit C, van Teijlingen E, Wrede S (eds) Birth by design: pregnancy, maternity care and midwifery in North America and Europe. Routledge, New York

43. Anderson T 2002 The misleading myth of choice: the continuing oppression of women in childbirth. MIDIRS Midwif Digest 12:405–407

44. Kirkham M, Stapleton H 2001 Informed choice in maternity care: an evaluation of evidence based leaflets. University of York NHS Centre for Reviews and Dissemination, York

45. Hodnett E D, Downe S, Edwards N et al 2005 Home-like versus conventional institutional settings for birth. Cochrane Database Syst Rev, Issue 1. Art. No.: CD000012. DOI: 10.1002/14651858.CD000012.pub2

46. Ontario Women's Health Council 2000 Attaining and maintaining best practices in the use of Caesarean sections: an analysis of four Ontario hospitals. Report of the Caesarean Section Working Group of the Women's Health Council. Online. Available: http://www.womenshealthcouncil.on.ca/English/Reports--Publications.html (accessed 30 August 2007)

47. Anderson T 2002 Peeling back the layers: a new look at midwifery interventions. MIDIRS Midwif Digest 12:207–210

48. Gould D 2000 Normal labour: a concept analysis. J Adv Nurs 31:418–427

49. Downe S 2000 A proposal for a new research and practice agenda for birth. MIDIRS Midwif Digest 10:337–341

50. Downe S 2001 Defining normal birth. MIDIRS Midwif Digest 11:S31–S33

51. Duff E 2002 Normal birth: 'commonplace', 'according to rule' or 'well-adjusted'? MIDIRS Midwif Digest 12:313–314

52. Skinner J 1999 Midwifery partnership: individualism, contractualism or feminist praxis? N Z Coll Midwiv J 21:14–17

53. Gilkison A, Holland D, Berman S 2005 Defining normal birth: a student perspective. NZ Coll Midwiv J 32:11–13

54. Skinner J, Lennox S 2006 Promoting normal birth: a case for birth centres. NZ Coll Midwiv J 34:15–18

Section **Three**

Evidence and debate

CHAPTERS

7

Rethinking risk and safety in maternity care

Denis Walsh, Amina M.R. El-Nemer and Soo Downe

Introduction

There is a story told about Nancy, a young aboriginal girl who lived near Kakado, a remote area of the Northern Territory in Australia. Nancy refused to go to the large maternity hospital to give birth. Healthcare workers were puzzled, as Nancy's sister and her baby had died in childbirth just 12 months earlier. Surely those events would convince her of the need for expert help. They wondered whether her reticence was because she wanted the company of her family, but when they arranged for them to accompany her, Nancy still refused to go. Despite their best efforts in pointing out the unsuitability of the impoverished conditions she currently lived in, Nancy was adamant. Then one of the women in Nancy's community let them in on a secret. The reason she was refusing was because aboriginal women think it is a very bad omen to give birth where previously babies have died or been very ill. As a nomadic people, they move on when such events occur. The healthcare workers immediately saw the perverse logic at work. Of course the big hospitals have deaths occurring within their walls because they encourage everyone to go there for birth, and, occasionally, a baby dies. And they began to understand from Nancy's perspective that the hospital was not the place of safety that the dominant discourse of contemporary childbirth said it was.

Similar stories emerged from a qualitative study of a free-standing birth centre in the UK.[1] When women were questioned as to why they chose the birth centre for birth as opposed to the nearby maternity hospital, they used language that redefined the birth centre as something quite different to hospital. They likened it to a 'bed & breakfast', 'small hotel', 'a health club', their 'own home' or 'my bedroom'. This naming framed the birth centre as a place of rest, relaxation, familiarity, unlike the maternity hospital which was perceived as busy, anxiety-provoking and impersonal.

These stories where there is an inversion of the accepted logic around place of birth and safety illustrates something of the ambivalence currently surrounding normal childbirth and the notion of risk.

This chapter examines risk and childbirth against a backdrop of changes in discourses over the past 25 years. The risk paradigm will be examined and critiqued in some detail. The discussion will be framed in two cultural contexts, that of the UK and that of Egypt. Finally, some recommendations will be made for resolving tensions around risk and childbirth.

The risk discourse

As Beck has observed in his seminal work on risk,[2] fear of adverse events appears all pervasive in contemporary society, despite unprecedented levels of prosperity and technological advance in the developed world. Beck notes that there is something of a paradox here: modern societies feel increasingly vulnerable to biological, environmental and technological developments, despite decreasing mortality and morbidity rates. Critics have analysed this phenomenon, particularly in relation to health care, and have proposed a number of factors that feature as part of this paradox. These factors herald significant departures from earlier societies' notions of risk and health. Two specific examples are outlined below.

First, the growth of a risk culture in health care is popularly held to be the result of the increasingly litigious environment in contemporary society. Various components of this trend have been identified. These include the high expectations that families have of modern health care, and the financial burden of caring for a relative with a long-term disability or illness.[3] More generally, McLaughlin tracks a movement from risk as a neutral concept to do with probabilities of an event happening or not happening, to risk framed only as negative or undesirable outcomes.[3] In relation to health, this movement has taken on a particular potency, fed by the discourse of evidence-based medicine.

Second, evidence-based medicine purports to reduce or eliminate risks by the appropriate use of diagnostic aids and the implementation of effective treatments. Procter, in her investigation of nursing development units in the UK,[4] argues that these processes of diagnosis and treatment are predicated on quantitative research methods only, rendering more experiential, interpretive research approaches to the margins. In this way, risk is constructed exclusively in clinical terms and its management becomes a scientific matter.[3] Horlick-Jones suggests this strips risk assessment of its context specific embeddedness and reifies the process as objective and rational.[5] Later it will be argued that context is essential in exploring the meaning of risk in maternity care.

Risk discourse and maternity care

In a number of ways, maternity care is an exemplar of the effects of the risk discourse on health. Childbirth straddles an ambiguous divide between what some perceive as an essentially physiological event and others as a pathology waiting to happen. These contrasting views have been conceptualized as emanating from differing models of care: a biomedical or technocratic model and a social model. Walsh & Newburn[6] proffer the characteristics of these models, based on the work of Davis-Floyd,[7] in Table 7.1.

The technocratic perspective sees birth as risky until proven otherwise. It aims to prevent the worst case scenario, regardless of the likelihood of that ever happening – an approach dubbed 'a maximum strategy' by Brady & Thomson.[8] This

Table 7.1 A comparison of the technocratic and social models of maternity care

Technocratic	Social
Body as machine	Whole person
Reductionism: powers, passages, passenger	Integration: physiology, psychosocial, spiritual
Control and subjugate	Respect and empower
Expertise/objective	Relational, subjective
Environment peripheral	Environment central
Anticipate pathology	Anticipate normality
Technology as master	Technology as servant
Homogenization	Celebrate difference
Evidence	Intuition
Safety	Self-actualization

requires adopting a low threshold for intervening and a highly sceptical view of labour physiology. The model supervalues morbidity and mortality outcomes over all others, especially the psychosocial, and monitors outcomes by measuring what goes wrong. It also casts labouring women as patients, dependent on medical interventions to rescue them from deviations from the norm. Professional expertise and knowledge is highly sought after in this model and is considered authoritative, based on positivistic notions of objectivity, generalizability and certainty, all of which are obtained through quantitative research findings.

Sociologists have typified these values as belonging to the techno-rational paradigm that views science as progressive and modern.[9,10] Techno-rationalism not only determines what counts as knowledge, but also supports an industrial model of productivity or work. Such a view endorses efficiency and bureaucracy as fundamental to work systems. Risk assessment becomes another tool to fine tune efficiency in labour care. Centralized provision for childbirth requires such a model and mimics assembly-line production.[1,11] This mainstream industrial model of maternity care in effect processes women through the phases of care. The organizational imperative to move women in at one end and out at the other end of hospital birth results in acute time pressures which, in themselves, could amplify risk. Later in this chapter, the invisibility of this organizational imperative to the risk assessment process will be explored. Labours have to be completed within a certain time frame and, therefore, they are frequently accelerated if perceived to have fallen behind the clock.

Manuals on the rationale for risk management and its operational mechanisms rarely explore the assumptions underlying it or its philosophical antecedents, all of which contribute seminally to what could be called a 'discourse of risk'.[12] Crawford develops his argument regarding a disjunction between the goal of health and the 'disordered experience of its attempted achievement'[12] (p 507) by identifying a number of characteristics in contemporary medical culture that contribute to a culture of fear. Some of these have strong resonance with current maternity care. Crawford writes of the growth in health education to assist individuals in their healthy lifestyle choices. These focus on risks to personal health and amount to a 'pedagogy of danger'. Information to newly pregnant women can resemble this: guidance on food and beverages to consume and avoid, drugs to avoid, behaviours to change (smoking, alcohol, stress-inducing activities), recommendations on safe places of birth (access to neonatal facilities, avoid home, avoid hospital) and early and regular contact with specialist maternity services (midwives, obstetricians). These reinforce the 'preciousness' of the pregnancy condition.

Crawford's second characteristic is the role of technologies in identifying risk factors and detecting early disease. This has spawned whole new categories of hidden pathology, predispositions and susceptibilities. Screening for fetal abnormality is a typical example. This has grown exponentially over the past 15 years on the back of increasing sophistication with ultrasound techniques. What began with early detection of neural tube defects has burgeoned into the identification of an apparently increasing number of genetic and/or hereditary conditions in utero. Unfortunately, in many cases, diagnosis is provisional and throws up relative rather than absolute risks. This is the phenomenon of 'soft markers'[13] which can generate anxiety and ambivalence in women who have to make vexed decisions about the appropriate course of action.[14] Shickle & Chadwick dub this trend as 'screeningitis' – the emotional inflammation and angst caused by the practice of inexact testing.[15]

Technologies applied in this way appear to be supervalued by clinical staff and have an almost transcendent, redemptive dimension. They contribute to the miracle stories of pregnancy and birth rescues reported in the media. But this masks some negative consequences. As a mediator of care, technologies can be dehumanizing and alienating, distancing patients from carers. Munro et al's survey of midwives' attitudes to electronic fetal monitoring demonstrated this.[16] Finally, technologies can consolidate and extend the professional hegemony of clinicians, disempowering childbearing women in the process.

Lauritzen & Sachs critique the advance of screening as the problematization of the normal, where everyone starts out normal but is unable to secure their healthiness.[10] Screening alerts them to the possibility of abnormality and the potential of a rare, but theoretical, risk of a future calamity. Everyone has a small chance of great misfortune and, in effect, becomes a 'not-yet-patient'. A cursory glance at maternity care notes reveals this potential. One UK maternity service lists over 60 risk factors for pregnancy in their history-taking page.[17] Evidence exists of the impact that a label of 'at risk' has on individual women, as Williams & Mackey's study of women treated for pre-term labour shows.[18] Heyman et al's more recent research highlighted the anxiety experienced by women deemed to be at risk.[19] The reality is that risk does not remain a statistic. It is 'experienced' by an individual and may well contribute towards the shaping of her identity.

The exponential growth of antenatal screening and the search for increasing numbers of risk factors has placed enormous pressure on midwives who have to introduce pregnant women to the complexity of these processes, and manage the intense feelings they can generate.

In Adelsward & Sachs' critique of the meaning of numeracy in epidemiology's identification of risk, they illustrate how population-based risks are translated inappropriately to individual risk by clinicians.[20] An individual, identified as having risk factors, becomes a 'not-yet-ill' patient. Pregnancy already has its share of symptomless illness, as mild pregnancy-induced hypertension and intrauterine growth retardation illustrate. The power of numeracy is that it is perceived as objective and 'true' and it therefore powerfully inscribes potential illness on the individual. The nuances of the risk discourse also invite dichotomous thinking, so a risk is either present or absent, leading to the implication that a risk-free state exists.[20] This kind of woolly thinking reinforces the notion in maternity care that 'high tech' hospitals are safer environments to give birth in because they can set in place measures to reduce the risk and rapidly treat its effects if they do occur.

Contextualizing risk

These critiques of how risk is conceptualized, particularly in maternity services, show how it is presented as a rational process, objectively undertaken for the greater good. This normative reading of risk obscures underlying values and beliefs that align it with scientific rationalism and the health specialism's professional projects.

Crawford makes the astute observation that the ritual of risk as realized in medical culture makes us fear the unlikely but be unconcerned about the truly dangerous.[12] Though paradoxical, this observation has resonance with how choices around place of birth and style of care are made in current maternity services. The discussion leads to the heart of contextualizing risk assessment. As Anderson insightfully argues, a number of known risks that operate on large labour wards are ignored by risk assessment procedures, which focus exclusively on the woman's own clinical features rather than organizational deficiencies.[21] These may include:

- lack of continuity of care and continuous support by midwives
- inexperienced doctors at the start of their rotation
- absence of expertise during the summer holidays, weekend night shifts, bank holidays
- disagreements between midwife and obstetrician
- inadequate handovers because of fatigue, intimidation.

She adds to these other incidental factors like unsupportive birth partners, bullying staff and a blame culture in completing her particular risk assessment for birthing on busy labour wards. The effects of a blame culture had been previously stressed by Ball and colleagues in their UK study, exploring why midwives leave the profession.[22] They found evidence of horizontal violence where many midwives felt under constant surveillance and feared reprisal if they made any errors. Stafford went further by suggesting that there is a current generation of 'what if' or 'just in case' midwives whose practice posture is defensive, linking this development to the ubiquity of risk.[23] Irony abounds here as current risk management strategies overtly emphasize a 'no blame' culture as an objective.

Anderson's contribution underscores the centrality of context in undertaking risk analysis.[21] If context is ignored, then its influences remain invisible though they may represent the 'truly dangerous' as opposed to the potential and rare risks associated with the woman's medical history.

Wagner articulates why contextual structural risks may be missed by risk assessors.[24] He writes of the 'fish can't see water' syndrome. If risk assessors are embedded within the organization where assessments are undertaken, then how the organization functions becomes normative. In effect, they are blinded to Anderson's factors.

Though Western childbirth appears to be dominated by a risk discourse, there are pockets of resistance. These tend to be expressed by practitioners who work in birth centres, or who provide home births, and by women and families who use these facilities. Later in this chapter, the birth centre narrative will be examined through the findings of an ethnographic study of a free-standing birth centre in England.[11] First, research from Egypt will examine risk and safety in the context of a society where maternal and infant mortality are high, and where the promise of safety offered by centralized resources may appear to be persuasive.

Safety in the context of Egyptian ways of birth

The study used for this section took the form of a feminist ethnographic account of hospital birth.[25,26] The participants comprised 21 women labouring in a busy hospital in a major city in Egypt. This hospital is affiliated to the local university and provides maternity services to women with diverse cultural backgrounds who live in both urban and rural areas. The number of births per month was on average 530 at the time of the study. Participants were selected on the basis of being in early labour each morning when the researcher arrived, and giving consent to inclusion. The participants included both primigravid and multigravid women. They were observed during their labours, and interviewed in the first few hours following birth. The nurses working in maternity care in the unit were also interviewed in focus groups. There were multiple findings from this study. Those related to maternal concepts of safety are explored here. Four specific aspects arising from the data are explored. These are set out in Box 7.1.

Box 7.1

Aspects of childbirth safety expressed by Egyptian women

1. The hospital's tempting promise of safety
2. Being done to and lack of self-control
3. Experiencing emotional safety: home birth and dayas
4. Rejecting the hospital's tempting promise of safety

The hospital's tempting promise of safety

Participants trusted that hospital was a good place for giving birth. They seemed to think that because the hospital had resources and technology, it would deliver good quality care. Eleven women out of 21 reported that they chose hospital birth because they believed that it was the safest place to be. The quotes below illustrate this initial expectation. They also indicate that, by the time the interviews were carried out, women had become more equivocal in their views.

I am an educated girl and I know that the university hospital has lots of resources, technology and professors so, for sure I will be safe. After my delivery I realized that in labour you do not need that technology as much as someone who cares for you. (Interview of Nona 4:4)

I refused to deliver by the daya and I told her it is safe there, in hospital they will give me glucose and vitamins but she said, 'it's better for you to deliver here at home'. (Interview of Nor 20:4)

The labour here is fine, there are machines and according to the condition of each woman, they will treat her. You feel that you are in a good hands but the doctors are very busy, they left us alone most of the time. (Interview of Rawan 15:4)

Being done to and lack of self-control

Women's postnatal accounts report multiple instances of being 'done to'. These accounts were reinforced by the observations of actual care given.

On numerous occasions, the processes women underwent were disempowering, unsafe and, in retrospect, apparently brutal. Women remembered being coerced, shouted at and having physical force applied to them, both to open their legs for delivery and to expedite the expulsion of the fetus by the dangerous practice of fundal pressure.

The doctor cut me, I felt the scissors cut through my body and then my baby came out. Then he stitched me. It was so painful and it hurts too much. (Interview of May 3:3)

Doctors at the delivery room screamed at me and slap me on my leg and the worker stretched out my legs by force and made a pressure on my abdomen and the nurse as well, until the baby is born. After that I didn't feel anything. They gave me anaesthesia I do not know why they gave it to me, I delivered and everything was ok. (Interview of Mary 12:3)

These accounts were typical of many others in the study, and illustrate that the integrity and humanity of women was systematically denied.

Beyond the obvious distress these experiences caused, there is fascinating evidence that the very discourse of safety which led these women to attend hospital was subverted by the unsafe nature of many of the practices carried out there. Women did not appear to note this consciously. However, they were very aware that they felt unsafe emotionally.

Experiencing emotional safety: home births and dayas

The data indicated that emotional safety played a vital role in determining the participants' satisfaction with hospital birth. They valued minimal technical intervention, and care which included reciprocal conversations, giving of information and clarification, kindness, smiling and supporting. However, participants could only express this by reflecting on the contrast between previous facilitative care they had experienced at home and their hospital experiences.

My first delivery was by the daya. She was helping me to sit on the floor, walk and to do what I wanted to do. She was warm. She delivered me sitting and she helped me moving around, sleeping, standing, and walking when I was like to do. (Interview of Zezy 6:4)

At home I have been walking during the pain. I was standing or sitting. The mobility was really helpful during my labours. My mother told me that the movement is helpful for the descent of the baby. At home I have been walking. When the pain came I was standing, sitting and walking. It was so helpful during my pain. (Interview of Wafa 8:3)

It was not the intention of this study to examine home birth experiences. However, it became evident in the analysis that they were intrinsic to women's narratives of their births. Participants' reflections about their past experiences of birth at home indicated that they were free and had control over their own labours and birth experiences. They used their own power and resources to deal with the stress of labour. They had freedom and choice about the conduct of birth. They experienced a perception of control over their position, mobilization, eating and drinking and companionship that they missed in their current hospital childbirth experiences. An important aspect of the experience was that women had confidence in the care provided by the daya, or traditional birth attendant. They felt both safe and cherished during the process of labour and during the birth of their babies.

It appeared that dayas used their personal and experiential knowledge to enable women to give birth naturally. Their role was mainly that of the wise carer who offered support, comfort and patience; in effect the 'sage-femme'. These data were tangential to the main area of interest for this study. Observation of dayas working at home births was not undertaken. However, they offer an interesting alternative qualitative perspective to studies of traditional birth attendants or dayas which attribute high maternal mortality rates to daya-attended births. In contrast to these accusatory reports, it has been claimed that, in reality, most maternal deaths occur in hospital as a result of complications following caesarean sections.[27] Whatever the truth of the matter, more qualitative work is needed on the nature of home birth in Egypt and other similar countries, and on the practice, values and beliefs of dayas.

Rejecting the hospital's tempting promise of safety

For many participants, their experiences led them to claim that they would never come to the hospital again, despite its supposed technical advantages. The following data highlight the consequences of the lack of emotional support within hospital care. The common impression can be summarized in the phrase: 'I will not deliver here again'.

I will not come to that hospital again. I will not deliver here again. It was very hard, hard, hard, I will never do it here again and if I will deliver again I will deliver at home. (Interview of Rawia 7:6)

Next time I will deliver in my home on my bed with my mother without cutting, I did not know that the delivery in hospital is lots of suffering. (Interview of Ward 11:3)

Do you know! If I will deliver again, I will deliver at home. Labour does not need hospital; my mother can help me better. (Interview of Zyzy 6:5)

Most of the women involved in the study had come to hospital because they saw it as the only suitable option they had. They felt that the hospital was the safest place to give birth because it had the medical expertise and the technology available and that these might be needed during childbirth. However, what women actually experienced during their hospital births led to a reappraisal of these views. Most of the participants found that more positive communication and interaction with service providers was preferable to the routine practices and care that they experienced during labour and delivery.

Women wanted more than just a physically healthy infant. As well as clinical safety, women desired a spiritually, psychologically and emotionally fulfilling experience. Ironically, procedures conducted by the hospital staff as part of their safety agenda were contrary to those shown to maximize the safety of childbirth. For instance, there is a body of literature indicating the benefits of social support in labour in terms of reduced length of labour and reduced need for instrumental or operative delivery.[28]

Even if safety was improved by hospital attendance, the participants did not expect to trade this benefit off against the loss of essential characteristics of support that the women experienced in their past birth experiences. They found, to their surprise and great distress in some cases, that they had to hand over the responsibility for their bodies and their babies to the professionals. Their own embodied knowledge was not relevant when set against the authoritative scientific knowledge of the hospital culture. The data imply that women felt useless, confused, punished and controlled by caregivers. Hospital care for most of the participants was provided through objectification. Women were treated as things rather than as humans with basic needs.

Safety in this context meant psychological as well as physical safety, where support, freedom and minimal interventions allowed them to experience childbirth as a positive and powerful life transition. The participants demonstrated that they recognized the difference between caring and uncaring experiences when they compared the care that they received at home with the 'daya' to their current hospital birth. They were able to level a critique against the system on the basis of their personal experiences and of those of their family and friends. This enabled them to reject the hospital's tempting promise of safety.

The experience of these Egyptian women is important to a critique of Western ways of birthing. The participants had personal experience of birth in two cultures, that of traditional Egyptian birthing with the daya, and that of the Western technological model. They were able to contextualize their unease with the latter through their embodied experiences of the former. This is of great importance to theorists who are trying to understand why the technological promise of safety has brought with it widespread unease about hospital-based ways of birth.

We now turn our attention back to Western childbirth and examine an alternative to large hospital birth. We will reframe the current risk discourse in a way that is empowering to women and supportive of physiological birth.

Re-visioning risk in normal childbirth

In attempting to sketch out an alternative approach to risk management in maternity services, the following discussion emanates from beliefs and values of a social model of care, mentioned at the beginning of this chapter. Deliberations are therefore based on a salutogenic or 'wellness' perspective of pregnancy and childbirth (see Ch. 1). A guiding principle becomes not the avoidance of risk but the promotion of well-being. A starting point can be what evidence-based medicine tells us about care that supports physiological birth. It is a peculiar irony that the same examination of evidence sources that has been used to identify sundry risks to childbirth can also inform as to what facilitates normal labour and birth. Even more startling is the fact that positivist research designs deliver this verdict, despite Procter's assertion of the limitation of evidence-based medicine when predicated solely on these methods.[4]

Systematic reviews and other quantitative studies conclude that birthing units existing alongside conventional labour wards, and as geographically separate facilities (free standing), appear to reduce labour interventions in women deemed to be at low risk.[29,30] Contributing to this low rate of intervention is probably the philosophy of carers in this setting which views labour and birth through a lens of normality. This focus on normality may also contribute to lower intervention rates in women deemed at be at higher risk, as a Canadian study showed.[31] In addition, women using these facilities are highly satisfied with their care. Researchers stress the centrality of a 'birth as normal' philosophy in achieving these outcomes.[31,32] Esposito tells a remarkable story of a New York birth centre in capturing the power of philosophy to affect outcome.[32] The birth centre explicitly adopted an 'active birth' approach to care that affirmed women's ability to birth without technology and medical interventions. Many of the women who came to the centre had previous negative experience of medicalized birth, but, over the course of their pregnancy, internalized a new vision. From a pessimistic disposition about the likelihood of experiencing a normal labour, they became expectant and positive and many went on to have very natural labours and births at the centre.

Alongside findings about the efficacy of birth centres, a substantial body of research has examined the style and type of care that contributes to non-interventionist, successful physiological birth. These findings emphasize the value of continuity of care,[33] of having a midwife as a lead carer[34] and of continuous support during labour.[35]

These characteristics of care echo what Nolan, a childbirth educator, believes to be fundamental to a proactive approach to risk management in maternity care.[36] Her work also uses as a starting point the promotion efficacy as opposed to identifying and avoiding risk. Her approach more aptly focuses on what women say are important themes in care provision, rather than what the professionals have researched. These have been identified many times by maternity service surveys and evaluations as the three Cs – choice, control and continuity. Government policy in the UK explicitly endorsed them in 1993,[37] 2004[38] and very recently in Maternity Matters.[39] Nolan urges us to build services around these themes as they actually represent a preventative strategy.[36] If combined with structural change to embrace birth centres and home birth, and the endorsement of a 'birth as normal' philosophy, then maternity services can create the conditions to realize efficacy.

An important adjunct to this re-fashioning of service priorities to address known benefits and efficacy of different models of care is the explicit acknowledgement that the current large-scale, all-purpose, industrial model of labour care is failing women who anticipate having normal labour and birth. The corollary of all the research findings is that this model predisposes women to intervention and the widespread use of labour and birth technologies. The model itself has become a risk to normal birth. Contextualizing risk assessment inevitably leads to this conclusion, yet there is little evidence that this is acknowledged or influences risk decisions.

Risk and safety in a birth centre

A recent ethnography of a free-standing birth centre in the UK revealed a contrasting language and meaning around the risk discourse.[11] The inversion of the current orthodoxy around this topic could be said to be subversive, as the following examples reveal.

Booking rationale

There were a number of striking features in the women's accounts around reasons for booking at the birth centre. One of the most obvious was the absence of references to the technocratic model of childbirth. Women did not raise concerns about 'risk' and 'safety' at the birth centre, at least not in the way that these terms are usually understood. They did not comment on an absence of doctors, epidural provision, electronic fetal monitoring, facilities for obstetric procedures like ventouse or caesarean deliveries, or an ambulance journey of at least 30 minutes if complications arose. Instead, women focused on the social (family and friends' recommendations, proximity for visiting), the environmental (calm, homely, small-scale, ease of parking, absence of busyness) and the personal (welcome, friendliness, helpfulness) aspects. In fact, their response to the technocratic model was negative when they had previous experiences of birth at larger consultant units.

It was clear that, for many, the first visit to the birth centre was very influential in their decisions to book there. In particular, the visit seemed to precipitate an immediate decision regarding the right place of birth for them. For many, this appeared to be an intuitive process that either simply felt right ('Yep – this is the sort of place') or could be visualized as the only appropriate place. As one woman said, 'I could picture myself at the Valley'. This response portrays the affective component of decision-making that is non-rational and non-scientific. It is immediate and 'right', rather than considered and weighed like probability-related decisions are. Sometimes idiosyncratic aspects of their lives influenced their considerations. The birth centre was seen as the best environment for a woman who was an insomniac. Another woman chose the centre because the nearest centralized maternity hospital was where her husband's mother had recently died of cancer.

All these examples serve to undermine the idea that evidence regarding the mortality and morbidity rates of different places of birth will be the dominant influence on women's decision making.

Nesting instinct

The study also revealed a shared preoccupation (for midwives and women) with the birth environment. The midwives were continually honing the physical environment through regular make-overs to optimize it for birthing. Though this was clearly important for the women, an additional dimension to environment emerged from the data – women's concern for the emotional ambience of the birth setting. This was illustrated by one woman's experience of visiting the unit. She was greeted at the door by a staff member holding a baby and she concluded that this was a baby-friendly place. It seemed to her 'the most natural thing in the world to find in an environment where babies are born', though it is uncommon in large hospitals where there is active discouragement of carrying babies around because of health and safety concerns. Women in the study were seeking a birth ambience characterized by compassion, warmth, nurture and love.

The focus on environmental and emotional ambience is interpreted in the study as characteristic of the nesting instinct. Human nesting instinct appears to seek out the right emotional ambience for childbearing, which is as integral to establishing a protective, safe place for birth as are the immediate physical surroundings. The links with the previous discussion on choosing the appropriate place of birth are clear: the non-rational immediacy of decision making when women visited the centre suggests an intuitive and rapid appraisal of emotional and environmental ambience. Similarly, it was the absence of the right emotional ambience in the other maternity units they visited (the more formal and depersonalized interactions with staff during their visits), together with their unsuitable physical environments that turned women against them.

As already mentioned, many of the women actually constructed meaning around the birth centre to redefine its purpose away from being a hospital or healthservice institution, using phrases like 'home', 'my bedroom', etc. These descriptions were attached to characteristics, sometimes juxtaposing their experience of a typical hospital with their experience of the birth centre. Clearly their thinking was unrelated to the traditional understanding of the risk discourse of childbirth safety. In fact, their thinking inverts the risk discourse's logic of protection and safety by deliberately choosing a non-medical environment for birth. For the women, protection and safety appeared to mean reducing the risk of iatrogenesis associated in their minds with hospital birth.

These findings don't actually challenge the alignment of risk and safety, for they seem to support an endorsement of the need for safety. It is the interpretation of what constitutes safety that is challenged here. Safety for these women had to do with their babies being protected rather than monitored, nurtured rather than managed and loved rather than cared for. For many, the traditional hospital was a threat to these aspirations, so much so that they took the radical step of deliberately redefining the facility as home-like.

It may be that if service users, as Nolan urges,[36] were the main arbiters of a risk strategy for maternity services, then these services would look very different from what is currently on offer. Along with the birth centre women in this study, they might rehabilitate the homely, the social and the interpersonal aspects of the childbirth event which have been largely dismantled by the technocratic and industrial approach. They might even change the process and outcome data, so targeted at the moment on interventions like epidurals and morbidities like caesarean section, to wellness markers like physiological labour, normal birth and personal empowerment.

Conclusions

The contributory factors to the evolution of a risk culture are complex. Technological innovations and obstetric specialization raise expectations with the implicit promise to reduce risk or eliminate it. Litigation is on the increase, and it fuels defensive practice. It also encourages a protocolized clinical service that is said to be based on the best available evidence. But huge inconsistencies remain. Much of the evidence around labour and birth is undermined by the technological context in which it was collected. Where high-quality evidence does exist, it supports non-institutional birth settings, diminished technical input and relational dimensions of care. But these models are conspicuous by their absence in current maternity services in the UK and across the world. In fact, to some extent the reverse is true – labour and birth are being increasingly centralized in mega units and intervention rates are escalating all the time. A vicious circle of iatrogenesis feeding yet more litigation and yet more defensive practice is becoming apparent.

If a change from this model is to be successful, we believe that midwives and other maternity care professionals need to respond as soon as possible. We must recognize the possibilities that exist for developing our practice and research so that, as a profession, midwifery can once again gain credence as the expert voice of normality during childbirth, and can use this position to enact change for women and babies. This needs to be aligned with an authentically collaborative relationship between the various professional and lay groups who support childbearing women, in pursuit of what we have termed 'skilled help from the heart'.[26] If this model of care can be exported to countries which are developing their maternity services in an attempt to reduce high maternal and infant mortality rates, there will be real hope for the women of the world to experience childbirth as a journey of transformation which is empowering and which offers physical, emotional, cultural, psychological and spiritual safety.

References

1. Walsh D 2006 Improving maternity services: small is beautiful – lessons from a birth centre. Radcliffe Publishing, London

2. Beck U 1992 The risk society: towards a new modernity. Sage, London

3. McLaughlin J 2001 EBM and risk: rhetorical resources in the articulation of professional identity. J Manag Med 15:352–363

4. Procter S 2002 Whose evidence? Agenda setting in multi-professional research: observations from a case study. Health Risk Soc 4:45–59

5. Horlick-Jones T 1998 Meaning and contextualisation in risk assessment. Reliability Engineering and System Safety 59:79–89

6. Walsh D, Newburn M 2002 Towards a social model of childbirth, Part 1. Br J Midwif 10:476–481

7. Davis-Floyd R 1992 Birth as an American rite of passage. University of California Press, Berkeley, CA

8. Brady H, Thompson J 1981 The maximum strategy in modern obstetrics. J Fam Pract 12:997–999

9. Fahy K 1998 Being a midwife or doing midwifery? Aust Coll Midwives Inc J 11:11–16

10. Lauritzen S, Sachs L 2001 Normality, risk and the future: implicit communication of threat in health surveillance. Sociol Health Illn 23:497–516

11. Martin E 1987 The woman in the body: a cultural analysis of reproduction. Open University Press, Milton Keynes

12. Crawford R 2004 Risk ritual and the management of control and anxiety in medical culture. Health: An Interdisciplinary Journal for the Social Study of Health, Illness and Medicine 8:505–528

13. Getz L, Kirkengen A 2003 Ultrasound screening in pregnancy: advancing technology, soft markers for fetal chromosomal aberrations and unacknowledged ethical dilemmas. Soc Sci Med 56:2045–2057

14. Filley R 2000 Obstetric sonography: the best way to terrify a pregnant woman. J Ultrasound Med 19:1–5

15. Shickle D, Chadwick R 1994 The ethics of screening: is 'screeningitis' an incurable disease? J Med Ethics 20:12–18

16. Munro J, Ford H, Scott A 2002 Action research project responding to midwives' views of different methods of fetal monitoring in labour. MIDIRS 12:492–495

17. Walsh D 2003 Birthwrite: maternity notes – a jaundiced account. Br J Midwif 11:268

18. Williams S, Mackey M 1999 Women's experience of pre-term labour: a feminist critique. Health Care Women Int 20:29–48

19. Heyman B, Hundt G, Sandall J et al 2006 On being at higher risk: a qualitative study of prenatal screening for chromosomal abnormalities. Soc Sci Med 62:2360–2372

20. Adelsward V, Sachs L 1996 The meaning of 6.8: numeracy and normality in health information talks. Soc Sci Med 43:1179–1187

21. Anderson T 2004 Conference presentation. The impact of the age of risk for antenatal education. NCT Conference, Coventry, 13 March 2004

22. Ball L, Curtis P, Kirkham M 2002 Why do midwives leave? Royal College of Midwives, London

23. Stafford S 2001 Is lack of autonomy a reason for leaving midwifery? Pract Midwife 4:46–47

24. Wagner M 1994 Pursuing the birth machine: the search for appropriate birth technology. Ace Graphics, Sydney

25. Rashad A 2003 Helping from the heart: a feminist ethnography of Egyptian women's childbirth experiences. PhD Thesis, University of Bradford, Bradford

26. El-Nemer A, Downe S, Small N 2006 'She would help me from the heart': an ethnography of Egyptian women in labour. Soc Sci Med 62:81–92

27. Kamal I 1998 The traditional birth attendant: a reality and a challenge. Int J Gynecol Obstet 63:S43–S52

28. Hodnett E D 2000 Continuity of caregivers for care during pregnancy and childbirth. Cochrane Database Syst Rev, Issue 1. Art. No.: CD000062. DOI: 10.1002/14651858. CD000062

29. Hodnett E D, Downe S, Edwards N et al 2005 Home-like versus conventional institutional settings for birth. Cochrane Database Syst Rev, Issue 1. Art. No.: CD000012. DOI: 10.1002/14651858.CD000012.pub2

30. Walsh D, Downe S 2004 Outcomes of free-standing, midwifery-led birth centres. Birth 31:222–229

31. Ontario Women's Health Council 2001 Attaining and maintaining best practices in the use of caesarean sections. Online. Available: http://www.womenshealthcouncil. on.ca/English/page-1–361–1.html (accessed 25 October 2007)

32. Esposito N W 1999 Marginalized women's comparisons of their hospital and freestanding birth center experiences: a contrast of inner-city birthing systems. Health Care Women Int 20:111–126

33. Coyle K, Hauck Y, Percival P et al 2001 Ongoing relationships with a personal focus: mother's perceptions of birth centre versus hospital care. Midwifery 17:171–181

34. Homer C, Davis G, Brodie P et al 2001 Collaboration in maternity care: a randomised trial comparing community-based continuity of care with standard hospital care. Br J Obstet Gynaecol 108:16–22

35. Hodnett E D, Gates S, Hofmeyr G J et al 2003 Continuous support for women during childbirth. Cochrane Database Syst Rev, Issue 3. Art. No.: CD003766. DOI: 10.1002/14651858.CD003766.pub2

36. Nolan M 2002 'The consumer view'. In: Wilson J, Symon A (eds) Clinical risk management in midwifery: the right to a perfect baby? Books for Midwives, Oxford, p 124–137

37. Department of Health 1993 Changing childbirth: report of the Expert Committee on Maternity Care. HMSO, London

38. Department of Health 2004 National Service Framework for children, young people and maternity services. Online. Available: http://www.dh.gov.uk/PolicyAndGuidance/ HealthAndSocialCareTopics/ChildrenServices/ ChildrenServicesInformation/fs/en (accessed 30 August 2007)

39. Department of Health 2007 Maternity matters: choice, access and continuity of care in a safe service. Department of Health, London

8

The early pushing urge: practice and discourse

Soo Downe, Trent Midwives Research Group,
Carol Young and Victoria Hall Moran

Chapter contents

Introduction

The nature of physiological childbirth is highly contested. As other authors in this book have illustrated, there is no agreement on the physiology of length of labour, on the nature of labour pain or on when to sever the umbilical cord. These are a few of the hundreds of questions that could be asked in this area. In 1958, the American obstetrician Thaddeus Montgomery stated: '... it is amazing how little of fact is known about the simplest phases of reproduction. The field for research here is widely open ...'.[1] It appears that this comment is still relevant half a century later. In Chapter 1, Soo Downe and Christine McCourt suggested that the very framing of the scientific endeavour in the area of health is antipathetic to an understanding of labour and birth. If this argument is accepted, it is hardly surprising that Montgomery's words still ring true. This chapter explores one particular area of childbirth in the context of three specific studies carried out in the UK. In doing this, it seeks to understand the myths and assumptions that surface in midwifery knowledge and expertise, dissonance between observed processes of labour, and the nature of authoritative knowledge in this area. This chapter is framed in our personal experiences, and in the way of seeing set out in Chapter 1. It looks again at midwifery practices in the area of the maternal urge to bear down before official diagnosis of full dilatation of the cervix.

In the argument we present here, the terms 'narrative', 'account' and 'discourse' are used with specific meanings. The narratives are the accounts given by the midwives: the content, events and actions of the stories they tell. We are not using the term 'discourse' in the sense understood by discourse analysts, where the linguistics and semiotics of story-telling are important. It is used in a loosely Foucaultian sense[2] as an operand: something that connects experience to the interpretation of that experience and which, in the process, indicates the nature of authoritative constructions of experience. Our use of the term is rooted in ways of communicating dominant and subsumed ideas, ideologies and below.

Why this topic?

This work arose from the experiences of one of us (SD) in the early 1980s. This section is expressed in the first person as an account of the events that underpinned the development of the research question.

My interest in this area of midwifery practice developed in the early 1980s when I was a direct entrant (non-nurse) student midwife studying in a hospital in the English Midlands. At the time, in the hospital where I was training, the early labour room was a Nightingale-style ward. The beds were separated only by curtains, and in the middle of the room a large table held all the notes for the currently labouring women. Women whose labours were induced were sometimes connected to electronic monitors with feedback systems. These entailed the use of a fetal scalp electrode, an intrauterine catheter and a tocographic belt. These devices were all wired up to the monitor, which assessed the strength of contractions and then delivered an intravenous dose of oxytocin (Syntocinon) titrated to these readings. Women stayed on the bed. If they wanted an epidural, if they were scheduled for a vaginal examination (which took place at least every four hours) or if they were deemed to be in second stage labour they were lifted onto a trolley and wheeled to the delivery room. Once there, they were lifted off the trolley onto the high narrow delivery table. The procedure, or the birth, then took place. In the case of anything other than a birth, this process was then repeated in reverse. All women laboured together in the first stage and listened to each other as they did so. First names were not normally used. Narcotic pain relief was often given with minimal or no explanation of the risks and benefits, and without formal consent.

While this rather bleak picture has now changed dramatically in the site concerned, it serves to illustrate the environment in which I began to observe the early pushing phenomena. It was not unique at the time as an environment for birth in Western contexts, as authors such as Suzanne Arms and Sheila Kitzinger have illustrated.[3,4]

The job of the direct entrant student midwife (a very junior member of staff) was to take routine observations from each of the encurtained women in turn and to write these in the notes on the central table. In casting my memory back to this, it seems like I was undertaking some kind of bizarre circular dance, in and out of the curtains and round the table. This took place with little opportunity to connect with the labouring women, especially since any conversation could be overheard by all those in the room. However, the system also meant that, for those who stayed in the room for any length of time (usually the students), the subtle nuances of a large number of women's labours could be heard and compared. I became increasingly baffled by a phenomenon that I heard and observed happening on numerous occasions. It would start with a woman beginning to make what I now know to be transitional noises. The attending midwife would come in, on hearing the noises herself or on being alerted to them by the student or the attending partner. Stereotypically the conversation would go something like this:

*Woman: 'I feel – really uncomfortable …
I … I think I want to push …'
Midwife: 'No Mrs X, you were only six
centimetres an hour ago, you can't be ready yet.
I'll get you some pethidine. Turn onto your side
and try to blow the pain away. If you push now
you may damage your cervix and your baby.'*

The midwife walks off. The woman puffs and groans a bit then starts grunting hard and bearing down. The midwife comes back with the pethidine drawn up, suddenly hears the grunting, rushes behind the curtains, takes one look and calls urgently for a trolley:

*Midwife: 'I can see the head! Can I have some
help here!'*

The trolley arrives post haste; the woman, still bearing down and out of control, is bodily carried onto it, rushed into the labour room by a flustered midwife and lifted onto the delivery bed. The women screams, the midwife urges her to pant, the baby is born. The midwife later reports 'a nice normal delivery'.

This is what first set me thinking – how can it be that a woman can be reported as having a cervical dilation of 6 cm (or 4 or 8) one minute, and the next she is pushing her baby out? How can it be that the midwives continued not to believe the women and their bodies? What exactly was happening, both physiologically and in terms of the apparent dissonance between what midwives saw and heard (and, probably, smelt) and what they said and did?

While my reflections on these events led me to a point where I was prepared to accept that maybe a woman could progress rapidly from the latter part of the first stage of labour to the point of bearing down, my next relevant experience, a few years later, took me further into apparently uncharted physiology. Newly qualified, I was allocated to a woman of Asian origin, who had had six previous babies and who did not speak any English. I approached her behind the curtains (which were still in existence at this time). She was gesturing that she was in pain and she thought the baby was coming. I undertook a vaginal examination, which was the subtly enforced but unwritten rule at the time, to find that her cervix was soft, long and barely dilated. Without seeking the consent of the woman, again as was common at that time, I set off to get her some pethidine. I was repeating the very same patterns of behaviour I had observed so critically a few years previously. I returned with the pethidine drawn up, opened the curtains – and was just in time to catch the baby as it slid gently onto the bed.

After this, I decided to trust my intuition more. Over the years, a new unit was built on the site, and I moved to a so-called 'delivery suite', which had single labour and birthing rooms for women, where first name terms were used and where partners stayed with the women. Anaesthetists were permanently on call, and use of epidural analgesia became more prevalent. I began to observe another phenomenon in this area. These observations were sketchier since they depended on being a second midwife in a room or on the decision of a colleague when I was on a break. It seemed that the discourse around women expressing a so-called 'premature' urge to push was being reconstructed by both women and midwives around the topic of epidural analgesia and maternal choice. A woman would become uncomfortable and would express this by demanding an epidural. Again, to use a stereotype to illustrate a point, the midwife would briefly discuss this with the woman and then go and get the anaesthetist. The woman, now focused on the epidural and not on her own inner resources, became increasingly agitated. This would cause the anaesthetist great difficulty in siting the epidural. Once it was sited (sometimes after a number of attempts), the woman would suddenly begin bearing down in an organized way, and the baby's head would appear. A flustered midwife would send the anaesthetist out, and get the woman pushing (usually using directed instructions). Sometimes this worked, and the baby would be born – another birth labelled a 'nice normal delivery'. Sometimes, however, the baby's head would still be high and, as the epidural took effect, the fetal head would fail to rotate on the woman's anaesthetized and relaxed pelvic floor; the baby would eventually be born by ventouse extraction or forceps.

As I have said, these are stereotypical cases. Often the woman concerned was very happy to have the epidural (or, earlier, the pethidine), and often the baby was born spontaneously and apparently well. However, all these observations set us thinking: what is the physiology of normal labour and birth? Following the work of anthropologists such as Bridget Jordan[5] and Robbie Davis-Floyd,[6] it is apparent that the dominant labour ward practices were based on local authoritative knowledge. Our question now was: do midwives really have two discourses in their heads, one born of observation and the other of this dominant knowledge? If so, what does this do to internalized conceptions of expertise and knowledge, or to the professional self-belief of midwives? How often does the early pushing phenomenon happen anyway? How did we learn to practise in the way we do around this phenomenon? What impact does this apparent dissonance have on physiological processes of labour and birth?

This chapter will not answer all these questions. It does, however, set out some empirical research we have undertaken that may point the way to further efforts to untangle some of the issues thrown up by the 'premature pushing urge', termed the early pushing urge (EPU) for the purposes of this chapter. We discuss the implications of the use of this term below.

The discussion also addresses more general issues around the nature and impact of dissonant discourses which midwives and women face when they try to work with ways of birth that respect physiological processes.

Background

The topic of pushing in labour has been the subject of debate in academic journals since at least the beginning of the 20th century. While much of the debate has been in the area of organized versus spontaneous pushing efforts,[7] or delayed versus immediate pushing following the diagnosis of full dilatation of the cervical os in the context of epidural analgesia,[8] there appears to have been less debate on the topic of women who feel an urge to push prior to the diagnosis of full dilatation of the cervical os.

It appears that fashions have changed with regard to the EPU since the 1960s, at least in the English language professional literature. Berkley and colleagues, writing in an obstetric textbook in 1931, seem to have been rather relaxed about the subject, at least when its occurrence was in the latter part of the first stage of labour: 'No good can be done by bearing down before the dilatation of the os is complete or nearly complete' (p 300).[9] Other authors have held that pushing prior to diagnosis of full dilatation of the cervix is harmful, even when they are apparently committed to a belief that labour is usually physiological. An example is a paper written by Constance Benyon, which was published around the same time as that of Thaddeus Montgomery, extolling the virtues of a relaxed, physiological, non-technical approach to the second stage of labour.[10] Constance Benyon was, and is, well known among critics of modernist technological childbirth for her belief in the essential normality of spontaneous labour. However, she states categorically in that paper: 'Everyone now accepts that pushing before full dilatation is both useless and harmful' and condemns it utterly.[10] Further to this, the paper was reprinted in full as a chapter in a book edited by Sheila Kitzinger and Penny Simkin on the subject of episiotomy and the second stage of labour.[11] The content of the book largely supports a relaxed approach to the second stage of labour, as does the article by Benyon. However, there is no attempt to contradict the firm view of the original Benyon article that pushing prior to full dilatation should not be supported.

Until recently, both professional and lay midwifery textbooks have generally presented the EPU as a phenomenon to be avoided through specific management strategies, such as changing maternal position and 'pant-blow' techniques.[12-14] More recent versions of these textbooks written by one of the authors of this chapter (SD) suggest that the evidence on the impact of EPU on maternal and fetal outcome is equivocal.[15,16] It is not clear what impact, if any, this has had on midwifery education or practice. The latest (2000) edition of the seminal evidence-based *Guide to Effective Care in Pregnancy and Childbirth* concludes: 'If … the cervix is less than 8 cm dilated the woman should be asked to … try to resist the urge to push … If there is only a rim of cervix left … it is unlikely that any harm will (occur) … as long as she does not exhaust herself' (p 290).[17] The evidence base for this assertion is not referenced.

The first fortuitous published findings in this area appear to be those of Yeates & Roberts, published in 1984.[18] This observational study set out to examine pushing techniques in two comparative groups, each of five women, in labour. Although the intention was to admit women to the study after diagnosis of full dilatation of the cervix, the authors found that nine of the ten women observed experienced the EPU. Following up this observation, Joyce Roberts et al undertook another research project, with the explicit aim of investigating this phenomenon.[19] It took the form of an observational study of 31 nulliparous women. All the women had an internal fetal monitor and intrauterine catheter in situ. They were all Black or Hispanic. The researchers found that 17 of the participants experienced early bearing-down urges at less than 9 cm of cervical dilatation. One woman in the early pushing group experienced cervical lacerations compared with two women in the group who reached full dilatation of the cervix prior to experiencing spontaneous bearing-down efforts.

An on-going systematic review of the English language literature undertaken by one of us (SD) has not located any published research focused on the EPU since the publication of this 1987 paper. While Joyce Roberts has since published descriptive reviews of evidence relating to the second stage of labour,[7,20] no new empirical evidence is cited in the sections on the EPU. In the absence of any other published studies in this area, this small, observational study, of women from two specific ethnic groups who experienced a series of technological interventions, is presumably the basis of the recommendations cited above. This overview of the current literature in the area of the EPU raises interesting questions about both its prevalence and its nature. The following section describes three empirical studies conducted by members of the Trent Regional Research Midwives Group, that were designed to further the evidence base in these areas.

Study 1: the incidence of the early pushing urge in one UK regional health authority

This study set out to establish the incidence of the EPU in one UK health authority using an anonymous incidence survey. The survey took place in two tertiary and two secondary level consultant maternity units during three randomly selected weeks in May 1999. The units were included because at least one of their midwifery staff was a member of the Trent Midwives Research Group. The sample included all women giving birth in these units during the three weeks, except those undergoing elective caesarean section.

The ethics committees were approached in each site. Since the survey was entirely anonymous beyond the woman and her attending midwife, none of the committees required a formal ethics submission. The forms were designed to maximize completion, so brevity was a priority. They were piloted for a week in each participating unit. After piloting, one question, relating to blood loss, was added at the midwives' request. The final survey comprised five questions (Box 8.1). The form was one page only, and no identifying details were noted other than the

Box 8.1

Questions for the incidence survey, study 1

1. What was the parity and gravidity of the woman?
2. Did this woman experience the early pushing urge?
3. If so, at what cervical dilatation was this noted by the midwife?
4. What type of birth did she experience?
5. Was the blood loss greater or less than 500 ml?

Trust in which the birth took place. Midwives in all collaborating units were asked to complete forms for each birth during the study weeks. The Trent Midwives Research Group member was responsible for coordination of the survey and for ensuring completeness of returns.

The forms were returned to the central office at the end of each study week. The data were scanned into a commercial character recognition system (Formic) that read the data from the questionnaires automatically. The data were then downloaded into SPSS. Simple descriptive and cross-tabulated analyses were employed.

Results

The annual statistics of the participating units in the year prior to the first survey are given in Table 8.1. The response rates by unit and the rates of reported EPU in the returned forms are given in Table 8.2.

The overall return rate was much lower than expected, at 42% (383/918). The parity and rates

Table 8.1 Incidence survey: annual birth statistics (1999) for units participating in study 1					
Unit	Total (n)	Percentage of all labouring women			
		Normal	Instrument use	Emergency caesarian section	Other
Consultant-led DGH	4255	73	14	13	0
Consultant-led tertiary	5148	67	16	15	2
Consultant-led DGH	1182	70	16	13	1
Consultant-led tertiary	5401	71	15	14	0

DGH, district general hospital.

Table 8.2 Incidence survey: return rates and reported rates of the early pushing urge, by unit

Unit	Survey response			Rates of the early pushing urge (EPU)	
	Eligible women	Response	Percentage response	EPU noted	Percentage EPU in responses
1	286	120	42	55	46
2	259	127	49	48	38
3	62	52	84	21	40
4	311	84	27	29	34
Total	918	383	42	153	40

of types of birth within the returned sample were similar to those of the whole population. The overall rate of early pushing was 40% (153/383) with an inter-unit range of 34–46%. Just about half of these women were reported as having wanted to push at 6–9 cm dilatation of the cervical os. An extreme assumption could be made that all those who did not respond did not want to push early. This would result in an extrapolated incidence of early pushing of 20% (153/765): one in five of all women labouring over the three weeks of the survey.

Blood loss was similar in both groups. When the data were subanalysed for women having their first baby, and for those whose urge to push was felt before 6 cm of cervical dilatation, the rate of early pushing and the average blood loss did not differ significantly from the findings across the whole sample. Normal birth was more prevalent among those women experiencing the EPU, but these findings may be a result of confounders. For example, epidural analgesia is associated with both a decrease in pelvic sensation and an increase in instrumental birth. Epidural usage was not recorded in the survey, so it is not possible to ascertain if this factor may have influenced the findings.

Discussion

The low response rate to this survey may militate against its generalizability. However, in terms of annual statistics, the units in which the work was undertaken were fairly typical of the range of such units across the UK. They also represented a range of models of practice, from total consultant care in

the largest of the units to a mixture of consultant and midwife-led care in one of the others. It may, therefore, be reasonable to assume that the picture gained from this study might be applicable in other sites across the country.

The estimate of 20% of women experiencing the EPU is probably artificially low because of adjustment for non-returns, and it is far lower than that found in the observational studies cited in the literature, as discussed above. However, it is still a significant proportion of women. In addition, the finding that the incidence was similar for women having a first or a subsequent baby, and that rates of normal birth did not appear to differ by parity or by the stage at which the EPU was experienced, was unexpected. These correlations need to be treated with a great deal of care, however, since the limitation of questions about confounders on the forms, and the low response rate, did not allow for formal statistical testing of any associations.

Although these data cannot be generalized, they provide a basis for hypothesizing that the EPU may be a common phenomenon in labour. This casts some doubt on the approach of most UK textbooks, which, as set out in the introduction, seem to recommend that the EPU should be prevented as far as possible. Equally, however, there is no clear evidence for the recommendations in the few sources that cautiously accept that the EPU may be physiological.

Given the prevalence of the EPU, the systematic review has located surprisingly little information on midwives' response to it. One exception is an extensive audit carried out in 1994–1995 prior to the implementation of the US Association of Women's

Health, Obstetric and Neonatal Nurses (AWHONN) second stage labor nursing management protocol project.[21] The audit generated returns from over 1500 nurse-midwives from 40 sites in the USA and Canada. One of the topics was the EPU. In the brief account of this element of the survey given in the paper, nearly 93% of respondents reported that they had witnessed the EPU in labouring women. Nearly half of the respondents (45.5%) said they would institute a 'no-push' policy in this context, with a 'pant-blow' technique being most commonly utilized. The major reason given for this response was to minimize the risk of cervical oedema and cervical damage.

No other accounts of the nature of, and rationale for, midwives' response to the EPU were located in the published literature. In order to assess this phenomenon in more detail in the UK context, two surveys were undertaken by one of the authors of this chapter (SD), separated by seven years. The next section reports both the quantitative and qualitative data generated by both these surveys.

Studies 2 and 3: exploring midwives' practices in relation to the early pushing urge

The two surveys were undertaken in the UK in 1994 and in 2001. In both cases, the participants were attendees at a study day run by the UK-based Midwives' Information and Resource Service (MIDIRS). MIDIRS study days typically attract a wide range of midwives, and this was the rationale for selecting this method of recruitment. The research took the form of an anonymous questionnaire survey, using a semistructured vignette-based[22–24] questionnaire. The questionnaire was designed to capture the topics shown in Box 8.2. The basic vignette is given in Box 8.3. Midwives were asked to write a free account of their response to this vignette, and to the three variations on this basic scenario. These variations were based on the findings in the literature and on the anecdotal observation that midwives were less concerned about early pushing if the woman was not having her first baby.

Box 8.2

Survey of midwives' views of the 'early pushing urge', 1994 and 2001: elements of the questionnaire

There were six sections.

1. Demographics: length of qualification as a midwife, years of midwifery experience and number of births attended as the lead midwife in the previous 12 months
2. Geographical location of respondents: to assess the spread of respondents and the potential for the findings to capture regional variations in midwifery practice
3. Vignettes: respondents' reaction, reasons for responses, to four situations (vignettes):
   - a primigravid woman bearing down at 7 cm of cervical dilatation
   - a primigravid woman bearing down at 9 cm of cervical dilatation
   - a multigravid woman bearing down at 7 cm of cervical dilatation
   - a multigravid woman bearing down at 9 cm of cervical dilatation
4. Influences on the midwives in relation to their response to this situation
5. Views of respondents' colleagues: an indication of how likely it was that the respondent's response would be similar to that of her colleagues
6. Changes over time: questions about whether the midwife felt her practice had changed since qualification, and, if so, how and why (2001 survey only).

Sections 1, 4 and 5 were closed questions. Section 3 comprised a series of open questions as a response to a basic vignette, which was subsequently elaborated in stages. The basic vignette used is given in Box 8.3. Section 6 comprised one closed and two open questions.[22–24]

In 1994, the questionnaire was tested for face validity with women and midwives based in one hospital. Pilot respondents were asked about the content and comprehensibility of the questionnaire, and about how long it took to complete. Minor amendments were made as a result of this exercise. The sequence of vignettes was ordered logically, based on the empirical evidence cited above. In order to minimize the possibility of response bias, the 2001 survey comprised two versions, between which the order of the vignettes was varied. These versions were placed in identical envelopes, then shuffled

Box 8.3

The basic vignette used in the survey of midwives' views of the early pushing urge

'Mary is a 25-year-old primigravida. There have been no problems with her pregnancy or labour so far. She has been in active labour for six hours. Her membranes have ruptured, and she is draining clear liquor. The fetal head is in the OA position, and it is well applied to the cervix. An hour ago, she was 6 cm dilated. She is now getting restless, grunting a little and saying she wants to push. You carry out a VE, and she is now 9 cm and beginning to push hard. How do you deal with this situation?'

Note: The abbreviations OA (for fetal occiput in the anterior position in relation to the mother) and VE (for vaginal examination) were in common use by UK midwives at the time.

together to minimize systematic bias in allocation, and subsequently distributed chronologically to the participants. Following some of the findings of the first survey, a section was added asking whether, why and how midwives' views had changed since qualification. In both years, the questionnaires were distributed on the day of the conference and returned to the central site using freepost envelopes.

In 1994, no reminders were sent. On this occasion, some of those receiving the forms also photocopied them for colleagues in their Trusts to complete. In 2001, two reminders were sent to the whole population of attendees by MIDIRS staff, and the respondents were asked not to copy the questionnaire for others.

Access was agreed in advance by the conference organizer. Ethics committee approval was not needed because the midwives were not approached by virtue of their NHS employment.

Simple content, descriptive and cross-tabulated analysis was employed. In 1994, the analysis was undertaken by hand. In 2001, the data were scanned into the Formic system and downloaded into SPSS for analysis.

Results

The first study day in 1994 was attended by 120 delegates. The demographics for the delegates were

not available. Of the 110 attending the second day in 2001, 72 were midwives. The rest were students or non-professionals. The geographic base of the respondents in both cases indicated that there was at least one respondent from each of the English regions, and a few (eight in 1994, six in 2001) from Scotland and Wales. This implies that, as anticipated, the respondents were based across a wide geographical area. The basic demographics for each year are given in Table 8.3. Because of liberal photocopying of questionnaires in 1994, the percentage response cannot be determined. Of the 132 responses, five were incomplete. The responses to these five were analysed with the complete responses where data were available. All percentages reported below are based on the total response to the particular question, unless stated otherwise.

In both surveys, the range of years qualified and practising ranged from students who were not yet qualified to midwives with over 30 years of experience. UK grades E and F are those awarded to newly qualified or experienced clinical midwives. Evidence collected by the Royal College of Midwives in 1992 indicated that the proportion of F and G grades in English regions in 1992 was 52.1%. This equates closely to the percentage of respondents in this band in 1994 (53%). In 2001, 64% of respondees were employed in E and F grade posts. Respondents in both years also reported being employed at G, H and I grades, which are

Table 8.3 Demographics of the midwives responding to the 1994 and 2001 surveys of the early pushing urge		
	1994 (study 1)	**2001 (study 2)**
Total No.	132	47
Percentage return	–	65.2[a]
Time qualified/ practised	2 months to 33 years	5 months to 33 years
No. births attended	0–200[b]	0–200 (range)
Time intrapartum: 'most' (%)	47	47
Percentage E or F grade	53	64

[a] Percentage of all midwives attending the study day.
[b] Excluding extreme outlier of 700.

those awarded to staff with additional clinical or managerial responsibilities. A few respondents in both years were teachers or students. Some service users and students also responded. Apart from the one student who responded in 1994, whose data could not be disaggregated from the analysis, data are not reported in this paper for these participants.

In both years, just under half of the respondents reported spending most of their clinical time in intrapartum care. The range of numbers of births attended as the lead midwife in the year prior to the surveys was similar, apart from an extreme outlier in 1994, who reported that she had attended 700 births. This midwife may well have misunderstood the question.

Response to the vignettes, 1994 survey

In 1994, there were 129 respondents to the basic vignette: 31 initial codes were used in the first analysis. Table 8.4 sets out these initial codes, and the final themes. Box 8.4 gives examples of data to support these themes.

As can be seen, 25 of the initial 31 codes or themes were for 'techniques to prevent or minimize pushing'. The great majority of respondents reported using such techniques (n = 124; 96% of responses). These included changing position (usually to the lateral), advising about breathing patterns, giving both pharmacological and alternative pain relief, giving information and supporting the labouring mother. Of these respondents, 56 wanted to prevent women from pushing under any circumstances (43%). It is of interest that this percentage response is very close to that reported in the AWHONN survey described above.[21] Sixty-eight (53%) respondents gave mixed responses and five gave answers that were coded to the theme 'follow maternal instinct' (4%).

Response to varying circumstances

Respondents were asked to specify how their management would change depending on varying circumstances, and the responses were categorized. Four clear categories, and some subcategories, emerged. All of these entailed the use of particular techniques. Numbers of midwives utilizing techniques in each category were accumulated with those who

Table 8.4 Initial vignette: early analytical codes and themes (1994 survey)

Techniques to avoid pushing	No action needed	Other codes
Information	Let her go with	Depends on
Change position	her body	women's wishes
Side	Wouldn't really worry	Depends on state
Knee	about involuntary	of cervix
All fours	pushing	Synto (oxytocin)
Standing/walking	It's a good sign	if no progress
Squatting		
Pain relief		
Breathing techniques		
Entonox		
Pethidine		
Epidural		
Bath		
Backrub		
Effleurage		
Massage		
Pool/bath		
Encourage support from partner		
Other techniques		
Empty bladder		
Push cervix away		
Tip head of bed down		
Assessment and observation		
Reassess after short time/1 hour		
Observe for signs of full dilatation		

said their practice would not change in these respects from their response to the original vignette. The total response is displayed in Table 8.5.

There seems to be a clear trend here from less use of pharmacological pain relief for a multigravid woman at 9 cm of dilatation of the cervical os than for a primigravid woman at 7 cm dilatation. To continue the conceptual stance taken elsewhere in this book, this phenomenon could be labelled a progression from a more 'physiological' to a more 'technocratic' approach.[25] The responses from the 2001 survey illustrate this point in more detail.

Box 8.4

Data supporting final themes, 1994 survey

1. Avoid pushing at all costs: 'If a woman is not fully dilated, why are you asking what a midwife would do, is there a question? I do not know what you are getting at. You would not try and let a woman push if she was 7–8–9 cm, primip or multip'. (587)

2. Try to avoid pushing, but if you can't it probably doesn't matter (the majority response): 'There is a need to use common sense and consider each situation independently depending on the needs and requests of the mother. Patience and support are key factors in this situation, but there is also a need to identify if a problem is arising'. (568) 'I was always trained that if a multip wanted to push you can't stop her, as she'll push anyway!' (574)

3. Follow maternal instinct: 'I feel the answer so often is to work with the woman and to encourage her to go with her feelings. Work with nature'. (510)

The numbers in parentheses refer to the field notes of the survey described in Chapter 6.

Box 8.5

Pre-analysis codes for the 2001 survey

1. Always use techniques to prevent early pushing
2. Always try to prevent early pushing
3. Adopt a physiological attitude in the short term when women express an early pushing urge
4. Never stop a woman from expressing the early pushing urge

in response. These new categories are given in Box 8.5. Although the code phrases were determined prior to detailed analysis, care was taken to note data that deviated from this schema. Two coders (SD and VHM) coded the responses separately, and interim decisions were reached by consensus. Minor changes to these codes were made by SD in the final analysis.

Impact of varying distribution of questionnaires

For all of the demographics except number of births in the last year (range 0–200 in 1994 and 3–100 in 2001), the demographics were similar for the respondents in each set of questionnaires. However, there was a marked variation in the distribution of the codes between the two groups, with one set of respondents taking a distinctly more physiological stance than the other. This variation was apparent from the initial vignette, which was the first one to

Response to the vignettes, 2001 survey

An initial review of the returns for the 2001 survey indicated that the responses on this occasion were more likely to be equivocal than most of those reported in 1994. A coding schema was devised prior to formal analysis, based on the 1994 data, but taking account of this apparently greater complexity

Table 8.5 Survey in 1994 of midwives' views of the early pushing urge: variation in response by gravida and cervical dilatation (1994)

	Multigravid woman (n (%))[a]		Primigravid woman (n (%))[a]
	9 cm dilatation	7 cm dilatation	7 cm dilatation
Change position	100 (76)	106 (80)	114 (86)
Breathing techniques	61 (46)	62 (47)	63 (48)
Pain relief			
Entonox	72 (54)	78 (59)	79 (60)
Narcotic	11 (8)	13 (10)	30 (23)
Epidural	5 (4)	7 (5)	30 (23)

[a] Percentages are of total response (n = 132).

be responded to in both questionnaires. The change in the ordering of the questions only occurred after this point. This suggests that it was not the ordering of the survey that led to the variation, but rather it was a random response bias between the groups. In both cases, responses were progressively more physiological, from Mary as a primigravid woman with a cervical dilatation of 7 cm to Mary as a multigravid woman with a cervical dilatation of 9 cm. The data were, therefore, amalgamated for the final analysis.

For the total sample, the spread between the more physiological and the more technological stances varied from that in 1994. Similar percentages of respondents generally supported the extreme physiological position (code 4 for 2001). Eleven respondents recorded this response for at least one of the vignettes (15%). The same percentage was coded to the extreme technological position (code 1). This was lower than in 1994. As in 1994, the vast majority of responses fell between these categories. The striking difference between the two surveys, however, was in the more equivocal nature of the responses in 2001 compared with 1994. The following response to the scenario of a primigravid woman whose cervical os was dilated to 7 cm demonstrates this tendency in the 2001 data: 'I would more strongly encourage Mary to breathe through urges to push ... however if the urge to push is overwhelming her body will bear down spontaneously and, in our experience, this causes no problems' (456 q11).

In order to see the underlying patterns in the complexity of the data, the multiple codes were amalgamated into four groups. Figure 8.1 shows the results as bar charts. As noted above, it can be seen that the trajectory of responses mirrors that of 1994, with decisions in the context of a multigravid woman at 9 cm of dilatation being more physiological than those of a primigravid woman at 7 cm of dilatation.

In parallel with this similarity in the trend, there were also similarities between the surveys in the techniques proposed to minimize pushing. The most commonly suggested technique in 2001 was changing position or mobilizing, which was noted by 37 respondents (79%). Breathing and distraction techniques were reported by 29 (62%). Entonox (nitrous oxide and oxygen) was suggested by 15, with an epidural suggested by 8 (17%). Eleven offered

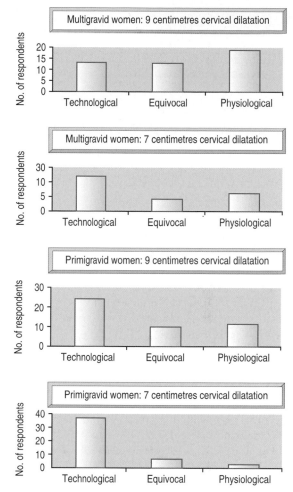

Fig 8.1 • Bar charts for responses to vignettes (amalgamated categories). Codes used for responses: 1, technological; 2, equivocal; 3, physiological.

information and a rationale for asking the women to stop pushing. Ten offered support, equally divided between support to stop pushing and support to 'go with her instincts'. Two suggested manual reduction of the cervical lip. A few respondents suggested techniques such as back massage, use of the bath and aromatherapy.

Response to the vignettes, both surveys

Reasons for response

The responses for all four vignettes were coded as one dataset for each cohort, and themes were developed. They are given in Box 8.6. In some cases,

Box 8.6

Reasons for response to vignettes (themes), 1994 and 2001

- To avoid oedema or trauma to the cervix: 54% (n = 71) in 1994; 47% (n = 22) in 2001
- To avoid delay, and stress to the mother or baby: 15% (n = 20) in 1994; 30% (n = 14) in 2001
- To aid dilatation: 5% (n = 6) in 1994; no responses fell into this category in 2001
- To support physiological processes: 9% (n = 12) in 1994; 32% (n = 15) in 2001

respondents gave multiple reasons. All responses were categorized to a theme. These are described in detail below. The percentages given in the box are based on the total number of respondents. As in the AWHONN survey mentioned above,[21] fear of cervical oedema or damage was the main driver for the midwives' responses.

Influences on midwives' decision making

Since the original literature review, undertaken in 1994, suggested that there was very little written information to help a midwife in making a decision about this area of care, midwives were asked in a multiple choice question to indicate sources of information and influence that had an effect on their practice in this area. Table 8.6 illustrates their responses. In each case, the percentages given are of

all respondents, since many ticked more than one category.

In both years, by far the most respondents indicated that 'observing women in labour' was the most powerful influence on their practice. The variation in midwives' response to the vignettes indicates that either women labour differently with different midwives or that midwives observing the same maternal behaviours draw different conclusions about their normality or pathology. These issues are explored further in the discussion below.

Anticipated response of colleagues

In order to overcome the potential selection bias created by the methods of recruitment, the respondents were asked if, in their view, their responses were the same as those that would be given by their colleagues. In 1994, the majority of respondents (67%; n = 89) said that they thought that their colleagues' response would be the same as their own; in 2001 this was 50% (n = 23).

This contrasts with the findings of Marianne Mead's study, described in Chapter 5, using a questionnaire with a very similar design to the one used in this survey, but focused on a variety of intrapartum techniques, which indicated that midwives thought their colleagues would be more interventionist in their approach. It is also intriguing that respondents to both of the EPU surveys apparently disagreed among themselves, while at the same time claiming that their colleagues' views were generally similar to their own.

Responses to the assumptions underlying the questionnaire

In 2001, 21 respondents (57% of all responding to this question) reported that they had changed their practice in this area over time. Most reported becoming more physiological in their approach. This may explain dissatisfaction expressed in the 2001 cohort about some of the assumptions underlying the vignettes:

I wouldn't have carried out the vaginal examination again so early. (14 q8)

It was quite difficult to answer the questions properly. As, often, I make decisions like these, having been with the women throughout the labour ... (224 q17)

Table 8.6	Influences on midwives in relation to maternal pushing prior to diagnosis of full dilatation (1994 and 2001)	
Source	1994 (n (%))	2001 (n (%))
Midwifery training	75 (57)	*
From mentors	45 (34)	22 (47)
From peers	77 (58)	31 (66)
Observing mothers in labour	111 (84)	40 (85)
Having own babies	24 (18)	14 (30)
Other	10 (7)	6 (13)

* Question not asked in 2001.

I have to add I wouldn't be doing all these VEs and would be relying on external signs. (32 q9)

These comments led to a more detailed content analysis of the narrative accounts given by respondents in 2001. The next section describes the results of this further analysis.

Qualitative analysis of responses in 2001

Many respondents to the 2001 survey used the opportunity of the open questions in the questionnaire to give thoughtful comments on the issues raised by the topic of early pushing in labour. These were subjected to simple thematic analysis. One overarching theme emerged, namely 'multiple discourses of midwifery'. As stated above, discourse is used in a particular way for this exposition. The nature of this interpretation is explored in the discussion below.

The five sub-themes relating to this are given in Box 8.7. Each is explained in more detail in the following sections.

Describing dissonance

A number of the respondents described situations that paralleled the stereotypical events set out at the beginning of this chapter. These descriptions were given from the perspective of the respondent as observer, as in the following quote (89 q20), and

Box 8.7

Key theme and sub-themes arising from qualitative responses to the 2001 questionnaire

Theme:
- multiple discourses of midwifery.

Sub-themes:
- describing dissonance
- unique normality
- determining the 'right' practice: the impact of anecdotal experience
- the nature of intervention
- proper pushing.

as an (occasionally reluctant) actor, as evidenced in later quotes in this section:

Observing women being left very frightened and midwife leaves to get medic/epidural, to find vx visible on her return!

For some of those who were more recently qualified, a sense of dissonance between observed events and their beliefs about midwifery care seemed to be acute. They described the discomfort of an obligation to adopt the practices that were acceptable at the ward level at the time, while believing that another approach was actually better.

I don't have much post-registration experience, so I feel obliged to fall back on 'traditional' practice (sometimes). I would very much like to see some real evidence to support this, however, as I don't really trust traditional practice where it so blatantly goes against what nature is trying to do … by shouting at women to push when they don't want to, and not to push when we don't want them to is disempowering and disruptive to the physiological event of birth, and undermines a woman's confidence in her body and possibly even her experience of parenting. (149 q17; midwife practising for 21 months)

I would anticipate that, as long as the position is definitely OA, and the head is well down, there would be no risk to Mary from pushing at 9 cm. However, this is from our own observation only, + I would find it difficult to justify if challenged, so I would probably still suggest to Mary that she 'breathe through' the contractions as much as she can. (84 q11; midwife practising for 2 years)

Later in the questionnaire, this same midwife goes on to say:

… however, as not pushing before full dilation is (I believe) officially accepted practice, I would find it difficult to justify going against this if challenged, as I feel I could be accused of being negligent towards the woman's interests. I am sure there are midwives … who have the confidence to practice differently, but as the dominant culture means they don't advertise the fact, there are limited opportunities to learn from them. (84 q17)

Another fairly newly qualified midwife echoes this confusion of discourses:

> ... *the pushing urge is so strong it can't be 'wrong' ... she'd probably push the cx out of the way ... I would go through the textbook motions of left lateral/entenox simply because I was taught that way ... (124 q9)*

All of them have difficulty because they are inclined to believe that the normal physiology of pushing in labour expresses itself in a range of maternal behaviours. In each case, their unease is related to a strong sense of a subtle set of authoritative knowledges operating at a local level. The clear sense in one account, that there may be a need to 'justify' alternative practice against an opposing set of accepted practices, may also be an underpinning feature of accounts. It is also of interest that respondent 84 confessed to a desire to learn differently, and a sense that a kind of 'underground' approach is being enacted by some midwives. This is seen as invisible to the ward-level authorities and, consequently, invisible to newly qualified midwives, some of whom appear to be very keen to find role models to help them to understand and live out their beliefs and values about physiological birth.

These accounts are of particular interest because, in Goffman's terms, they are narratives of practitioners who are not fully skilled at riding the professional 'rocking horse'.[26] In this almost liminal state, these respondents can see both discourses clearly, and they are hesitating between them. This means that they may be unable to practise fluently – one of the respondents recounts later in her response that she often calls in more senior midwives to help her because she is not confident in which approach she should take.

It is possible that more experienced midwives have made a decision to overcome this sense of dissonance by adopting either one approach or the other. However, barriers may still be in place if the practice adopted contradicts that of the dominant discourse at the ward level – if it is seen as 'deviant'. For example, one midwife with 19 years' experience stated that she is 'aware that nature is far more efficient than the controlling urge of midwives and obstetricians' (98 q19). However, she gave one of the main reasons for having a 'concern over premature pushing' as 'time constraints of delivery suite protocol' (98 q17).

Midwifery practice in out-of-hospital births has been firmly associated with women-centred individual care, respect for maternal physiology and a 'hands-off' approach from the midwife. The account of one respondent is of interest in this context. In relation to her usual practice, she said: 'as a community midwife delivering babies at home our policy is to keep mothers mobile and upright as long as possible, keep well hydrated ... well informed ... encourage partners to massage etc., and wait for nature to take its course without "clock watching"' (100 q17). However, her response to the question about the primigravid woman at 7 cm of cervical dilatation was in striking opposition to this assertion: 'Review analgesia and discuss. Possibly top up epidural or IM [intramuscular] injection' (100 q10).

It is hard to explain the variation between her stated philosophy of birth and this specific response. The question of impact of place of birth on midwives' practice may be an important factor to explore.

For some respondents, non-adherence to subtle rules was a powerful method of circumventing other rules that were more heavily enforced: 'it is much better not to confirm full dilatation by VE if you are confident with your own recognition skills, particularly in units where there is a "time limit" on the second stage of labour, as you then find yourself clock watching' (31 q17). This may be one of the skills practised by the invisible 'deviant' practitioners; however, this was impossible to evaluate in this particular survey.

It can be hypothesized that recently qualified midwives who adopt the approach that agrees with that operating as authoritative knowledge at ward level will become visible reinforcers of that knowledge. If they adopt the alternative stance, they will become the invisible practitioners who are sought by at least one of the respondents above, and, at least in the settings experienced by these respondents, they will operate in opposition to the accepted norms. These suppositions remain to be tested in more detailed studies in the future.

Unique normality

The concept of a unique normality in childbirth, which was discussed in Chapter 1, was evident in the accounts of midwives responding to this survey. To illustrate this, the specific case of the fetal occipito-posterior (OP) position is described initially in this section. More generalized instances follow on from this.

As the literature review illustrates, the situation of the OP position has been seen as a cardinal indication not to allow women to push when they feel a spontaneous desire to do so. The word 'allow' is used deliberately in this context. The general sense is that pushing in the absence of a fully dilated cervical os is very likely to cause morbidity, and so, for their own sake, women must be supported in avoiding this situation. Since the vignettes specified that the fetal occiput was in the anterior position, few respondents made reference to this eventuality. However, where reference was made, it was unexpectedly to question the assumptions underlying the authoritative source. In one case, these assumptions are described, but the account is framed in the third person: 'It is generally understood to be more of a problem with the OP baby. In this instance some colleagues (+ doctors) would recommend an epidural' (124 q17). Some of the personal accounts given by respondents contradicted this position: 'Own experience of childbirth: VE at 7p.m. = 7 cms the cervix well applied OP. Urge to push intermittent used entonox. Finally pushed without another VE for 45 minutes delivered face to pubes at home, 8.28p.m.' (103 q19). This example of a situation that contradicted the received knowledge in this area was framed by generalizations about unique normality.

I don't think there are hard and fast rules regarding this topic. Experience has taught me each situation is unique … (297 q17)

… I sometimes feel that this type of practice (preventing women from pushing) ignores the individuality of women and their labours; that there is somehow a 'textbook' procedure that we can 'make' women fit into. (465 q17)

With experience, midwives learn to recognize deviations from … 'normal' progress. Some women will progress when pushing early whatever direction is given, but some will develop problems … the skill is to support women pushing early but without progress … (417 q17)

'Every labour different for every woman' principle. (231, q10)

It is of interest to note that, despite the sentiments expressed in the final quote above, this particular respondent gave very similar responses to each of the vignettes given in the survey (all categorized to 2). This illustrates one of the problems of taking self-report accounts alone and not examining actual practice. However, the accounts do express what the respondents believe, if not what they do. In fact, in some cases, specific practice-based instances that deviated from received knowledge in this area were also cited, for example '… have cared for a P0 who wanted to push from 4 cms thick cx loosely applied membranes intact who progressed normally and delivered normally …' (262 q9).

As discussed below under the impact of anecdotal experience, seminal events ('critical incidents' in Schon's terminology)[27] could push respondents either towards accepting the EPU as a physiological expression of unique normality or towards rejecting it as a universally pathological phenomenon. More subtly, some respondents saw the expression of variations in the EPU as the context for a decision about which kind of intervention to suggest to women to stop them pushing. In this case, the rhetoric of individuality was expressed only in the range of interventions that could be chosen, or in the differential ability to cope with not pushing, and not in a decision about intervention or not. This was sometimes framed by an assertion of maternal choice in the context of specific interventions:

… pushing will slow delivery – but hopefully instigating an epidural is not needed – the minuses outweigh the plusses – but I'm always led by the patient's wishes – wherever possible. (426 q30)

Depends on decent [sic] of head and thinness of cx + Marys abilities to cope with pain and managing to stop pushing. Each patient is different – this is where midwife's experience is useful. (426 q9)

Where respondents showed a faith in the uniqueness of women and their bodies, there were no firm rules against which they could judge the 'correctness' or otherwise of their response in relation to local authoritative knowledge. The question arises as to the basis on which these respondents constructed their practice. In many cases, this was in a loose sense of 'rightness': 'if she feels this way then it probably is "right"' (51 q9), or a call on intuition or instinct: 'Trust a woman's instincts – Books aren't always right. Experience tells you when pushing may be causing harm. Not sure how I know – instinct' (295 q19). This last comment raises the issue of the subtleties around midwives' responses to women's behaviours. The concept of instinctive professional nursing and midwifery behaviours has become a topic of interest since the 1980s.[28,29] The value of instinct may be fundamentally questioned by the data above. Where responses to the EPU are highly divergent, which instinct is 'right'? It is notable from the data that respondents who championed unique normality in the context of the individuality of women's bodies (as opposed to a professional management of those bodies) were more likely to use intuition as an explanation for, or even defence of, their response. There are a number of questions here, including whether midwives who are invisible in the dominant discourse need to refer to 'unscientific' explanations for their response. The next theme addresses the impact of anecdotal experience; the formative observations that stand out for practitioners and which underpin their attitudes and responses in the future.

Determining the 'right' practice: the impact of anecdotal experience

It was apparent in reading the questionnaires that the approach of a number of respondents was crystallized by a particular single experience, or critical incident, especially if this was subsequently repeated. One individual with a relatively technological approach commented that she responds this way 'after seeing women who, after pushing too early, had a cervix that became swollen and which led to an EmLSCS [emergency lower segment caesarian section] for failure to progress. This problem only seems to occur in primipara' (91 q9). The mixture of singular and plural is as recorded by the respondent and suggests an interesting elision between one experience and a set of similar experiences. Later in the questionnaire she goes on to say: 'As a student we were told "let" women push when they felt the urge ... however,

I have discovered through experience ... that many primiparous women have an urge to push (from rectal pressure) long before full cervical dilation. If left to push and cervix swells then the risk of C/S is much higher' (91 q19). A contrary experience has led another respondent to state that she is now 'more relaxed, more trusting of women's ability to labour without examination. As yet never found an oedematous cx!'.

For this last midwife, the increased trust seems to have been built up through not observing adverse effects. Similar comments relating to never having seen side effects of early pushing are recorded by other respondents. This raises a question. What would happen if these midwives did come across this phenomenon? Would it change their practice or would it be integrated into the overall schema of the 'rightness' of nature? Another respondent gives some indication of how experiences that contradict a set of prior beliefs can be integrated into a particular personal position in this area. She describes a situation where she encouraged pushing in a primigravid woman who experienced the EPU, after confirming apparent full cervical dilatation with a vaginal examination. After 45 minutes of pushing, the baby's head was visible, along with a swollen lip of cervix. The respondent recounts:

It had a profound effect on me ... it did make me reluctant to support instinctive pushing ... However, having gained a lot of experience in normal labour, I have relaxed my views, and am much more likely to look at all factors ... I now offer encouragement and support for the women who, for the vast majority, know instinctively how to push ... (15 q17)

In this case, the critical incident had led the respondent to question profoundly her prior beliefs. However, this was mitigated over time by a different set of experiences, which she uses 'for the vast majority'. By logical deduction, she does not do this for a certain minority of women. This indicates that she has used her experience to take a more complex approach to this issue than she had before.

The nature of intervention

This theme explores the nature of midwifery intervention with specific emphasis on cervical reduction. The general midwifery discourse in countries with low maternal and infant mortality tends to assume that doctors interfere and that midwives support, although some have disputed this interpretation (see, for example, Marianne Mead's work in Ch. 5). Techniques such as the use of pharmacological pain relief and oxytocin for augmentation of labour are seen to fit into the (perjorative) category of interventions. However, practices used by midwives, such as massage to provide pain relief, or nipple stimulation or membrane sweeping to start or augment labour, are seen as woman centred and supportive. Tricia Anderson has raised a question around this apparently uncritical dichotomy[30] and proposed an alternative approach, where midwifery practices are placed on a scale with a gradually increasing level of intervention attached to them. Some of the data from this survey support the 'problematization' of the midwifery account of supportive practices:

... I do not think midwifes [sic] should interfere, as much as they do, with the process of childbirth. I would not have assessed after only 1 Hour to check for full dilation ... (465 q9)

This respondent was one of the few whose responses over the span of the survey were coded to the whole span of themes from 1 to 4. This indicates a great deal of flexibility in her approach to the EPU. However, she does recommend using breathing techniques, mobilization, change of position and back massage. How are these practices weighed against the 'interference' that she condemns in other midwives? Another account gives an even more dramatic example:

... eg, 1 A primip – labouring instinctively, no ve's performed throughout labour; 2, P4 – cx was 'holding back' baby's head at 9 cms. Woman was instinctively pushing hard with no progress (in kneeling position). With permission I pushed cx back, baby born with next push. (297 q17)

This respondent later commented that she had experienced cervical reduction personally, and she found it very painful and would rarely use it for women. Her comment was not the only account of this technique. The questions raised by Tricia Anderson and echoed in these quotes challenge

the dichotomous discourse about intervention that is apparently deeply held by the midwifery profession.

'Proper' pushing

The final theme in the data illustrated the complexity of the respondents' analysis of the EPU. Some noted different types of pushing, which they responded to differently:

I feel that women who are pushing too early – you can hear it in the noises they make and the pushes they give (in my experience). (458 q17)

Many women with the urge to push find they are unable to push effectively if they are not yet ready to actively push. Instead of an expulsive push you get a throaty grunt with little expulsive action. (103 q8)

One midwife reported her personal experience of being informed after five hours of labour that her cervical os was only 1 cm dilated, and then, one hour later, being in second stage labour. She commented:

At 4 cm dilated my pushing urges began, and being curious I allowed my body to do what it wanted. The pushes were not second stage pushes, but presumably encouraged the fast dilatation of my cervix.' (28 q20)

These three accounts illustrate subtle variations on this theme. In the first two, the midwives are claiming the expertise to differentiate between effective and ineffective pushing. In the third quote, while acknowledging that the pushes were different from 'second stage pushes', the midwife used her personal birth experience to reflect on the possibility that the instinctive behaviours she was expressing were of value in their own right.

On a different note, one respondent recounted observations of women who, when prevented from pushing early (in a way deemed as ineffective), were then subsequently unable to push (in the way expected by caregivers) when given permission to do so.

My views have changed through observing the distress women often seem to feel when they want

*to push and can't. I am not sure I am doing the
right thing in denying such a strong urge …
sometimes when women are asked not to push
when they want to, they then find it hard to push
when they are deemed ready – they have lost
touch with what their bodies are telling them …
(84 q17; midwife practising for 2 years)*

This last observation is echoed in incidental findings
in two published papers, where women in US
settings who were prevented from pushing when it
was deemed to be 'early' (maybe when the midwives
felt the noises they were making were not 'second
stage pushes') found themselves unable to do so
when officially sanctioned as 'complete' (with full
cervical dilatation).[31,32]

Multiple discourses of midwifery

As we noted above, we are using the term *discourse*
as a transactional term rather than a linguistic one.
We draw on Kendall & Wickham's interpretation
of Foucault's methods for this usage.[2] Discourse in
this sense is a calculation, a discursive operation,
which produces something concrete (so-called
'materiality'). In this case, the concrete construction
is notions of midwifery practice. Foucaultian thinking
would not fix normality or physiology, but it provides
a legitimate space for conscious reflection on these
concepts. Kendall & Wickham provide steps for the
use of discourse (p 42):[2]

1. The recognition of discourse as a 'corpus' of
   statements whose organization is regular and
   systematic
2. The identification of rules of the production
   of statements
3. The identification of rules that delimit the
   sayable
4. The identification of rules that create the
   spaces in which 'new' statements can be made
5. The identification of rules to ensure that practice
   is material and discursive at the same time.

We do not claim to have followed these rules in
depth in our analysis. However, we propose the
synthesis in this section in an attempt to understand
how the discourses used by the midwives both define
and delimit the space in which they act as midwives.

We see the dissonances experienced by some of the
respondents as the result of 'delineations of the
sayable' (and thus the doable) and as the spaces
in which new constructions of midwifery and of
normality can be found.

The sub-themes set out above link to the overall
theme of multiple discourses in midwifery in the
context of the EPU. They raise questions about
a number of aspects of the midwifery discourse.
They illustrate that it is not singular, and that it
is contested. From a post-modernist perspective,
this is not surprising. However, these multiple
approaches are framed in a system that does not
acknowledge multiplicity. This generates a state
of dissonance for some respondents. In exploring
dissonance between the discourses of the EPU,
the issue of deviance arises. Deviance in midwifery
has been raised before, notably in Mavis Kirkham's
ethnography of midwifery practices in the settings
of a consultant unit and a free-standing birth centre.[33]
In each setting, one midwife was observed to
be deviant. This deviance took different forms in
each setting, and each was in contradistinction to
the authoritative discourse of practice prevalent
in the settings. In the case of the midwife in the
hospital setting, this resulted in her resignation, after
she found it impossible to practise as she wanted
against the hostility of the other midwives.

While the responses to this survey do not indicate
such a dramatic schism between midwives, they do
indicate that, in a context in which authoritative
knowledge tends to be linear and certain, as
described in Chapter 1, multiple discourses can
cause confusion and unease. While some of the
midwives whose voices are represented here can
clearly operate within complexity and flex their
care according to a woman's unique circumstances,
even if this contradicts the ward-level authoritative
approach, many find this difficult. Techniques to
resolve the difficulty may include adoption of a way
of practising that does not contradict the dominant
practices, or a kind of invisibility in which the least
acceptable practices can be undertaken away from
the gaze of the enforcers of the dominant discourse.

In some cases, multiple discourses are more
acceptable than in other circumstances. Recognition
of different noises made at different stages of pushing
does not seem to raise concerns over conflicted

practice in those who describe them. Constructions of intervention are also relatively unproblematic. Examination of the interface between discourses and dissonance may reveal interesting facets of midwives' construction of midwifery and of normal ways of birthing.

Further discussion of findings from the surveys

The issue of midwives' own birth experiences on their attitudes to birthing women have not been widely explored. In the analysis of the 2001 data, where midwives gave their personal birth story, there was evidence that it inclined them towards recognition of the EPU as a physiological concept. However, this is unlikely to be the full range of midwifery experience of this phenomenon, and many others that make up a labour experience. If personal beliefs and values are accepted as a fundamental component of birth attitude, understanding midwives' own birth stories may be an instinctive part of any movement to refocus on the potential for physiological birth for many women.

We were intrigued by the similarities in the findings between our work and that of the AWHONN survey,[21] despite the lack of formal evidence in this area. Recently, we have conducted a survey into UK midwives' responses to the management of the nuchal cord, another area with little data to support practice.[34] Again, we found striking similarities between our findings and those of a survey of members of the American College of Nurse Midwives.[35] As a consequence, we have suggested that theories of diffusion of innovation may explain some of these findings.[34] This hypothesis requires more investigation.

Beyond these specific aspects of the data, the qualitative analysis also casts the term 'early' into some doubt. We chose to use this term in opposition to the pathological assumptions underlying the term 'premature pushing urge' which is often employed in this context. However, early and, by logical deduction, late also imply some kind of deviation from the norm of 'on time'. Current approaches to childbirth are saturated with the concept of time.[36] Chronology provides the basis for a number of terms used to describe processes that deviate from the accepted norm. These terms include premature rupture of membranes, post-dates, post-maturity, prolonged labour, late decelerations and delay in second stage labour. The use of chronology as an indicator of normality implies a linear perception of labour. Accepting an approach to birth based on complexity may imply that this simple linearity should be challenged. This would imply a radical reassessment of phenomena such as that termed the EPU in this chapter.

Conclusions

The literature review discussed at the beginning of this chapter indicated that there is little published evidence around the incidence and nature of the EPU, or on midwives' response to it. The empirical work described here provides an insight into some of these aspects. In the process, questions have also been posed about the existence of multiple midwifery discourses. Some insight has been gained into the ways by which midwives might deal with the dissonance engendered by these discourses, in this area specifically and possibly in the more general context of intrapartum care. Specifically in the area of EPU, there is a great deal more work to do in analysing the nuances of this phenomenon and in addressing the views and experiences of women. More generally, work is needed on the nature and impact of multiple discourses in midwifery. This chapter is one small part of that much larger work.

References

1. Montgomery T L 1958 Physiologic considerations in labor and the puerperium. Am J Obstet Gynaecol 76:706–715

2. Kendall G, Wickham G 2000 Using Foucault's methods, 2nd edn. Sage, London

3. Arms S 1975 Immaculate deception: a new look at women and childbirth. Bantam Books, New York

4. Kitzinger S 1987 The experience of childbirth, 5th edn. Penguin, Harmondsworth

5. Jordan B 1993 Birth in four cultures: a cross-cultural investigation of childbirth in Yucatan, Holland, Sweden and the United States. Waveland Press, Champaign, IL

6. Davis-Floyd RE, Sargent CF (eds) 1997 Childbirth and authoritative knowledge: cross-cultural perspectives. University of California Press, Berkeley, CA

7. Roberts J, Hanson L 2007 Best practices in second stage labor care: maternal bearing down and positioning. J Midwifery Womens Health 52:238–245

8. Roberts C L, Torvaldsen S, Cameron C A et al 2004 Delayed versus early pushing in women with epidural analgesia: a systematic review and meta-analysis. BJOG 111:1333–1340

9. Berkeley C, Fairbairn J S, White C 1931 Midwifery, 4th edn. Arnold, London

10. Benyon C 1957 (Reprinted 1990) The normal second stage of labor: a plea for reform in its conduct. In: Kitzinger S, Simkin P (eds) Episiotomy and the second stage of labor, 2nd edn. Pennypress, Seattle, WA

11. Kitzinger S, Simkin P (eds) 1990 Episiotomy and the second stage of labor, 2nd edn. Pennypress, Seattle, WA

12. Davis E, Arms S, Harrison L 2004 Heart and hands: a midwife's guide to pregnancy and birth, 4th edn. Celestial Arts, Berkeley, CA, p 74

13. Varney H, Kriebs J M, Gegor C L (eds) 2004 Varneys midwifery, 4th edn. Jones and Bartlett, Boston, p 1244

14. Bennett V R, Brown L K (eds) 1993 Myles textbook for midwives, 12th edn. Churchill Livingstone, Edinburgh, p 453, 885

15. Downe S 2003 Transition and the second stage of labour. In: Fraser D, Cooper M (eds) Myles textbook for midwives, 14th edn. Harcourt Health Sciences, London

16. Downe S 2004 Transition and the second stage of labour: In: Henderson C, MacDonald S (eds) Mayes' midwifery, 13th edn. Harcourt Health Sciences, London

17. Enkin M, Keirse M J N C, Neilson J et al (eds) 2000 A guide to effective care in pregnancy and childbirth, 3rd edn. Oxford University Press, Oxford

18. Yeates D A, Roberts J E 1984 A comparison of two bearing down techniques during the second stage of labor. J Nurs Midwifery 29:3–11

19. Roberts J E, Goldstein S A, Gruener J S et al 1987 A descriptive analysis of involuntary bearing-down efforts during the expulsive phase of labour. J Obstet Gynecol Nurs 16:48–55

20. Roberts J E 2002 The 'push for evidence': management of the second stage. J Midwif Womens Health 47:2–15

21. Petersen L, Besuner P 1997 Pushing techniques during labor: issues and controversies. J Obstet Gynaecol Neonat Nurs 26:719–726

22. Finch J 1987 The vignette technique in survey research. Sociology 21:105–114

23. Polit H 1997 Essentials of nursing research: methods, appraisal, and utilization, 4th edn. Barnes and Noble, New York

24. Hughes R, Huby M 2002 The application of vignettes in social and nursing research. J Adv Nurs 37:382–386

25. Davis-Floyd R 1994 The technocratic body: American childbirth as cultural expression. Soc Sci Med 38: 1125–1140

26. Goffman E 1959 Performances. In: Goffman E (ed.) The presentation of the self in everyday life. Doubleday, New York, p 17–34

27. Schon D A 1983 The reflective practitioner: how practitioners think in action. Basic Books, New York

28. Benner P, Tanner C A, Chesla C A 1996 Expertise in nursing practice: caring, clinical judgement and ethics. Springer, New York

29. Davis-Floyd R, Arvidson P S 1997 Intuition: the inside story. Interdisciplinary perspectives. Routledge, New York

30. Anderson T 2002 Peeling back the layers: a new look at midwifery interventions. MIDIRS Midwif Digest 12:207–210

31. Bergstrom L, Seidel J, Skillman-Hull L et al 1997 'I gotta push. Please let me push!' Social interactions during the change from first to second stage labor. Birth 24:173–180

32. McKay S, Barrows T, Roberts J 1990 Women's views of second-stage labor as assessed by interviews and videotapes. Birth 17:192–198

33. Kirkham M 1987 Basic supportive care in labour; interaction with and around labouring women. PhD Thesis, Manchester University, Manchester

34. Jackson H, Melvin C, Downe S 2007 Midwives and the fetal nuchal cord: a survey of practices and perceptions. J Midwifery Womens Health 52:49–55

35. Mercer J S, Skovgaard R L, Peareara-Eaves J et al 2005 Nuchal cord management and nurse-midwifery practice. J Midwifery Womens Health 50:373–379

36. Simonds W 2002 Watching the clock: keeping time during pregnancy, birth, and postpartum experiences. Soc Sci Med 55:559–570

Fetal to neonatal transition: first, do no harm

Judith Mercer, Rebecca Skovgaard and
Debra Erickson-Owens

Introduction

The moment of birth is profound. For humans, it is a moment of deep spirituality and renewed hope. For a labouring woman, it is a moment of accomplishment and vast relief. For a newborn, it is a moment of physiological change so extreme that nothing short of death approaches it. Clinical practices and traditions surrounding the moment of birth should acknowledge and support its profundity. In the last century, as birth moved from home to the hospital, much of the respect for the moment – its spiritual aspect, its power and its physiological processes – was lost to practical goals of efficiency and expedience. But the medicalization of childbirth was unsatisfactory to many women and families, and counter movements grew. These included natural childbirth, family-centred care and a rebirth of midwifery.

One practice, developed for simple expedience and without study or careful regard for the physiological processes at work, persists in many hospital settings. That is the immediate clamping of the umbilical cord at the time of birth. For a few minutes after birth, the newborn continues to receive oxygenated blood through the umbilical cord. A delay in clamping the cord facilitates a gentle, physiological transition that likely benefits all neonates and may be critical to especially vulnerable infants.

This chapter examines the issue of the timing of cord clamping within the context of a reconceptualization of the processes at work in the early moments

149

of neonatal transition. The theory described places due emphasis on the importance of a transfusion of blood from the placenta to the neonate.[1] Clinical situations in which protecting placental blood flow is of particular importance are addressed, and practical solutions provided. The benefits of such practice, including potential effects on newborn complications for which aetiological factors are uncertain, are discussed. Recommendations for practice and issues requiring further research are identified. All ideas are supported with evidence.

Evidence regarding cord clamping practices

Interest in the optimal time for cord clamping can be found in early medical literature.[2] The first high-quality controlled trials were carried out at the Karolinska Institute by William Oh, Alice Yao and others under the direction of John Lind, and are reviewed elsewhere.[3] These studies provide much of the basic physiological knowledge used currently. Between 1980 and early 2007, eight randomized controlled trials[4-11] and five controlled trials[12-16]

have been completed on early versus delayed cord clamping in full-term infants (see Appendix). Two recent reviews of studies of delayed versus immediate cord clamping found reduced rates of anaemia in infancy, and no evidence of harm for the babies randomized to the delayed clamping group.[17,18] Sixteen randomized controlled trials on pre-term infants with delays varying from 30 seconds to three minutes have found benefits for pre-term infants without evidence of harm.[19-34] A review done in 2004 concludes that a delay in clamping the cord by 30 to 120 seconds appears to be associated with less intraventricular haemorrhage and less need for blood transfusion in pre-term infants.[35]

A review of neonatal transition physiology provides a basis for these findings. The fetal–placental circulation contains 110–115 ml/kg of whole blood throughout gestation.[36] The volume of blood found within the infant's body after birth varies by cord clamping practices (Fig. 9.1).[37] Term infants with immediate cord clamping have approximately 70 ml/kg blood at birth while those infants with delayed clamping have approximately 90 ml/kg or more, an increase of 30% in blood volume. In a 3000 g infant, this results in a cross-cord transfusion of approximately 210 ml

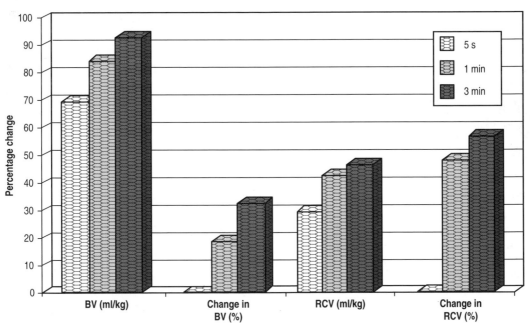

Fig 9.1 • Percentage change in blood volume (BV) and red cell volume (RCV) by cord clamping time. (Adapted from Yao et al.[37])

whole blood when cord clamping is immediate versus 270 ml when clamping is delayed.

Yao and colleagues found that infants with a delay in cord clamping of three minutes obtain approximately 50% more red blood cells.[37] Red blood cells play a critical role in oxygen and carbon dioxide transport. Jones estimated that infants need approximately 45 mg/kg red blood cells for adequate oxygen-carrying capacity.[38] The only infants in the study of Yao and colleagues who obtained 45 mg/kg red blood cells were those infants whose clamping was delayed for 3 minutes while they were held at the level of the perineum.[37]

It is worth noting that accurate measurement of blood volume and red cell volume is notoriously difficult. The haematocrit level, being simple to obtain, is most commonly used. But it can be unreliable in circumstances of trauma or stress. In a study involving 259 infants admitted to a high-risk newborn unit, Faxelius et al measured red cell volume by tagging the red blood cells with non-radioactive chromium.[39] With this more accurate assessment, they found that infants with a history of asphyxia often had a low red cell volume even if no signs of blood loss were present. More importantly, there was only a 60% correlation when haematocrit was plotted against red cell volume, indicating that haematocrit is not always a good predictor of red cell volume.

Other studies comparing delayed cord clamping with early clamping have provided evidence for the physiological outcomes of increased red cell volume. These include higher haematocrit level,[40,41] more cutaneous perfusion and higher skin temperature,[42,43] less hypovolaemia[3,37,44] and a 12–20% increased red blood cell flow to the brain and gut.[14] An infant with an adequate blood volume stays warmer and is better perfused.[42,43] Increased renal blood flow and the resulting increase in urine output is another important finding.[45] Hypovolaemia and red blood cell flow are issues in infants who have failed resuscitation. Poor renal output is an issue in infants with seizures and hypoxic-ischaemic encephalopathy (HIE).[46] The greater pulmonary vasodilatation found in late-clamped infants[14] should raise flags about the possibility of hypovolaemia in those infants with oxygen-dependent illnesses such as persistent pulmonary hypertension.

In the most recent systematic review and meta-analysis of controlled trials on late versus early cord clamping in full-term neonates, Hutton & Hassan present the results of their review of eight randomized trials and seven controlled trials.[18] They found that delaying the cord clamping for a minimum of two minutes is beneficial to the newborn (prevents anaemia) and that those benefits extend into infancy (reduces anaemia of infancy up to six months of age). Their review included two large randomized controlled trials completed in Argentina and Mexico published in 2006 and involving more than 600 infants.[10,11] The trial done in Mexico City included the intervention of a two minute delay in cord clamping versus immediate cord clamping, and followed a sample of 358 children over six months in order to assess iron status and ferritin concentrations. While there was no difference in haematocrit and haemoglobin at six months, they found a signficant difference in iron stores and ferritin levels ($50.7 \mu g$/L versus $34.4 \mu g$/L, $p = 0.0002$). The study completed in Argentina included 276 newborns with cord clamping done either immediately, at one minute or at three minutes after birth. The authors report less neonatal anaemia in both delayed groups. While there was an increase in polycythaemia (>65%) among the infants who were randomized to the delayed groups, the infants remained asymptomatic and no treatment was necessary.

Polycythaemia and hyperbilirubinaemia

The greatest obstacle to the clinical application of delayed cord clamping at birth has been the persistent belief that it causes polycythaemia and hyperbilirubinaemia.[47,48] Reports of 'symptomatic' polycythaemia from delayed cord clamping are based on a secondary analysis of a previous study published by Saigal & Usher in 1977.[48] Although the authors identified 11 babies with symptomatic polycythaemia, only two term infants had a haematocrit level above 70% and none of the pre-term infants had an elevated haematocrit. Saigal & Usher did not address other causes of polycythaemia such as maternal diabetes,[49] small for gestational age infants,[50] hypertension in the mother,[51] maternal smoking[52] and other conditions causing erythropoiesis in the fetus that were unknown at the time. The impact of this publication on clinical practice has been disproportionately significant. The study suffers from two major weaknesses. Maternal factors which influence neonatal polycythaemia are not addressed, and some infants with 'classical respiratory distress' were removed from the final analysis without identification of which cord clamping group they belonged to. Conclusions drawn from this paper therefore need closer examination.

In their meta-analysis, Hutton & Hassan[18] report no significant differences in mean serum bilirubin levels at 24 and 72 hours of life between infants with immediate or delayed cord clamping. The idea that delayed cord clamping causes hyperbilirubinaemia was also propounded by Saigal and colleagues in 1972.[47] Data from randomized and non-randomized controlled trials between 1980 and 2006 do not support this hypothesis.[18] The evidence from the randomized trials challenges the myth that delayed cord clamping causes harm to newborns and calls for a re-evaluation of the practice of immediate cord clamping.

The need for re-evaluation of current practice

We believe that immediate clamping of the umbilical cord is an intervention in the normal process of birth that was introduced without adequate study of its potential impact on neonatal transition and infancy outcomes. Our hypothesis is that immediate cord clamping can cause hypovolaemia leading to poor capillary perfusion, resulting in inflammation and ischaemia during the neonatal period in vulnerable

infants (Fig. 9.2). The ischaemia may result in subtle to overt damage to newborn organs, including the brain. We suspect that this damage may lead to morbidities and developmental impairments in the child. We offer examples of relevant cases, related evidence and a theory to support our hypothesis and to encourage rethinking of the current practice.

The stimulus for the authors' interest in this area of study arose from clinical experiences and from discussions with colleagues and peers. Case history 9.1 offers a dramatic example of resuscitation with an intact cord and engendered the first author's interest in the process of transition from fetus to newborn.

In most hospital settings, the birth of an infant such as the one described in Case history 9.1 would lead to immediate clamping and cutting of the cord in order to accommodate resuscitation by neonatal staff at an infant warmer. Indeed, guidelines for neonatal resuscitation such as those provided by the American Academy of Pediatrics routinely presume immediate cord clamping.[53] Yet this case amply demonstrates the value of the placenta as a source of blood transfusion for a volume-depleted newborn. In Case history 9.1, immediate clamping of the cord may have inflicted harm by preventing the reperfusion of this pale, lifeless infant. This case prompted a review of the literature on delayed cord clamping and a survey of colleagues to investigate cord clamping practices.

Prior to the current decade, there was little evidence-based evaluation of the issue of cord clamping. Routine practice has typically been based on tradition and convenience.[54] Our survey of

CLAMPING	PLACENTAL TRANSFUSION	BLOOD VOLUME	CAPILLARY PERFUSION	TISSUE EFFECT	OUTCOMES	DEVELOPMENT
Delayed; Infant lowered or cord milked	Good	Euvolaemic Normotensive (More red blood and stem cells)	Normal; Good capillary distension and erection	Normal tissue perfusion	Physiological stability Normal organs	Normal development, health, normal motor function
Immediate	Little or none	Hypovolaemic Hypotensive (Less red blood cell and stem cell volume)	Poor; Little capillary distension and erection	Inflammation leading to subtle to overt structural and functional damage	Physiological fragility Organ/system damage	Increased health concerns More motor dysfunction and other delayed aspects of development

Fig 9.2 • Theoretical pathway for cascade effects of placental transfusion.

Case history 9.1

Baby with tight double nuchal cord (home birth, 1979)

The labouring woman had requested that her membranes not be ruptured because of a traumatic first birth experience during which this had been done against her wishes. She progressed rapidly to full dilatation with intact membranes. During second stage, the fetus descended to +3 station with each push, but slipped back high into the pelvis after each contraction. After 30 minutes, the mother agreed to artificial rupture of the membranes (AROM). The infant descended, crowned and was born in one contraction after AROM. A tight double nuchal cord was unwound immediately. The infant was extremely pale white with no tone, reflexes or respiratory effort, though his heart rate was above 100 beats/minute. The baby was placed on the bed between the mother's legs where the care provider bulb suctioned, dried and stimulated the infant. A second check of the heart rate revealed that it remained over 100 beats/minute. The cord, which initially felt pulseless, began to pulsate forcefully and the infant's body rapidly gained colour. The provider continued to stimulate the baby and the parents encouraged and touched the infant. At approximately 1.5 to 2 minutes (time was not recorded), the baby, now pink, moved his left arm upon his chest, opened his eyes and took an easy breath. He immediately flexed the other extremities and continued with quiet shallow breaths. This baby never vocalized a screaming cry in spite of strong stimulation but continued gentle, even, shallow respirations. He was placed skin to skin, proceeded to breastfeed well and had a normal neonatal course.

American nurse-midwives identified a wide variety in practices and beliefs with regard to newborn management during transition.[55]

Survey of American nurse-midwives' practices and beliefs regarding cord clamping

In informal discussions with midwives and other providers, we found a wide variation in practice and beliefs among practitioners in different settings and around the world. As a result, we surveyed members of the American College of Nurse-Midwives (ACNM) in 1998 to confirm the absence of a standard practice for cord clamping and the underlying rationale.[55] One-third of respondents reported clamping the cord after pulsations cease, in the belief that the continued circulation provides additional blood and oxygen for the infant and assists with a gentle neonatal transition. Thirty-six per cent clamped between one and three minutes, largely believing that cord clamping time is insignificant, but were willing to clamp later at the request of parents. Twenty-six per cent reported clamping immediately or before one minute, with the thought that immediate clamping facilitates management of the newborn and prevents jaundice.

The respondents were also asked to describe their practice in particular clinical situations. In the case of a pale infant with poor tone at birth, 51% reported that they would cut the cord and take the infant to a warmer, 28% said they would place the infant on the maternal abdomen and stimulate, and 10% stated they would resuscitate at the perineum without clamping the cord. For the scenario of nuchal cord management, 57% reported that they would cut and clamp a nuchal cord only when very tight, and 40% reported the use of the somersault manoeuvre to avoid cutting the cord.[56] For management of meconium-stained amniotic fluid, 53% reportedly cut and clamp immediately while 47% delay clamping, preferring to manage meconium at the perineum. These results demonstrate significant differences in cord clamping and neonatal management among this group of practitioners.

The survey did not specifically assess differences in management by birth settings. However, additional comments the midwives wrote on the questionnaire implied that the setting for the birth might influence providers' practice. One midwife who practices at home, birth centre and hospital reported that she felt great pressure in the hospital to clamp the cord and pass the baby to others, whereas she was very satisfied with the success of her methods of supporting the neonate's transition with an intact cord in the other settings.

When asked about the evidence for their practice, 75% of survey respondents offered no specific references for their cord clamping practices, or only very general references such as basic midwifery or obstetrics textbooks. At the time of the survey, the last review of the literature on this topic had been published in 1982.[3] This observation led us to publish a subsequent review, which included all the randomized and non-randomized controlled trials found on cord clamping from 1980 to 2000.[54]

Uncertain aetiology for many newborn and infant problems

Another reason to carefully examine practices related to neonatal transition is that the aetiology of many newborn and infant problems is uncertain. Meconium aspiration syndrome (MAS),[57] persistent pulmonary hypertension,[58] hypoxic-ischaemic encephalopathy (HIE) and seizures in the immediate newborn period[59] and learning disabilities, developmental delay, cerebral palsy (CP)[60] and autism[61] in older children remain unexplained. Hankins et al stated that 'most cases of CP occur as the result of multi-factorial and unpreventable causes that occur either during fetal development or in the newborn after delivery' (p 11).[46] However, Cowan et al performed magnetic resonance imaging on infants with HIE and newborn seizures and found evidence of pre-birth damage in only 1% of the infants.[59] They stated: 'our data strongly suggest that events in the immediate perinatal period are most important' (p 736).[59] The debate in this area is spirited.

As shown in Figure 9.1, major differences in the composition and the volume of blood are seen in relationship to the time of cord clamping. An infant's blood volume can be increased by 30% and red cell volume by as much as 50% by delayed cord clamping.[37] Though there are currently no studies that examine long-term outcomes of children who have been subjected to immediate cord clamping, an increasing body of knowledge documents short-term effects. Evidence relating long-term health and developmental issues to circumstances of early life is increasing.

Anaemia and developmental outcomes

Delayed cord clamping effects a physiological increase in newborn haematocrit values.[18] At least in developing countries, infants with delayed cord clamping have a lower incidence of anaemia at three months of age[5] and better iron stores at six months.[10] These findings have led to recommendations for delayed cord clamping in resource-poor areas.[62] The issue of anaemia takes on additional significance when one reviews the work of Lozoff and colleagues.[63–65] They have demonstrated a clear relationship between anaemia and poorer developmental outcomes. They found that the harm persisted even when the anaemia was successfully treated in infancy, and persisted at 19 years of age.[66]

Cord blood transfusion as protection against inflammatory response

A newborn inflammatory response has been associated with adverse outcomes such as CP.[67] An iatrogenic reduction in normal neonatal blood volume (due to immediate cord clamping) may play a role in the initiation of the cascade of events associated with the newborn inflammatory response. In a study of the effects of haemorrhage on the mammalian body, Rajnik and colleagues used a juvenile (6–8 weeks) mouse model to measure cytokines as evidence of an inflammatory response.*[68,69] Study mice had 25% of their blood volume removed. Within three hours, pro-inflammatory cytokines (interleukins 6 and 10, tumour necrosis factor alpha and Toll-like receptor 2) showed marked upregulation in both liver and lung samples. Their conclusion was that loss of 25% of blood volume initiated a cytokine response in the organs with symptoms similar to that of adult respiratory distress syndrome and multiple organ failure (preceding any resuscitative measures or reperfusion).

This response to diminished blood volume may also play a role in the development of intraventricular haemorrhage (IVH) in pre-term infants. In a randomized, controlled study comparing immediate and delayed cord clamping among very pre-term

---

* The authors understand that animal experimentation may be ethically problematic for some readers. This study's importance is that it is the only study to show an inflammatory response to blood volume loss alone. As seen in Figure 9.1, some infants with immediate cord clamping may have 25% or more loss of circulating blood volume with which to begin life, which may contribute to an inflammatory process. It is an important area of inquiry.

infants, Mercer et al found that delayed cord clamping in this group protects against IVH.[20]

A possible role for cord blood progenitor (stem) cells

The same study by Mercer et al also showed a reduction in late-onset sepsis among pre-term infants with delayed clamping.[20] Haneline et al documented that the cord blood of very pre-term infants is especially high in primitive haematopoietic progenitor cells,[70] leading Mercer et al to speculate that these cells may confer an immunoprotective effect for pre-term neonates.

Human cord blood (HCB) is now used to treat a multitude of conditions.[71] Evidence is building that HCB may help prevent long-term injury from perinatal hypoxia. Meier et al documented that human cord blood mononuclear cells injected into rat pups that had suffered an ischaemic brain injury prevented the development of associated spastic paresis (cerebral palsy). The cells were incorporated into the area of inflammation that caused the brain injury and alleviated symptoms of cerebral palsy.[72] No stem cells were noted in the non-damaged part of the brain.

If a provider is convinced of the benefits of delayed cord clamping, how might it alter one's practice? How does delaying cord clamping affect the neonatal transition and the management of the infant at birth? In order for a provider to re-evaluate the current practice of immediate cord clamping, basic information about neonatal transition must be reviewed to understand how delayed cord clamping impacts neonatal transition.

The blood volume theory of neonatal transition

Traditionally, the focus at birth, and particularly during a newborn resuscitation, has been on providing oxygen. A good cry reassures everyone present at a birth and the administration of oxygen under positive pressure is the mainstay of resuscitation. This focus on the breath, and specifically the use of positive pressure oxygen, discounts critical physiological processes that occur with birth. These processes are driven by blood volume, not oxygen (Case history 9.2).[1]

Case history 9.2

Infant with hypoxic-ischaemic encephalopathy who survived with cerebral palsy (level I institution)

A birth that was videotaped offered a unique opportunity to view this baby at birth and as resuscitation occurred. Review of the videotape and all of the mother's records revealed no obvious or predisposing risk factors. The tracing was not ominous, although it suggested marked variable decelerations during late second stage with widening variable decelerations going from 80–90 bpm to 150–160 bpm and back down again. The mother was encouraged to push using maximum force. The baby was toneless and pale at birth. The provider cut the umbilical cord immediately and rushed the baby to the warmer where resuscitation was started and assistance was requested. It was noted at one point that the infant's heart rate was above 100 bpm. The baby responded very slowly and later had a seizure and developed hypoxic-ischaemic encephalopathy. Paediatric admission notes on this baby mentioned 'extreme paleness'. The infant developed severe cerebral palsy.

Case histories 9.1 and 9.2 present remarkably similar situations – depressed, volume-depleted infants – with extreme differences in treatment approaches and outcome. These differences pose a question about the critical role of blood volume in neonatal stabilization and outcome.

The blood volume theory of neonatal transition, described fully elsewhere[1] is depicted in Figure 9.3. It represents a paradigm shift in thinking about transitional physiology and highlights the value of maintaining placental circulation as a way of supporting optimal transition. The momentous physiological transition at birth is the process of weaning from the placenta as the site of gas exchange and transferring that function to the newborn lung. Because that process has traditionally been thought of as abrupt (and, with immediate cord clamping, is in fact made abrupt), there develops an urgency about seeing that the lungs are filled with air or, presumably even better, oxygen. This explains the high value placed on a lusty newborn cry and the quick intervention of positive pressure ventilation

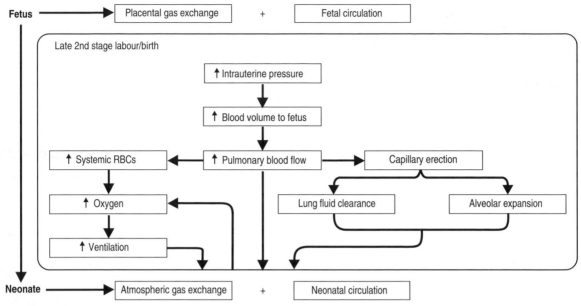

Fig 9.3 • The blood volume model of neonatal transition.[1]

when there is perceived to be a lack of 'vigorousness' in the newborn.

Yet air is more than readily available. The lungs, as they expand for the first time, have nothing but air with which to fill. The presence of air is not at issue. It is interesting to note that recent changes in recommendations for adult cardiopulmonary resuscitation reflect more emphasis on blood flow with the importance placed on chest compressions rather than rescue (mouth to mouth) breathing.[73] Some experts in resuscitation advocate dispensing with ventilation entirely.[74]

The critical elements are establishing effective gas transfer at the site of the alveoli and the availability of red blood cells for delivery of oxygen from the air to the essential organs. These elements depend upon adequate neonatal blood volume.

In the fetal–placental unit, there is a limited amount of blood (on average 110 ml/kg) and it is the only blood that is available to the fetus/neonate.[36] The fetus begins making blood during the yolk sac phase and develops a circulatory system with a beating heart by 21 days' gestation. At term, a third of the blood volume is in the placenta at any one time and two-thirds is in the fetus. Earlier in fetal life, fully half of the blood volume is in the placenta. This reflects the importance of the placental role in gas and nutrient/waste exchange.

Circulation, and comcomitant blood volume, within the fetus has as its purpose the transport of gas and nutrients. The ratio of cardiac output to various sites demonstrates this. In fetal life, 8% of the cardiac output goes to the lung, 20% to the brain and 15% to the gut, while 45–50% goes to the placenta.[75]

Birth brings about necessary, drastic changes as the lung assumes the role of gas exchange. Immediately after birth, 50% of the cardiac output must flow to and through the lungs as significant pulmonary circulation is established for the first time. Perfusion of the pulmonary capillary bed now requires a volume of blood (50% of cardiac output) that was not needed in the fetal state (8% of cardiac output).

In fact, the volume of blood devoted to gas exchange for the fetus resides in the placenta. In most mammalian births, circulation from the placenta persists for a few minutes after birth. This allows for a physiological transfer of blood volume from the placenta to the fetus. When the cord ceases pulsating (or is artificially clamped), the volume of blood within the newborn becomes fixed. If the blood volume needed to expand the lung has not come from the placenta, then it must be sacrificed from other organ systems and the general circulation in the neonate's body.

Several papers have documented that blood continues to flow through the placenta to the infant in the first few minutes of life.[76-80] A study from the 1950s showed this in a simple manner.[80] Immediately after birth, an infant was placed into a basin on a scale that continuously recorded the infant's weight over 20 minutes. The infant gained a total of 100 g, beginning immediately at birth and continuing for 15 minutes until the weight stabilized. This demonstrated that the infant continued to receive additional placental transfusion as the mother's uterus contracted during the same period.

The infant continues to get oxygen from the placenta for at least a few minutes after birth. Case histories 9.1 and 9.3 illustrate this. Indeed, the advent of the EXIT (ex utero intrapartum treatment) procedure verifies it dramatically. In these cases, surgical repair of a fetal anomaly, such as

Case history 9.3

Infant with a congenital anomaly (hospital birth centre)

A young mother gave birth spontaneously to an infant who did very well for three to four minutes while the umbilical cord was routinely left intact. Then the infant began to struggle with his breathing and turned blue. The midwife cut the cord and took him to the warmer. He had significant retractions and was unable to breathe well. Paediatric staff had difficulty suctioning his nose and considered a possible coanal atresia. They placed an oral airway and subsequently the newborn breathed easily. Later testing revealed a tumour at the base of the brain, compressing the nasopharynx and interfering with respiration. A tracheostomy was placed and the infant eventually had successful surgery. This infant's Apgar scores were 9[1], 5[5], 9[10]. He did well for the time that he was supported by placental circulation. When the umbilical vessels closed, he lost that source of oxygen and was unable to establish his own until the oral airway was placed.

an obstructive tumour in the neck, takes place after an infant is partially delivered by caesarean section, but before the umbilical cord is cut. Support of the infant by the placenta has been maintained for as long as an hour.[81]

The role of blood in fetus-to-neonate transition

Blood plays an essential role in the body by transporting oxygen and carbon dioxide, nutrients, waste products, hormones and stem cells. In addition, it helps to protect against disease and is involved in temperature, fluid and electrolyte regulation.

At the time of birth, blood has two additional essential functions. One is to effect the opening of the alveoli[82,83] and the other is to clear the lung fluid from the alveoli immediately after birth.[1] Physical changes in the lung occur with tremendous speed in the minutes after birth, when the lung takes over the job of gas exchange from the placenta. Alveoli during fetal life are not closed but are filled with lung fluid. However, they are small and not expanded, as they will be after birth. A capillary plexus surrounds each alveolus and is cemented in place by the intracellular matrix.[84]

At birth, the capillaries fill fully with blood for the first time. During this process, the capillaries expand, become erect and actively open the alveoli, a process labelled *recruitment*. Sheets of these blood-filled capillaries completely surround each alveolus, and it is the distension of these vessels that provides the 'scaffolding' structure to keep the alveoli open.[1,85] If pulmonary blood flow is low, structural support for the lung tissue diminishes and can result in collapse of the newborn lung, or 'derecruitment' with each breath.[86] Air pressure does not keep the lungs open; lungs have no more than atmospheric pressure. They do not collapse with exhalation because of the hydrostatic exoskeleton generated by this capillary network.

Minimal separation between air and blood is critical for effective diffusion of gases. In most areas, the respiratory membrane consists of only three thin tissue layers – the capillary endothelium attached to the basement membrane attached to the alveolar epithelium.[84] Supportive architecture, designed any other way, would come at the cost of rapid gas exchange.

A second important function of blood at birth is to clear the alveoli of fluid as the lung expands. The fetus produces approximately 200 ml/kg/day of lung fluid. Structurally, immediately at birth, the lung must change from a fluid-filled organ to one filled with air. Functionally, it must change from an organ of fluid production to an organ of gas exchange. Suctioning at birth may clear the airway but it will not clear the fluid deep in the alveoli. The squeeze during a vaginal birth also does not, as some have suggested, adequately clear lung fluid.[87] Lung fluid is not absorbed into 'lung tissue' as there is no extraneous tissue in this area of active gas exchange. The only way lung fluid can clear is through the intricate circulation established within the lung tissue immediately at birth. The higher colloidal osmotic pressure of the blood in the capillaries surrounding each alveolus draws the fluid from the lung.

Professor Jaykka at the University of Tirku in Finland first coined the term 'capillary erection' in 1958 and documented its importance.[82] Normal aerated lung tissue is mostly air and space (like a sponge), with a mass of capillaries outlining each alveolus. This tissue is buoyant. This piqued Jaykka's curiosity about what causes the expansion of the lung at birth. To achieve this effect in the lab, he performed his first experiment by blowing air into a lung. Using fetal lamb or cadaverous human tissue, he began by blowing room air into isolated but intact lungs. He noted that the process required high air pressures. Microscopic sections of these lungs showed overdistended alveoli alternating with areas of atelectasis where the lung did not expand properly. This tissue was not buoyant and most likely was not effective for normal respiration.

In the next experiment, he infused fluid through the pulmonary artery in order to mimic the action of blood flow. He then filled the lung with air and the air flowed in easily and the lungs became buoyant. The thin sections of these lungs resembled normal aerated lung tissue.

Upon close examination, the septa between the alveoli seen by Jaykka were thicker than those in adult lung tissue (adult septa are one capillary wide). Wasowicz et al demonstrated that the architecture of the lung continues to change from the saccular phase at birth to the alveolar phase in early neonatal life.[85] They produced revealing electron microscopic slides of rat lung tissue at 2 and 21 days of age. At 2 days, the interalveolar septa have a diameter of two to four capillaries. As the lung matures, the septa decrease in width to a single capillary. This wider structural support immediately at birth would offer more assistance to maintain the newborn lung during transition. Theoretically, this structure would require more blood volume and, fully expanded, would account for differences of higher pulmonary resistance, lower lung capacity and slightly increased respiratory rate seen in newborns after a physiological transition with an intact placental circulation.

These findings demanded a new theory for explaining physiological fetal-to-neonate transition. We developed the blood volume theory to explain what most likely occurs during a physiological transition.[1] The following summarizes the critical aspects of the theory (see Fig. 9.3).

High intrauterine pressures of late second stage and early third stage labour effect a transfer of blood from the placenta to the fetus.[88] That volume of blood is one of the essential components for establishing normal pulmonary blood flow. Infants with immediate cord clamping generally establish normal pulmonary blood flow, but we believe that this may occur with some sacrifice of blood flow to other organs.[89] Providing the extra blood volume helps to support capillary bed expansion in the lung and to maintain normal blood volume for the systemic circulation. Increased pulmonary blood flow opens the capillary bed, effects capillary erection, causing the alveoli to expand, and subsequently clears the lung fluid. Ventilation begins through the lung. Atmospheric gas exchange is established. As respiration continues, higher levels of systemic oxygen stimulate the respiratory centre of the brain and the baby goes on to continue normal neonatal respiration.[55,87,90]

Protecting placental circulation

Immediate cord clamping is an intervention that was accepted without study but now bears the heavy weight of institutional tradition. This has persisted to the point that delaying cord clamping is seen as an intervention which needs to be proven, one for which institutional practices should not have to accommodate.

In fact, placental circulation can be supported in any setting and in any circumstance. This possibility is addressed in the following situations, typical of those in which immediated cord clamping has been traditionally thought necessary.

Management of an infant with a nuchal umbilical cord

Nuchal cord, or cord around the neck, is a condition that often leads to premature interruption of the placental circulation. Nuchal cords can appear and disappear throughout gestation. They can be seen on ultrasound, then disappear by the time the infant is born, or vice versa.[91] Cords grow longer with fetal movement. Fetuses that move a lot have longer cords and are more likely to form entanglements.[91]

There is a particularly good reason not to immediately clamp and cut nuchal cords even though they present themselves easily. When the cord is compressed, it sets up a process for transfer of blood from the fetus to the placenta. Blood flowing in the umbilical vein to the fetus from the placenta is sacrificed first when the cord is compressed. The umbilical vein is a large, thin-walled, floppy, low-pressure structure that is easily subject to compression. The thicker-walled, muscular, high-pressure umbilical arteries are not so easily compressed. In fact, there is physiological evidence of that every time there is a variable deceleration. The primary acceleration is the compression of the umbilical vein. The fetus receives less blood flow back from the placenta so the blood pressure falls and the fetus compensates by speeding up the heart rate. If cord compression continues, the umbilical arteries are compressed as well, the fetus loses the low-pressure circulation to the placenta and the heart rate drops to compensate for that increased blood pressure. The secondary acceleration occurs when the blood flows again through the umbilical arteries.

Several case reports demonstrate neonatal anaemia and hypovolaemia with tight nuchal cords at birth.[92,93] Additionally, a large Canadian study documents that nuchal cords affect birth weight.[94] Records of 10 000 births were examined, and 20%

of infants had a nuchal cord at birth. These infants weighed approximately 60 g less than babies without nuchal cords. The authors' theory was that babies with nuchal cords weighed less because they did not get enough nutrients or oxygen. Because the 60 g was similar to the amount of blood that an infant would not get if the cord is clamped immediately, we contacted them to enquire about management at birth. They stated that the protocol was to cut and clamp the cord before the body of the baby is born. We think that these infants lost about 60 ml of blood due to pre-birth cord clamping.

There are two options for managing nuchal cords without cutting them. The first is to slip the cord over the head or down around the shoulders and slide the baby through it. The other option is the somersault manoeuvre, first described by Schorn & Blanco.[56] It involves delivering the baby slowly and bringing the head as it is born back towards the mother (up into the mother's thigh or symphysis pubis). The baby is kept tucked near the perineum so that it rolls out and the feet are away from the mother with the head still up towards the introitus (Fig. 9.4).

With either method, it is particularly important to avoid cutting the nuchal cord immediately after the birth, no matter how depressed the infant appears. The dynamics of cord compression will likely result in an increased transfer of blood to the placenta. Pale colour or poor tone of the infant would indicate this. A delay in cord clamping is needed for the blood volume to equalize. This may be a situation in which keeping the baby below the level of the placenta is useful. *Nuchal cord management should be the same in any setting.*

Shoulder dystocia

The possibility of shoulder dystocia is an underlying concern at any birth. An infant who has experienced shoulder dystocia may also have had a terminal bradycardia and is apt to appear shocked, stunned, cyanotic, white and floppy. The infant who appears this way needs volume expansion, especially if the body is white or mottled blue-white with a weak pulse. Volume expansion is available in any setting if the placental circulation is not interrupted. A full resuscitation can be done at the mother's perineum if indicated.

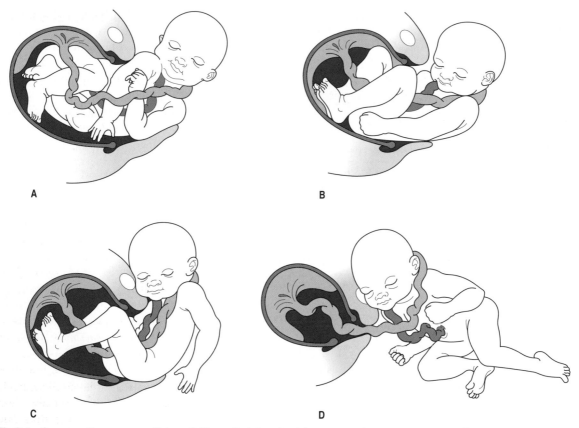

Fig 9.4 • Somersault manoeuvre: Schorn & Blanco first described the somersault manoeuvre in 1991.[56] The head is delivered normally but, as the body is being born, the head is raised towards the symphysis pubis and the body is moved away from the perineum. This allows for minimum tension on the cord; the midwife can more easily unwrap it and allow the infant to reperfuse.[56]

Shoulder dystocia may place infants at particular risk of hypovolaemia. The squeeze of a tight fit through the birth canal may cause more of the fetal blood than usual to be extruded into the placenta. This may account for the poor condition of many of these infants at birth – worse than would be anticipated from a few minutes of hypoxia, from which a healthy fetus would be expected to recover.[95] Rapid cutting of the cord to facilitate resuscitation of these depressed infants may, in fact, be a critically harmful intervention.

Explaining to parents before the birth what one will do if the infant needs assistance is extremely important, and especially so when the infant will be positioned between the mother's legs. Parents are involved and most often will verbally encourage the infant to breathe (Case history 9.4).

Resuscitating an infant at the perineum requires that all the equipment is ready and in reach at the time of the birth. If positive pressure ventilation is indicated, it may be initiated with room air, as this is safe and effective, and may alleviate practical difficulties.[96]

Shoulder dystocia and the presence of a nuchal cord can be especially dangerous for a newborn. Iffy and colleagues published two reviews of nine cases of shoulder dystocia where the nuchal cord was cut before the birth.[97,98] All births occurred three to seven minutes after the birth of the head. Six infants developed cerebral palsy. All women had normal second stages. Two infants were born by vacuum extraction and one with forceps. Only one showed any distress before birth. All had poor Apgar scores.

Case history 9.4

Maternal involvement in the resuscitation of an infant with shoulder dystocia and a true knot in the cord (home birth)

A woman having her fourth baby experienced shoulder dystocia with an infant who had terminal bradycardia and was born very depressed. The midwife placed the infant between the mother's legs and proceeded with a full resuscitation including mask and bagging. As the midwife was bagging the infant, the mother sat up and saw that there was a true knot in the cord. She instinctively reached down and loosened the knot. As soon as she had loosened it, the baby started reperfusing and breathed immediately. The infant and mother had a normal postpartum/newborn course.

Flamm reported the birth of an infant where he almost cut the nuchal cord before he was assured that the infant would be born.[99] He was able to slip the cord over the head. However, he was unable to deliver the baby vaginally. He used the Zavanelli manoeuvre to replace the head. The infant was born by caesarean section and had Apgar scores of 3^1, 7^5 and 9^{10}.

The usual occurrence of shoulder dystocia is approximately 1.7% of all births, while nuchal cords occur in 20–33%; both phenomena are often unpredictable.[97] Cutting a nuchal cord prior to the birth of the shoulders may increase an infant's risk of asphyxia and even death if there is a severe shoulder dystocia.[97,99]

Management of infants with meconium-stained amniotic fluid (MSAF) at birth

Management of an infant with MSAF usually involves immediate clamping, although this is an area where typical practice and the evidence have been inconsistent until very recently.[100] In the 1970s, paediatric and obstetric experts proposed an approach to prevent meconium aspiration syndrome (MAS). It was based on the assumption that MAS is caused by aspiration of meconium at the time of birth. This approach involved DeLee suctioning on the perineum, immediate cord clamping and passing the baby to paediatric staff for laryngoscopy

and suctioning below the cords. Unfortunately, this approach failed to effect a significant decrease in morbidity. It has become clear that the aetiology of MAS is a more complicated process.[101]

Normal healthy fetuses have mechanisms to cope with the challenge of meconium. Meconium is typically passed as a physiological process and the fetus has physiological processes to deal with it.[102] Normal healthy fetuses make breathing movements, drawing fluid into their lungs; therefore, if meconium is present in the fluid, it would be present in the lung. However, most babies who have meconium in the amniotic fluid do not have meconium in the lungs because they clear it through the process of lung fluid production. Fetuses typically produce approximately 200 ml/kg fluid per day, which is extruded into the amniotic fluid, in essence flushing out the lung. In addition, they can clear their amniotic fluid through a filtering process involving fetal swallowing and urination. Fetuses swallow approximately one litre of fluid per day and pass approximately one litre of urine per day, essentially filtering amniotic fluid.

Meconium is probably passed more often than is observed at birth. It is seen during amniocentesis throughout gestation.[101] It should normally clear over the course of a number of days, suggesting that some fetuses who look as if they had clear fluid have, some time during the gestation, passed meconium. This supposition is reinforced by the fact that meconium can be seen microscopically in the amnion and in the lungs of babies who had clear fluid. Light or moderate meconium is not an ominous sign. In fact, it suggests that a fetus urinates and swallows normally and has a normal fluid volume.

Meconium is, however, worrisome when it is thick. This does not happen because some fetuses have more meconium than others. The problem stems from inadequate dilution and filtration. That is, fetuses with thick or particulate meconium do not have the normal amount of fluid volume they need to dilute it or the normal physiological processes for its clearance. Therefore, a fetus with thick meconium is somewhat compromised.

Awareness of fetal mechanisms for clearing MSAF raises the questions of what goes wrong when neonates have MAS. Thureen et al looked at postmortem and pathology findings of babies who died of MAS.[103] They failed to find big areas of atelectasis where a bronchus had been clogged by meconium or any presence of large deposits of meconium. They did find thickening of the arterial walls in the lung that is exactly similar to what is seen with persistent pulmonary hypertension. We suggest that adequate blood volume after birth supports normal lung functioning and clearance of wastes, including meconium, from the lung.

Thureen et al recommended looking at pre-birth strategies for prevention of meconium aspiration.[103] These measures would include surveillance for issues that lead to chronic fetal hypoxia and to institute labour management that supports the physiological adaptation of the fetus (see Case history 9.5).

Recent changes in guidelines for management of neonates with MSAF reflect these observations. DeLee suctioning and routine intubation are no longer recommended.[104] Policies are important because addressing how one manages MSAF in any setting is something that needs to be negotiated with all stakeholders, including nurses and consultant medical staff. The current evidence indicates that, with MSAF, the only babies who should be intubated and resuscitated are those who are not vigorous at the time of birth.[100] Institutional policies which demand that all babies get passed to paediatricians immediately are no longer necessary. If MSAF occurs during an out-of-hospital birth, many practitioners feel that there is a case for transfer to the hospital for birth, with the caveat 'if they can do so safely'. Unless membranes are routinely ruptured early (contrary to physiological management of labour), then, in many cases, thick MSAF would not be diagnosed until it is too late to transfer. It is essential to pay close attention to the biological markers which indicate that babies are healthy in labour. These include fetal movement and fetal heart rate accelerations, which can be documented with a fetascope in any setting.

Case history 9.5 describes a situation where a midwife works with the neonatologist to care for an infant with thick MSAF while keeping the placental circulation intact.

For thick MSAF, the process by which the infant will be managed at the time of birth needs to be negotiated, as many hospital settings have a policy about who needs to be present for suctioning and intubation of the infant.

Case history 9.5

Infant with particulate meconium staining (level II hospital)

Labour progressed with evidence of particulate meconium. There were some unremarkable variable decelerations in the later part of labour and during second stage. The neonatologist was in attendance and had agreed to visualize the infant's vocal cords at the bedside, if indicated, with the umbilical cord left intact after birth. After birth of the head, the nares and mouth were suctioned and about 3 ml of meconium-stained fluid were obtained. After birth, the infant appeared somewhat depressed (there was some lack of tone but good heart rate). The infant was born in the bed and was placed on dry pads at a 90° angle to the perineum. As the neonatologist touched the infant's face, she began to cry. The neonatologist decided that the infant was vigorous and did not proceed to visualize the cords. The infant was placed on her side, dried and then moved to her mother's abdomen with the cord still intact. She nursed very well and had an uneventful neonatal course.

Infants that are slow to start

It is difficult to differentiate between a slow-to-start baby and one that is going to need a more full resuscitation. There may be contributing factors such as a terminal bradycardia, a long crowning and/or a tight fit, or if the water is too warm at a water birth (Tracey Bowman, personal communication, 2003). Precipitously birthed babies can be stunned

Case history 9.6

Slow-to-start infant (home birth)

A 39-year-old woman in her first pregnancy with an eight hour labour had been pushing for two hours. She gave birth spontaneously and immediately picked up her infant, who was slightly stunned, holding the infant against her chest. After the initial gasp, the infant did not breathe for over a minute and had mediocre tone, although her heart rate was above 100 bpm. The midwife took the infant from the mother's arms and lowered the baby below the placenta. With very little stimulation, the infant breathed, cried and regained tone immediately.

and slow to start. In Case history 9.6, lowering the infant below the level of the placenta helped to begin breathing and normalized the transition.

If an infant is placed on the maternal abdomen and then does not proceed to have a normal transition, there is a greater likelihood that, in the hospital, the cord will be cut and the infant taken to the warmer. When the infant's problem is hypovolaemia, it is preferable to keep the baby at the level of the mother's perineum for assessment and continue resuscitation with the cord intact. This will allow continued placental–infant transfusion and enhance oxygenation. The resuscitation can be performed at the perineum if the cord is still pulsating or, if necessary, the cord can be cut and the infant taken to the warmer for a full resuscitation.

Management of an infant needing full resuscitation

An infant who needs a full resuscitation is most likely hypovolaemic. Dawes & Mott[105] and Brace[106] have all documented that blood volume is shifted to the placenta when a fetus experiences hypoxia. Using a fetal sheep model, Brace found that not only does the fetus shift blood to the placenta, but also it takes 30 minutes for the blood volume to return to normal once the hypoxic insult is removed.

Providers should be prepared for a full resuscitation at every birth, but it is more likely that an infant with a suspicious tracing will need a full resuscitation. These infants will be extremely floppy, pale, with wide open eyes (owing to poor tone) and sometimes with a significant bradycardia. If the baby is born at a traditional delivery table, the infant can be lowered significantly while being dried, stimulated and assessed. Lowering the infant or milking the cord (see below) facilitates faster volume expansion for these infants.

Babies with delayed cord clamping do take longer to breathe,[89] reflecting the gradual process of a natural transition. A lusty cry may not be heard and is not necessary at all. Observation of heart rate, cord pulsations, colour and tone can reassure that the transition is progressing well.

Infants with an Apgar score of 0 (who had a pulse in utero) are most likely so hypovolaemic that there is not adequate volume to perfuse the coronary arteries or to stimulate the heart to beat. Morley

and others advised that milking or stripping of the cord towards the infant in this case may be life saving.[107,108] If the cord is flat and bloodless, as it is in some cases of extreme fetal distress where there has been fetal–placental vasoconstriction, it may be necessary to clamp and cut the cord and prepare for immediate fluid replacement.[107] Fortunately, this is a very rare occurrence.

Milking or stripping the umbilical cord

Although a rare occurrence, delayed cord clamping is not always feasible at the time of birth. Milking or stripping the umbilical cord can offer a viable alternative in those situations when speed and time are critical factors. In eight controlled trials and one randomized controlled trial involving over 803 babies[44,108-115] cord milking has been shown to facilitate the rapid transfer of blood and red cell volume to the infant without causing harm. Hosono and colleagues[115] suggest that milking the cord is a safe, advantageous technique for pre-term infants. In their small preliminary study, 40 very-low-birth-weight infants were randomized into either an immediate cord clamping or cord milking group. The infants who received the cord milking had higher initial haemoglobins and were less likely to need a red cell transfusion during their hospital stay. Colozzi compared a group of 25 term infants who had cord milking after birth with a group of 25 term infants who were held at the level of the maternal perineum and had cord clamping after pulsations ceased.[108] Each infant in the cord milking group was placed below the level of the placenta and the cord was milked until it was limp and bloodless. This required four to eight slow methodical milkings. The group with cord milking had an average haemoglobin level of 18.6 g/dl at 24 hours while those in the delayed group had an average level of 17.5 g/dl. No adverse outcomes were reported in any of the infants. In this study, Colozzi described infants with 'asphyxia pallida' (asphyxiated and pale) on whom he performed cord milking with excellent results. If one is confronted with a pale, listless infant, then lowering the infant for 30 seconds or milking the cord may provide some volume expansion for the infant first before immediate clamping of the cord and rushing to the warmer (Case history 9.7).

Case history 9.7

Milking the cord (level II hospital)

A 37-year-old woman in her first pregnancy had a long labour with many mild variable decelerations and slow descent of the fetal head. Light to moderate meconium was suspected. After two hours of pushing, her epidural was lightened and she was positioned on a birthing stool for pushing. The infant descended rapidly, accompanied by a long deceleration down into the 80s. The mother was immediately assisted back to bed and placed on her hands and knees. The infant's head was born quickly and the nares and mouth were suctioned with a DeLee catheter. The infant was born spontaneously and was placed on a dry, clean pad between the mother's legs. The baby's vocal cords were visualized at the bedside and no meconium was seen. The midwife dried and stimulated the infant, whose heart beat was above 100 bpm; but the baby remained pale and toneless. The umbilical cord was extremely long and was not pulsating. After assessing that this infant was hypovolaemic and recognizing that the cord was not pulsating, the midwife milked the cord from the mother's introitus to the infant's umbilicus one time only. The infant immediately flexed all extremities, cried and became pink. The mother turned onto her back and the infant was placed skin-to-skin on the maternal abdomen with an intact cord. The infant proceeded to have an uneventful neonatal course, nursed very well and was thriving at four years of age. This was the first time the midwife had stripped a cord in over 20 years of practice.

Management of an infant who needs resuscitation at a water birth

Unresponsive infants at water births present some challenges that can be overcome creatively. One certified nurse-midwife who does births in water mentioned that she resuscitates at a water birth by having a small table next to the tub. If the baby is not responsive, she has the mother stand and then resuscitates the infant at the table with the cord intact. On the table, the infant is lower than the mother, which allows gravity to assist in the placental transfusion. Another person who teaches neonatal resuscitation stated that she trains those attending her courses to be able to use the bag and mask without necessarily having the infant on a flat surface. Bowman recommends holding the infant

with the face down just after birth so that fluids can drain, and wiping the face as a swimmer would coming out of the water (T. Bowman, personal communication, 2003).

Prevention of hypothermia

While prevention of hypothermia is an important part of neonatal resuscitation, it should not be used as an excuse or reason for immediate cord clamping. Infants with a full placental transfusion have been shown to have more stable temperatures than those with immediate clamping.[41] Infants maintain their temperature on the maternal abdomen as well as, or better than, in a warmer or isolette and there are many other benefits.[116] In some instances, concern about hypothermia is allowed to supersede all other considerations about a newborn. As a routine practice, separating the infant and mother may have undesired effects on other aspects of birth and infancy, including initiation of breastfeeding, parent–infant bonding and normal bacterial colonization that occurs with skin-to-skin contact.

Placement of the infant on the maternal abdomen

Many practitioners worry about blood loss or flow back into the placenta if they place an infant on the maternal abdomen. Figure 9.5 shows the amount of blood remaining in the placenta after delaying cord clamping for various times and holding the infant at different levels.[117] At three minutes after birth, an infant at the level of the maternal abdomen (10–20 cm above the perineum in a supine position) has received most of its placental transfusion if the uterus has contracted appropriately. Colozzi found that a group of infants placed on the maternal abdomen with the cord clamping delayed until pulsations ceased had the same haemoglobin levels at 24 hours (17.4 g/dl) and 72 hours (17.1 g/dl) as those infants kept at the maternal perineum until pulsations ceased.[108] However, there is one study that raised a concern for early cord clamping when the infant is placed on the maternal abdomen. Grisaru (et al) found that when the umbilical cord was cut at 30 seconds, he was able to collect more blood for harvesting if the infant was on the maternal abdomen than if the infant was below the level of

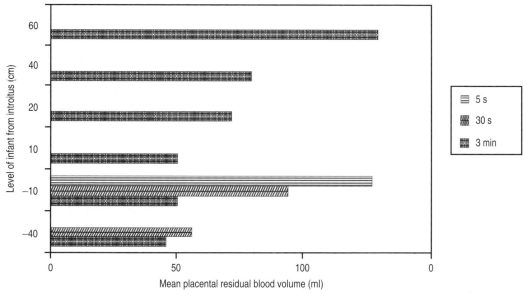

Fig 9.5 • Effect of gravity on placental transfusion at normal vaginal births.[117]

the introitus.[118] This is our rationale for not placing pale, toneless infants on the maternal abdomen immediately. Instead we recommend resuscitation at the perineum and placing the infant skin to skin when good tone, colour and breathing are present.

Active management of the third stage of labour

Recent evidence recommends active management of the third stage of labour (AMTSL) for the prevention of postpartum haemorrhage in the mother. Active management has been the routine use of uterotonics, controlled cord traction and the immediate cutting and clamping of the umbilical cord. The perceived conflict between delayed cord clamping and AMTSL is unnecessary and a realistic option is offered. The World Health Organization (WHO) has recently published recommendations to support a less rigid management of third stage in regards to cord clamping time.[119] Their recommendation states that, in AMTSL, 'the cord should not be clamped earlier than necessary for applying cord traction' (p 15).[119] For those care providers committed to AMTSL, this means a delay in cord clamping of approximately three minutes, which offers not only benefit to the baby but allows

an expeditious delivery of the placenta to avoid postpartum haemorrhage.

The concern that delayed cord clamping may lead to overtransfusing of the infant after administering a uterotonic in the third stage of labour is unsupported. Yao & Lind[78] demonstrated that the infant receives a maximum of 90 ml/kg (normal physiological volume) within the first few minutes after a uterotonic is administered, no matter how long the cord clamping is delayed.

The usual practice of immediate cord clamping as part of the active management of third stage has potential to cause harm by increasing the risk of anaemia of infancy. Delayed cord clamping is endorsed by the WHO and can easily be incorporated into any provider's practice of active management, resulting in benefit for both mother and infant.

Caring, healing and infant interaction issues

As parents will testify, infants come into the world with their own personalities. Not all scream or cry immediately. In fact, those with a gentle transition often do not cry (see Case history 9.1).[120] Some may be slower than others to face their new world.

As long as there is a good, strong heartbeat, it is safe to allow an infant some individuality at the time of transition. Newborns should be handled with a reassuringly strong but gentle touch and be comforted with calm soothing voices, including those of the parents. The fact that parents' voices encourage the baby's movement and its responses to the new environment has been witnessed by the authors and demonstrated by Condon & Sander.[121] They found that infants responded to the human voice with dance-like movements. Providers can teach parents about the importance of their voices to the infants at all times, but especially during resuscitation. If one has to do a full resuscitation, the infant will need comforting during its recovery time. This is best done at the breast. If the baby is not ready to nurse, he or she can be observed in the mother's arms or preferably skin to skin on the chest of either parent.[122] This can be done with monitors attached if indicated.

Cord blood gases: if and when to obtain the specimen

Arguments have been made for routine collection of cord blood gases as a risk management procedure.[123] Some European midwives have reported to the UK midwifery research electronic discussion list that local risk management policies require them to obtain cord blood gases at every birth. However, if the cord is cut to obtain gases, this measure may be counterproductive.[107] In fact, cord clamping for this purpose may increase the likelihood of a poor outcome by increasing the infant's risk of hypovolaemia, as it prevents the infant from obtaining blood volume and stem cells shown in animal studies to produce healing. If mandated, blood for gases can be obtained with a fine needle in an artery while the cord is still pulsing.[107] Venous blood can be obtained later when the cord is cut. Research is needed to document the process of blood gas equilibration over the first few minutes as the infant takes on independent life with an intact cord.

Cord blood harvesting

The American Academy of Pediatrics recommends cord blood harvesting only if there is a family member with a current or potential need for stem cell transplantation.[123] The initial policy also pointed out that immediate cord clamping may place an infant at risk of anaemia and deprivation of its placental transfusion, resulting in low blood volume. Parents should be informed of the value of delayed cord clamping and its potential impact on cord blood collection. Since there is evidence that haematopoietic stem cells produce dramatic healing in animal models, more research is needed on the value of retaining them in the infant's body at birth.

The need for suctioning at birth

Routine suctioning of the oropharynx and the stomach is another birth intervention adopted without adequate evidence. One study by Estol et al examined the routine suctioning of normal newborns.[124] They found that the quantity of suctioned fluid is minimal and far less than the total the infant needs to clear from the lungs. The study looked at respiratory resistance and lung compliance in babies at 10, 30 and 120 minutes after birth, and through hospital stay, and found no differences between the group suctioned versus the group not suctioned. They did find some risks associated with routine suctioning, which include bradycardia and cardiac rhythm disturbances. The issue of unnecessary cost was raised. Their findings show no evidence that routine suctioning of normal babies is beneficial. Lactation consultants question the practice of routine suctioning and find that vigorous suctioning can interfere with breastfeeding.

Conclusion

Immediate clamping of the umbilical cord is an intervention that disrupts the normal physiological processes that occur at birth. Adopted as a matter of convenience and without adequate consideration, it has the potential to cause harm. Immediate cord clamping can cause an unnecessarily abrupt and traumatic transition for the newborn. It limits the supply of blood that is vital to a successful transition and can lead to anaemia in infancy. Additionally, newborns are deprived of stem cells and other factors in the blood that may protect them from illness, injury or in yet unknown ways which may promote their normal, best potential development.

We contend that delaying cord clamping is the best practice until proven otherwise. Furthermore, we believe that it is a rare or even non-existent circumstance in which proper care of the newborn could not take place with the cord still intact. Difficulties caused by artificial assignations of turf and responsibilities should not be excused when, certainly, all parties have the benefit of the newborn most in mind.

Increasingly, the effects of hypovolaemia on newborn transition have and will become more evident. New insights into the value of stem cells and other factors present in blood will also help shape the final answer. As the potential for preventing harm is vast, research is critically needed to establish best practice. In the meantime, where evidence for practice is lacking, common sense, the value of maintaining normalcy and respect for the normal processes of birth and life must prevail.

References

1. Mercer J, Skovgaard R 2002 Neonatal transitional physiology: a new paradigm. J Perinat Neonatal Nurs 15:56–75

2. Darwin E 1801 Zoonomia, 3rd edn, vol III. Johnson, London, p 302

3. Linderkamp O L 1982 Placental transfusion: determinants and effects. Clin Perinatol 9:599

4. Grajeda R, Perez-Escamilla R, Dewey K G 1997 Delayed clamping of the umbilical cord improves hematologic status of Guatemalan infants at 2 mo of age. Am J Clin Nutr 65:425–431

5. Gupta R, Ramji S 2002 Effect of delayed cord clamping on iron stores in infants born to anemic mothers: a randomized controlled trial. Indian Pediatr 39:130–135

6. Geethanath R M, Ramji S, Thirupuram S et al 1997 Effect of timing of cord clamping on the iron status of infants at 3 months. Ind Pediatr 34:103–106

7. Oxford Midwives Research Group 1991 A study of the relationship between the delivery to cord clamping interval and the time of cord separation. Oxford Midwives Research Group. Midwifery 7:167–176

8. Nelson N, Enkin N W, Saigal S et al 1980 A randomized trial of the Leboyer approach to childbirth. New Engl J Med 302:655–660

9. Emhamed M O, van Rheenen P, Brabin B J 2004 The early effects of delayed cord clamping in term infants born to Libyan mothers. Trop Doct 34:218–222

10. Chaparro C M, Neufeld L M, Tena Alavez G et al 2006 Effect of timing of umbilical cord clamping on iron status in Mexican infants: a randomised controlled trial. Lancet 367:1997–2004

11. Cernadas J M C, Carroli G, Pellegrini L 2006 The effect of timing of cord clamping on neonatal venous hematocrit values and clinical outcome at term: a randomized controlled trial. Obstet Gynecol Surv 61:564–565

12. Nelle M, Zilow E P, Kraus M et al 1993 The effect of Leboyer delivery on blood viscosity and other hemorheologic parameters in term neonates. Am J Obstet Gynecol 169:189–193

13. Nelle M, Zilow E P, Bastert G et al 1995 Effect of Leboyer childbirth on cardiac output, cerebral and gastrointestinal blood flow velocities in full-term neonates. Am J Perinatol 12:212–216

14. Nelle M, Kraus M, Bastert G et al 1996 Effects of Leboyer childbirth on left- and right systolic time intervals in healthy term neonates. J Perinat Med 24:513–520

15. Linderkamp O, Nelle M, Kraus M et al 1992 The effect of early and late cord-clamping on blood viscosity and other hemorheological parameters in full-term neonates. Acta Paediatr 81:745–750

16. Kliot D, Silverstein L 1984 Changing maternal and newborn care: a study of the Leboyer approach to childbirth management. N Y State J Med 84:169–174

17. van Rheenen P, Brabin B J 2004 Late umbilical cord-clamping as an intervention for reducing iron deficiency anaemia in term infants in developing and industrialised countries: a systematic review. Ann Trop Paediatr 24:3–16

18. Hutton E K, Hassan E S 2007 Late vs early clamping of the umbilical cord in full-term neonates: systematic review and meta-analysis of controlled trials. JAMA 297:1241–1252

19. Mercer J, McGrath M M, Hensman A et al 2003 Immediate and delayed cord clamping in infants born between 24 and 32 weeks: a pilot randomized controlled trial. J Perinatol 23:466–472

20. Mercer J S, Vohr B R, McGrath M M et al 2006 Delayed cord clamping in very preterm infants reduces the incidence of intraventricular hemorrhage and late-onset sepsis: a randomized, controlled trial. Pediatrics 117:1235–1242

21. Aladangady N, McHugh S, Aitchison T C et al 2006 Infants' blood volume in a controlled trial of placental transfusion at preterm delivery. Pediatrics 117:93–98

22. Baenziger O, Stolkin F, Keel M et al 2007 The influence of the timing of cord clamping on postnatal cerebral oxygenation in preterm neonates: a randomized, controlled trial. Pediatrics 119:455–459

23. Ultee K, Swart J, van der Deure H et al 2007 Delayed cord clamping in preterm infants delivered at 34 to 36 weeks gestation: a randomized controlled trial. Arch Dis Child Fetal Neonatal Ed; Feb 16:[Epub]

24. Strauss R G, Mock D M, Johnson K et al 2003 Circulating RBC volume, measured with biotinylated RBCs, is superior to the Hct to document the hematologic effects of delayed versus immediate umbilical cord clamping in preterm neonates. Transfusion 43:1168–1172

25. Oh W , Carlo W A, Fanaroff A A et al 2002 Delayed cord clamping in extremely low birth weight infants – a pilot randomized controlled trial. Pediatr Res 51:365–366

26. Ibrahim H M, Krouskop R W, Lewis D F et al 2000 Placental transfusion: umbilical cord clamping and preterm infants. J Perinatol 20:351–354

27. Rabe H, Wacker A, Hulskamp G et al 2000 A randomised controlled trial of delayed cord clamping in very low birth weight preterm infants. Eur J Pediatr 159:775–777

28. Nelle M, Fischer S, Conze S et al 1998 Effects of later cord clamping on circulation in prematures [abstract]. Pediatr Res 44:420

29. Rabe H, Wacker A, Hulskamp G et al 1998 Late cord clamping benefits extrauterine adaptation. Pediatr Res 44:454

30. Narenda A, Beckett C A T, Kyle E et al 1998 Is it possible to promote placental transfusion at preterm delivery? Pediatr Res 44:453

31. McDonnell M, Henderson-Smart D J 1997 Delayed umbilical cord clamping in preterm infants: a feasibility study. J Paediatr Child Health 33:308–310

32. Kinmond S, Aitchison T C, Holland B M et al 1993 Umbilical cord clamping and preterm infants: a randomized trial. BMJ 306:172–175

33. Hofmeyr G J, Bolton K D, Bowen D C et al 1988 Periventricular/intraventricular haemorrhage and umbilical cord clamping. Findings and hypothesis. S Afr Med J 73:104–106

34. Hofmeyr G J, Gobetz L, Bex P J et al 1993 Periventricular/intraventricular hemorrhage following early and delayed umbilical cord clamping. A randomized controlled trial. Online J Curr Clin Trials; Doc No 110:[2002 words; 26 paragraphs]

35. Rabe H, Reynolds G, Diaz-Rossello J 2004 Early versus delayed umbilical cord clamping in preterm infants. Cochrane Database Syst Rev, Issue 4. Art. No.: CD003248. DOI: 10.1002/14651858.CD003248.pub2

36. Wardrop C A J, Holland B M 1995 The roles and vital importance of placental blood to the newborn infant. J Perinat Med 23:139–143

37. Yao A C, Moinian M, Lind J 1969 Distribution of blood between infant and placenta after birth. Lancet 2(7626):871–873

38. Jones J G, Holland B M, Hudson I R et al 1990 Total circulating red cells versus haematocrit as the primary descriptor of oxygen transport by the blood. Br J Haematol 76:288–294

39. Faxelius G, Raye J, Gutberlet R et al 1977 Red cell volume measurements and acute blood loss in high-risk newborn infants. J Pediatr 90:273–281

40. Buckels L J, Usher R 1965 Cardiopulmonary effects of placental transfusion. J Pediatr 67:239–246

41. Oh W, Lind J 1966 Venous and capillary hematocrit in newborn infants and placental transfusion. Acta Paediatr Scand 55:38–48

42. Oh W, Lind J 1967 Body temperature of the newborn infant in relation to placental transfusion. Acta Paediatr Scand 172S:137–145

43. Pietra G G, D'Amodio M D, Leventhall M M et al 1968 Electron microscopy of cutaneous capillaries of newborn infants: effects of placental transfusion. Pediatrics 42:678–683

44. Usher R, Shephard M, Lind J 1963 The blood volume of the newborn infant and placental transfusion. Acta Paediatr 52:497–512

45. Oh W, Oh M A, Lind J 1966 Renal function and blood volume in newborn infants related to placental transfusion. Acta Paediatr Scand 55:197–210

46. Hankins G D, Loen S, Fei A F et al 2000 Neonatal organ system injury in acute birth asphyxia sufficient to result in neonatal encephalopathy. Obstet Gynecol 99:668–691

47. Saigal S, O'Neill A, Surainder Y et al 1972 Placental transfusion and hyperbilirubinemia in the premature. Pediatrics 49:406–419

48. Saigal S, Usher R H 1977 Symptomatic neonatal plethora. Biol Neonate 32:62–72

49. Cordero L, Treuer S H, Landon M B et al 1998 Management of infants of diabetic mothers. Arch Pediatr Adolesc Med 152:249–254

50. Tenovuo A 1988 Neonatal complications in small-for-gestational-age neonates. J Perinat Med 16(3):197–203

51. Kurlat I, Sola A 1992 Neonatal polycythemia in appropriately grown infants of hypertensive mothers. Acta Pediatr 81:662–664

52. Rao R, Tkac I, Townsend E L et al 2006 Perinatal iron deficiency predisposes the developing rat hippocampus to greater injury from mild to moderate hypoxia-ischemia. J Cereb Blood Flow Metab 27:729–740

53. Kattwinkel J (ed.) 2006 Textbook of neonatal resuscitation, 5th edn. American Academy of Pediatrics and American Heart Association, Washington, DC

54. Mercer J 2001 Best evidence: a review of the literature on umbilical cord clamping. J Midwifery Womens Health 46:402–414

55. Mercer J, Nelson C, Skovgaard R 2000 Umbilical cord clamping: beliefs and practices of American nurse-midwives. J Midwifery Womens Health 45:58–66

56. Schorn M N, Blanco J D 1991 Management of the nuchal cord. J Nurse Midwifery 36:131–132

57. Wiswell T E, Gannon C M, Jacob J et al 2000 Delivery room management of the apparently vigorous meconium-stained neonate: results of the multicenter, international collaborative trial. Pediatrics 105:1–7

58. Walsh-Sukys M C, Tyson J E, Wright L L et al 2000 Persistent pulmonary hypertension of the newborn in the era before nitric oxide: practice variation and outcomes. Pediatrics 105:14–20

59. Cowan F, Rutherford M, Groenendaal F et al 2003 Origin and timing of brain lesions in term infants with neonatal encephalopathy. Lancet 361:736–742

60. Nelson K B, Grether J K 1998 Potentially asphyxiating conditions and spastic cerebral palsy in infants of normal birth weight. Am J Obstet Gynecol 179:507–513

61. Anon 2003 Autism: the number of children afflicted has increased tenfold in the last 10 years. The Providence Sunday Journal, 9 Feb

62. Singhal N, Niermeyer S 2006 Neonatal resuscitation where resources are limited. Clin Perinatol 33:219–228, x–xi

63. Algarin C, Peirano P, Garrido M et al 2003 Iron deficiency anemia in infancy: long-lasting effects on auditory and visual system functioning. Pediatr Res 53:217–223

64. Lozoff B, Beard J, Connor J et al 2006 Long-lasting neural and behavioral effects of iron deficiency in infancy. Nutr Rev 64:S34–43, discussion S72–91

65. Felt B T, Beard J L, Schallert T et al 2006 Persistent neurochemical and behavioral abnormalities in adulthood despite early iron supplementation for perinatal iron deficiency anemia in rats. Behav Brain Res 171: 261–270

66. Lozoff B, Georgieff M K 2006 Iron deficiency and brain development. Semin Pediatr Neurol 13:158–165

67. Nelson K B, Dambrosia J M, Grether J K et al 1998 Neonatal cytokines and coagulation factors in children with cerebral palsy. Ann Neurol 44:665–675

68. Rajnik M, 2001 Early cytokine expression induced by hemorrhagic shock in a non-resuscitated rat model. Pediatr Res 49:44A

69. Rajnik M, Salkowski C A, Thomas K E et al 2002 Induction of early inflammatory gene expression in a murine model of nonresuscitated, fixed-volume hemorrhage. Shock 17:322–328

70. Haneline L S, Marshall K P, Clapp D W 1996 The highest concentration of primitive hematopoietic progenitor cells in cord blood is found in extremely premature infants. Pediatr Res 39:820–825

71. Moise K J Jr 2005 Umbilical cord stem cells. Obstet Gynecol 106:1393–1407

72. Meier C, Middelanis J, Wasielewski B et al 2006 Spastic paresis after perinatal brain damage in rats is reduced by human cord blood mononuclear cells. Pediatr Res 59:244–249

73. American Heart Association 2005 American Heart Association guidelines for cardiopulmonary resuscitation and emergency cardiovascular care. Circulation 112:1–203

74. Ewy G A, Kern K B, Sanders A B et al 2006 Cardiocerebral resuscitation for cardiac arrest. Am J Med 119:6–9

75. Teitel D 1998 Physiologic development of the cardiovascular system in the fetus. In: Polin R A, Fox W (eds) Fetal and neonatal physiology. W B Saunders, Philadephia, PA

76. Stembera Z K, Hodr J, Janda J 1965 Umbilical blood flow in healthy newborn infants during the first minutes after birth. Am J Obstet Gynecol 91:568–574

77. Stembera Z K, Hodr J, Janda J 1968 Umbilical blood flow in newborn infants who suffered intrauterine hypoxia. Am J Obstet Gynecol 101:546–553

78. Yao A C, Hirvensalo M, Lind J 1968 Placental transfusion-rate and uterine contraction. Lancet 1(7539):380–383

79. Yao A C, Lind J 1974 Blood flow in the umbilical vessels during the third stage of labor. Biol Neonate 25: 186–193

80. Gunther M 1957 The transfusion between baby and placenta in the minutes after birth. Lancet ii:505–508

81. Bouchard S, Johnson M P, Flake A W et al 2002 The EXIT procedure: experience and outcome in 31 cases. J Pediatr Surg 37:418–426

82. Jaykka S 1958 Capillary erection and the structural appearance of fetal and neonatal lungs. Acta Paediatr 47:484–500

83. Jaykka S 1957 Capillary erection and lung expansion; an experimental study of the effect of liquid pressure applied to the capillary network of excised fetal lungs. Acta Paediatr 46(suppl 112):1–91

84. Dunsmore S E, Rannels D E 1996 Extracellular matrix biology in the lung. Am J Physiol 270:L3–L27

85. Wasowicz M, Biczysko W, Marszalek A et al 1998 Ultrastructural studies on selected elements of the extracellular matrix in the developing rat lung alveolus. Folia Histochem Cytobiol 36:3–13

86. Clark R, Slutsky A, Gertsmann D 2000 Lung protective strategies of ventilation in the neonate: what are they? Pediatrics 105:112–114

87. Rigatto H 1998 Control of breathing in fetal life and onset and control of breathing in the neonate. In: Polin R, Fox W (eds) Fetal and neonatal physiology, 2nd edn. W B Saunders, Philadelphia, PA

88. Caldeyro-Barcia R, Alvarez H, Reynolds S 1950 A better understanding of uterine contractility through simultaneous recording with an internal and a seven channel external method. Surg Gynecol Obstet 91:641–646

89. Oh W, Lind J, Gessner I H 1966 The circulatory and respiratory adaptation to early and late cord clamping in newborn infants. Acta Paediatr Scand 55:17–25

90. Baier R J, Hasan S U, Cates D B et al 1990 Effects of various concentrations of O2 and umbilical cord occlusion on fetal breathing and behavior. J Appl Physiol 68:1597–1604

91. Larson J D, Rayburn W F, Harlan V L 1997 Nuchal cord entanglements and gestational age. Am J Perinatol 14:555–557

92. Cashore W J, Usher R 1973 Hypovolemia resulting from a tight nuchal cord at birth. Pediatr Res 7:399

93. Shepherd A J, Richardson C J, Brown J P 1985 Nuchal cord as a cause of neonatal anemia. Am J Dis Child 139:71–73

94. Osak R, Webster K M, Bocking A D et al 1997 Nuchal cord evident at birth impacts on fetal size relative to that of the placenta. Early Hum Dev 49:193–202

95. Hope P, Breslin S, Lamont L et al 1998 Fatal shoulder dystocia: a review of 56 cases reported to the Confidential Enquiry into Stillbirths and Deaths in Infancy. Br J Obstet Gynaecol 105:1256–1261

96. Corff K E, McCann D L 2005 Room air resuscitation versus oxygen resuscitation in the delivery room. J Perinat Neonatal Nurs 19:379–390

97. Iffy L, Varadi V 1994 Cerebral palsy following cutting of the nuchal cord before delivery. Med Law 13:323–330

98. Iffy L, Varadi V, Papp E 2001 Untoward neonatal sequelae deriving from cutting of the umbilical cord before delivery. Med Law 20:627–634

99. Flamm B L 1999 Tight nuchal cord and shoulder dystocia: a potentially catastrophic combination. Obstet Gynecol 94:853

100. Halliday H L, Sweet D 2001 Endotracheal intubation at birth for preventing morbidity and mortality in vigorous, meconium-stained infants born at term. Cochrane Database Syst Rev, Issue 1. Art. No.: CD000500. DOI: 10.1002/14651858.CD000500

101. Ghidini A, Spong C T 2001 Severe meconium aspiration syndrome is not caused by aspiration of meconium. Am J Obstet Gynecol 185:931–938

102. Kizilican F, Karnak F, Tanyel C et al 1994 In utero defecation of the nondistressed fetus: roentgen study in the goat. J Pediatr Surg 29:1487–1490

103. Thureen P J, Hall D M, Hoffenberg A et al 1997 Fatal meconium aspiration in spite of appropriate perinatal airway management: pulmonary and placental evidence of prenatal disease. Am J Obstet Gynecol 176:967–975

104. Velaphi S, Vidyasagar D 2006 Intrapartum and postdelivery management of infants born to mothers with meconium-stained amniotic fluid: evidence-based recommendations. Clin Perinatol 33:29–42, v–vi

105. Dawes G S, Mott J C 1964 Changes in O2 distribution and consumption in foetal lambs with variations in umbilical blood flow. J Physiol 170:524–540

106. Brace R A 1986 Fetal blood volume responses to acute fetal hypoxia. Am J Obstet Gynecol 155:889–893

107. Morley G M 1998 Cord closure: can hasty clamping injure the newborn? OBG Management 7:29–36

108. Colozzi A 1954 Clamping of the umbilical cord: its effect on the placental transfusion. New Engl J Med 250:629–632

109. McCausland A, Holmes F, Schumann W 1949 Management of cord and placental blood and its effect upon the newborn: Part 1. California Medicine 71:190–196

110. Siddall R, Crissey R, Knapp W 1952 Effects of cesarean section babies of stripping or milking of the umbilical cord. Am J Obstet Gynecol 63:1059–1064

111. Siddall R S, Richardson R P 1953 Milking or stripping the umbilical cord; effect on vaginally delivered babies. Obstet Gynecol 1:230–233

112. Whipple G A, Sisson T R, Lund C J 1957 Delayed ligation of the umbilical cord; its influence on the blood volume of the newborn. Obstet Gynecol 10:603–610

113. Lanzkowsky P 1960 Effects of early and late clamping of umbilical cord on infant's haemoglobin level. Br Med J 5215:1777–1782

114. Walsh S Z 1969 Early clamping versus stripping of cord: comparative study of electrocardiogram in neonatal period. Br Heart J 31:122–126

115. Hosono S, Mugishima H, Fujita H et al 2007 Umbilical cord milking reduces the need for red cell transfusions and improves neonatal adaptation in infants born less than 29 weeks' gestation: a randomized controlled trial. Arch Dis Child Fetal Neonatal Ed, 29 Jan:[Epub]

116. Fardig J 1980 A comparison of skin-to-skin contact and radiant heaters in promoting neonatal thermoregulation. J Nurse Midwifery 25:19–28

117. Yao A C, Lind J 1969 Effect of gravity on placental transfusion. Lancet 2(7619):505–508

118. Grisaru D, Deutsch V, Pick M et al 1999 Placing the newborn on the maternal abdomen after delivery increases the volume and CD34 cell content in the umbilical cord blood collected: an old maneuver with new applications. Am J Obstet Gynecol 180:1240–1243

119. World Health Organization 2007 Recommendations for the prevention of postpartum haemorrhage. World Health Organization, Geneva

120. Leboyer F 2002 Birth without violence. Revised edition of the classic. Healing Arts Press, Rochester, VT

121. Condon W S, Sander L W 1974 Synchrony demonstrated between movements of the neonate and adult speech. Child Dev 45:456–462

122. Anderson G C, Dombrowski M A, Swinth J Y 2001 Kangaroo care: not just for stable preemies anymore. Reflect Nurs Leadersh 27:32–34, 45

123. American Academy of Pediatrics 1999 Cord blood banking for potential future transplantation: subject review. Pediatrics 104:116–118

124. Estol P C, Piriz H, Basalo S et al 1992 Oro-naso-pharyngeal suction at birth: effects on respiratory adaptation of normal term vaginally born infants. J Perinatal Med 20:297–305

Level IA. Systematic reviews: 2 found

Hutton & Hassan 2007[18]

Concluded that delayed cord clamping of at least two minutes resulted in improved iron stores at six months of age and that the polycythaemia that may occur as a result of delayed cord clamping is benign.

van Rheenen & Brabin 2004[17]

Concluded that delayed cord clamping in term infants increases haemoglobin at two to three months of age and reduces the risk of anaemia without increasing perinatal complications.

Level IB. Randomized controlled trials: 8 found

Authors, year	Study population	Cord management, placement of infant	Sample size	Significant results	Comments
Chaparro et al 2006[10] (Mexico)	Women 37 to 42 weeks, early labour, singleton pregnancy, vaginal birth, normal pregnancies, plan to breastfeed for 6 months, no smokers, no IUGR or major anomalies (excluded after birth)	EC: at 10s (x = 16.5s) DC: at 2 min (x = 94s) Level: at the uterus	171 187	Primary outcome: at 6mo, DC infants had higher MCV (79.5 fl vs. 81 fl, $p = 0.001$), ferritin (51 µg/L vs. 34 µg/L, $p = 0.0002$) and total body iron (48mg/kg vs. 44mg/kg, $p = 0.0003$) than EC infants	Largest study to date to look at any long-term outcomes. Conservative in that they used only a two minute delay. No significant differences in Hgb or Hct at 6mo although differences evident in the newborn period (Hct 60% vs. 62%, $p = .003$). Significantly higher ferritin and total body iron at 6mo of age. No harmful effects seen
Cernadas et al 2006[11] (Argentina)	Term infants, no complications Normal pregnancies with vag and C/Sec births	EC: within 15 s IC: at 1 min DC: 3 min	93 91 92	Hct > 70: EC 8% vs. DC 13%, $p < 0.15$. Jaundice: EC 14% vs. DC 17%, $p \le 0.36$. Venous Hcts at 6h were: EC 53.5%, IC 57% and DC 59%. Hct < 45 higher with EC (9%). At 24–48h, 16.9% of infants with EC had Hct < 45% (RR 0.13–0.2)	No harmful effects were seen. Hct > 65 was highest in DC (14.1%) but no clinical symptoms

171

Level IB. Randomized controlled trials: 8 found

Authors, year	Study population	Cord management, placement of infant	Sample size	Significant results	Comments
Emhamed et al 2004[9] (Libya)	BW > 2500 g, 37–42 weeks, singletons, excluded for major congenital anomalies, maternal complications, tight nuchal cord, need for resuscitation	EC: immediate DC: after cord stopped pulsating Oxytocic after CC	45 57	DC infants had significantly higher Hct (53% vs. 49%, $p = 0.004$) and Hgb (17.1 g/dl vs. 18.5 g/dl, $p = 0.0005$) Three DC infants had polycythaemia with no symptoms; two EC infants needed phototherapy	No perinatal complications from DC in this study
Gupta & Ramji 2002[5] (India)	Infants born to anaemic mothers (Hgb < 10 g/dl), vag delivery, no resuscitation needed at birth, no major congenital anomalies	EC: immediately LC: when placenta descended into vagina Infant held 0–10 cm below introitus	53 49	29 infants in each group followed to 3 months of age (58 total) At 3 months of age, infants with LC had higher serum ferritin levels (118 (g/L vs. 73 g/L, $p = 0.001$) OR for anaemia at 3 mo was 7.7 times higher for the EC group	EC infants weighed 2707 g, LC infants 2743 g Iron stores in neonates born to anaemic mothers can be improved by LC (BR and polycythaemia not addressed)
Grajeda et al 1997[4] (Guatemala)	≥37 weeks, ≥2000 g, singleton vaginal deliveries, no GD, AP haemorrhage, CPD or other anomalies	EC: immediately LC: at end of pulsation, infant at level of placenta LC: after pulsations, infant held below introitus	21 26 22	At 2 mo, 88% of infants with delayed CC had Hct > 0.33 versus 42% in the early group ($p = 0.001$) No differences between two late groups	Recommends delay in CC as a feasible low-cost intervention that can reduce anaemia in developing countries No differences in polycythaemia or jaundice Two babies with Hct > 70% were asymptomatic
Geethanath et al 1997[6] (India)	Term, vaginal births, mothers with Hgb > 10 g/dl	EC: immediately LC: after placenta in vagina; infant lowered < 10 cm	48 59	Mean ferritin higher in LC: 73.6 ng/ml vs. 55.7 ng/ml but did not reach significance level as set by PI	Set difference for significance at 30 ng/ml of ferritin Did not report other variables

Level IB. Randomized controlled trials: 8 found

Authors, year	Study population	Cord management, placement of infant	Sample size	Significant results	Comments
Oxford Midwives Research Group 1991[7] (England)	37–42 weeks, vertex, vag delivery, no AP complications	EC: stat or ≤1 min LC: after 3 min or when pulsations stopped, infant on abdomen	256 296	No significant difference in any variable except higher rates of continued BF at 10–12 days among mothers in LC group ($p = 0.05$)	Largest sample studied No significant difference in jaundice Highest BR levels = 12 mg/dl 32 babies in LC group had early clamping (intent-to-treat analysis)
Nelson et al 1980[8] (Canada)	Low OB risk, > 37 weeks, wanted Leboyer birth, would attend prenatal classes	EC: < 60 s LC: after pulsations ceased, baby on maternal abdomen	26 28	No differences in any variable except mothers' opinion at 8 mo that the birth influenced the child's behaviour ($p = 0.05$)	Found that Leboyer method was not unsafe Found no differences in polycythaemia or jaundice

AP, antepartum; BF, breastfeeding; BR, bilirubin; BW, birth weight; CC, cord clamping; CPD, cephalopelvic disproportion; C/Sec, caesarean section; DC, delayed clamping; EC, early clamping; GD, gestational diabetes; Hct, haematocrit; Hgb, haemoglobin; IC, immediate cord clamping; IUGR, intrauterine growth restriction; LC, late clamping; MCV, mean corpuscular volume; OB, obstetric; OR, odds ratio; PI, principal investigator; RR, relative risk; vag, vaginal.

Level IIa. Well-designed controlled studies: 5 found

Authors, year	Study population	Cord management, placement of infant	Sample size	Significant results	Comments
Nelle et al 1996[14]	30 FT neonates from normal pregnancies and labours, vag births	EC: < 10 s LC: > 3 min, infant on maternal abdomen	15 15	Hcts were higher in LC ($p < 0.05$) Pre-ejection period ratios indicated higher systemic and pulmonary resistance on day 1 and same as EC babies on day 5	Findings suggest more pronounced pulmonary vasodilatation in the LC group in the first 5 days
Nelle et al 1995[13]	30 FT neonates from normal pregnancies and labours, vag births	EC: < 10 s LC: > 3 min, infant on maternal abdomen	15 15	LC: BV 32% higher Blood viscosity increased at 4h by 32%, vascular hindrance 25% lower, RBC flow to brain and intestines 25% higher on day 1 and 10% higher on day 5	Higher viscosity offset by lower vascular hindrance (marked vasodilatation) Authors state EC deprives infants of placental transfusions and increases risk of hypovolaemia and anaemia

Level IIa. Well-designed controlled studies: 5 found

Authors, year	Study population	Cord management, placement of infant	Sample size	Significant results	Comments
Nelle et al 1993[12]	Healthy, term, vag deliveries, pH ≥ 7.25, Apgar scores 9/10, all breastfed	EC: <10 s	15	RPBV higher in EC infants	Example: for 3 kg infant: EC = 135 ml in placenta, 210 ml in baby
		LC: > 3 min, infant on maternal abdomen (Leboyer method)	15	Hct rose from 49% at birth to 58% at 2 h, 56% at 24 h, and 54% at 120 h	LC = 75 ml in placenta, 270 ml in baby
					(See Nelle et al 1995 above for discussion of viscosity)
				Viscosity increased by 32% in LC at 2 h with no further change	
Linderkamp et al 1992[15]	39–40 weeks, normal	EC: <10 s	15	RPBV = 15 vs. 47 ml/kg in EC	LC results in marked rise of blood viscosity due to fluid shifting out of vascular space
	EFM, vag delivery, pH > 7.25, Apgars 9/10, AGA, 3390–3620 g	LC: at 3 min, infant held at introitus	15	Hct increased at 2 h	No infants developed any clinical symptoms
				Blood viscosity at 2 h 40% higher	(See Nelle et al 1995 above for discussion of viscosity)
				3/15 with elevated BR over 15 mg/dl	
				All breastfed	
Kliot & Silverstein 1984[16]	Normal FT infants, vag births, from private practice	EC: < 60 s and on maternal abdomen	39	No significant difference in temperature, heart rate, Hct, BR, pH, Apgar scores or other variables	Completed random assignment to two Leboyer groups
		LC: > 10 min and on maternal abdomen	40		Validated safety of Leboyer-type delivery
		Control: CC < 60 s			

AGA, average gestational age; BR, bilirubin; BV, blood volume; CC, cord clamping; EC, early clamping; EFM, electronic fetal monitoring; FT, full term; Hct, haematocrit; LC, late clamping; RBC, red blood cell; RPBV, residual placental blood volume; vag, vaginal.

Promoting normal birth: weighing the evidence

Denis Walsh

Chapter contents

Introduction

This chapter will first examine the contemporary context of childbirth in which evidence is applied, tracing some seminal influences and trends over the past 30 years. The evidence on the contribution that providers and processes of care make to promote normal birth will then be discussed in some detail, focusing on aspects where a range of good quality evidence currently exists, or where significant questions remain to be answered. This includes the organization of midwifery care; belief systems about childbirth; place of birth; response to the latent phase of labour; approaches to the pushing/bearing down phase of labour; and systematic approaches to improving childbirth.

What is happening to childbearing women?

Recent surveys of low-risk primigravid women across the developed world reveal high rates of childbirth interventions. In the UK, Downe et al's survey of low-risk first time mothers showed that only 17% could be said to have laboured physiologically[1] and Mead's review of midwife-led cases found wide discrepancies in epidural rates (14–51%) and labour augmentation rates (38–57%) among maternity units in different geographical settings.[2]

In the USA, a major survey of women discovered excessive rates of electronic fetal monitoring (93%) and epidural analgesia (63%).[3] In addition, 71% laboured on beds and vaginal birth rates were as low as 64%, with a caesarean rate approaching 30%.

Finally, in Australia, less than 50% of women in the public system give birth without labour interventions and less than 25% in the private system.[4]

This is, in part, because of the wide scale hospitalization of birth across the Western world and the almost universal adoption of monitoring and intervention technologies. In recent decades, the assumption that the increased use of technology has been responsible for a decline in mortality rates has been challenged.[5,6] In the field of maternity care, there has been a long history of critique.[7-10] By the late 1980s, an accumulating body of research evidence in the Cochrane Collaboration Database highlighted the benefits and hazards of routine maternity interventions.[11] In 1985, The World Health Organization expressed concerns about rising intervention rates in childbirth[12] and developed standards to achieve normal birth.[13]

In addition, over many years women have complained about impersonal care, lack of continuity of carer, long waiting times,[14] unnecessary use of interventions and lack of explanation in labour.[15,16] As Chalmers et al pointed out, obstetricians were particularly vulnerable to lay criticism, as pregnant women were less willing to adopt the sick role.[17]

There has been a long sad history of unevaluated interventions in the area of reproductive health. Specific examples include the link between X-rays in early pregnancy and childhood leukaemia, and that of disease in the children of diethylstilbestrol.[16] Simultaneously, along with technological change, there is an increasing public mistrust of these developments and of professional expertise. Consumer groups in the UK express concern that technological interventions in childbirth are increasing at a relentless pace, in spite of government policy advocating otherwise, both in the UK[18] and in North America.[19]

Maternity pressure groups and midwifery interest groups have highlighted a number of factors in the context of these changes. For example, the UK Association for Improvements in Maternity Services (AIMS) has reported that some student midwives have come to the end of their training without seeing a normal birth. In Chapter 4 of this work, Beverley Lawrence Beech of AIMS and Belinda Phipps of the National Childbirth Trust set out women's perceptions of the importance of straightforward birth. Central to this debate is the concept of 'normality'. As they discuss, there have been a number of reports and initiatives on normal birth from official bodies such as the World Health Organization and the UK Royal College of Midwives. The definition of normality varies across these documents. The account given in Chapter 4 also notes that women are often categorized as having a normal birth despite experiencing several major childbirth interventions, including induction and augmentation of labour, artificial rupture of membranes, epidural analgesia and episiotomy. It appears that the vast majority of women are not experiencing physiological birth in the UK today. It is likely that this is a feature of technocratic childbirth across the world. The next section addresses the implications of this phenomenon.

The impact of childbirth on mothers, their babies and their families

Women remember what happened to them during childbirth,[20] either with joy and a sense of empowerment, or of dread and disempowerment.[21] Some women suffer the after-effects of post-traumatic stress.[22] Higher levels of obstetric intervention have been shown to be an important factor in predicting a negative experience.[23] While there have been some systematic attempts to measure the relationship between obstetric interventions and psychological morbidity,[24] findings tend to vary, with some studies identifying an association with depression and anxiety and a poor relationship with the baby, and others showing no such effect. This could be due to different outcome measures, timing of measurement, the demographics of the population studied, sample size and women's perceptions of the intrusiveness of the intervention. In addition, it seems to be important to include women's views of how they feel about an intervention, rather than just assuming that technology is always unwelcome.

One level of critique has been aimed at the differing philosophical underpinning of normal and technological birth, conceptualized as a social versus biomedical model. Among others, Davis-Floyd has summarized contrasting attributes of these models (Box 10.1).[25]

Box 10.1

Models of childbirth

Technocratic model of birth	Holistic model of birth
Male perspective	Female perspective
Woman = object	Woman = subject
Classifying, separate approach	Holistic, integrated approach
Body = machine	Body = organism
Female body = defective machine	Female body = healthy organism
Pregnancy and birth inherently pathological	Pregnancy and birth inherently healthy
Hospital = factory	Home = nurturing environment
Baby = product	Mother/baby inseparable unit
Fetus is separate from mother	Baby and mother are one
Best interests of mother and baby antagonistic	Good for mother = good for baby
Supremacy of technology	Sufficiency of nature
Institution = significant social unit	Family = essential social unit
Action based on facts, measurements	Action based on body/intuition
Only technical knowledge is valued	Experiential and emotional knowledge valued as highly
Labour = mechanical process	Labour = a flow of experience
Time is important; adherence to time charts during labour is essential	Time is irrelevant; the flow of a woman's experience is important
Once labour begins, it should progress steadily, if it does not, intervention is necessary	Labour can stop and start, follow its own rhythms of speeding or slowing
Medical intervention necessary in all births	Facilitation (food, positioning, support) is appropriate, medical intervention is usually inappropriate
Environmental ambience is not relevant	Environmental ambience is key to safe birth
Woman in bed hooked up to machines with frequent exams by staff is appropriate	Woman doing what she feels like (movement, sexual play, eating, sleeping) is appropriate
Labour pain is problematic and unacceptable	Labour pain is acceptable, normal
Analgesia/anaesthesia for pain during labour	Mind/body integration, labour support for pain
Birth = a service medicine owns and supplies to society	Birth = an activity a woman does that brings new life
Obstetrician = supervisor/manager/skilled technician, responsibility is the doctor's	Midwife = skilled guide, responsibility is the mother's
The doctor/midwife delivers the baby	The mother births the baby

(Davis-Floyd, p 160–161)[26]

Though articulating contrasting models may help to tease out why practitioners and systems of care render care in the way they do, it is too inflexible as an analysis for explaining increasing intervention rates. Individuals and systems are more complex than that. Recent years have seen an increasing criticism of binary classification made in this way.[27]

It is far more helpful to examine the research on place of birth, style of care, beliefs/philosophies and practices to ascertain what they tell us about how care should be organized and implemented. The rest of this chapter will review the evidence in these areas. But first, some introductory comments shall be made about the nature of evidence.

The evidence paradigm

Evidence is commonly held to be about the application of research findings to practice in the main, though its original exponents acknowledged that clinical experience and patient preferences also played a part in clinical decision making.[28] Less common is the view that anthropology, archaeology, common sense and organizational scale could contribute to evidence. These sources will be alluded to during the forthcoming discussion. They are included because decision making in practice is a complex affair and it is misleading to reduce it to a linear process between research findings and practice (see Ch. 1).

Organization of midwifery care

Continuity during birth

The term *continuity* is multi-layered. It has been used to mean: [29]

- a stated commitment to a shared philosophy of care (continuity of care)
- a commitment to streamline information processes so that all providers have access to relevant client data and history (informational continuity)
- the actual provision of care by the same caregiver or small group of caregivers (continuity of carer)
- consistent place of care (situational continuity).

The research findings are muddied by using these terms interchangeably and mixing these models together in evaluation studies and reviews. It is probably most helpful to start with schemes that deliver care by the same caregiver or small group of caregivers (continuity of carer) in tightly defined ways. Continuous support during labour and birth falls into this category.

Organizationally, studies in this area are relatively straightforward to set up as randomized controlled trials (RCTs), as the independent variable is the presence or not of a labour companion from the beginning to the end of the labour. Some women in published studies of continuity of care in labour also received care from midwives, nurses or doctors other than their lead caregiver. These individuals conducted observations and undertook labour procedures if these were indicated. However, they were only intermittently present to the women.

Over the past 25 years, many RCTs have been done in this area. The relevant Cochrane review notes a number of positive findings, with one consistent result across studies, namely a reduction in caesarean section rates for women randomized to the continuity of carer arm.[30] The only exception to this was Hodnett et al's study of nine north American hospitals which had extremely interventionist practices.[31] The effect of these on the birth environment, it was concluded by the researchers, confounded results. Although continuous support for labour remains one of the few forms of care that demonstrably lowers caesarean section rates, Hodnett's study suggests that unsupportive contexts may mediate the strength of this effect.

Another important dimension to the labour support studies was the finding that continuity of carer provided by untrained (lay) females seemed more effective than care from medically trained attendants, suggesting both gender and professionalizing influences on effectiveness.[32]

Recently, the numbers of carers a woman has during her period of continuous support has been shown to be relevant to outcomes. The caesarean section rate appears to increase in direct line with increasing number of carers.[33] The researchers recommend keeping the number of changes of labour support persons to a minimum.

Continuity during pregnancy, labour and birth

Caseload schemes

The second category of studies that measure the fairly discrete organizational feature of continuity of carer are those assessing caseload schemes. The core philosophy of these models is the importance of the relationship between women and a small number of carers (usually two or three) who deliver care throughout the antenatal, intrapartum and postnatal spheres of care. There are no RCTs of caseload practice and the nature of the organizational model makes trials extremely difficult to mount. However, there are a number of prospective cohort studies that measured clinical interventions and outcomes. These showed that, when compared to women with a similar profile who gave birth in a consultant unit with a more fragmented care arrangement, women booking with caseload schemes appear to experience: [34-37]

- fewer caesarean sections, epidurals, episiotomies
- fewer augmented and induced labours
- more normal birth, intact perineum
- more home birth, birth centre births
- greater maternal satisfaction.

In a qualitative study of caseload practice, women expressed clear preference for being cared for by a midwife with whom they had developed a relationship during the antenatal period. These accounts contain a number of anecdotes of women apparently timing their labours so that their caseload midwife would be available to care for them.[38]

In addition, Sandall had earlier shown that caseload schemes result in less burnout for midwives.[39] For the participating midwives, positive aspects of this way of providing care included control over their working lives, high levels of social and professional support and the freedom to develop meaningful relationships with women.

It can be concluded from the caseload evaluations that providing an opportunity for women to actually get to know midwives during the pregnancy, rather than simply meeting them, is a critical factor in their success.

Team midwifery schemes

There have been a number of randomized trials of team midwifery. This model is differentiated from caseload schemes by involving more midwives (up to six or eight per team). Only two studies were included in the original Cochrane review by Hodnett[40] which has been superseded by the 'home-like' birth setting review[41] and a new protocol for midwife-led care.[42] Since then, additional trials have been done in the UK[43,44] and Australia.[45,46] In summary, these studies on team midwifery show:

- a reduction in antenatal admissions and increase in attendance at antenatal education classes

- a reduction in epidural and other pharmacological interventions
- a reduction in electronic fetal monitoring and the need for neonatal resuscitation
- that women were better prepared and supported during labour
- a lower caesarean section, as was reported in the Homer et al study.[45]

Midwife-led care

Finally, there are a few trials of midwife-led care as opposed to routine obstetric involvement in normal labour care, but these did not necessarily build in continuity of care as an objective. The studies which took place in Canada[47] and Australia[48] confirmed what the later team and continuity studies showed – a reduction in labour and birth interventions. It is also worth noting that Tracy & Tracy found that midwife-mediated care was less expensive than obstetric care.[49]

Before leaving the research on continuity, it is worthwhile stating that, at one level, continuity underpins the idea of relationship. That women want to get to know their carers during this pivotal time of their lives would have seemed axiomatic to indigenous cultures[50] and, historically, it is likely that earlier civilizations would have prioritized this aspect of care.[51] In other words, there is a certain element of 'common sense' or simply thoughtful, compassionate care in the notion of prioritizing relationship in childbirth care. It may be only relatively recently that maternity service providers have had to be convinced through research studies of the benefit of this fundamental aspect of care.

Place of birth

Home

It is now acknowledged by the most influential sources of evidence that there is no risk-based justification for requiring all women to give birth in hospital and, furthermore, that women should be offered an explicit choice when they become pregnant over where they want to have their baby.[18,52] Tew argues that the perinatal mortality rate for planned home birth is actually better at home than in hospital, though she is reliant on retrospective analysis of data.[53] Nevertheless, her scholarship has been in-depth and meticulous. It was thought to be almost impossible to undertake a prospective RCT in this area because of the large numbers required to establish statistical significance on perinatal mortality, and because it is a topic that most women are not neutral about. In other words, they may be reluctant to be randomized to either hospital or home. However, Dowswell and colleagues mounted a small RCT of high quality to show it may be possible to investigate outcomes apart from mortality.[54] Their study showed no differences between home and hospital apart from the women who gave birth in hospital expressing disappointment as to their allocation. The size of the study indicates wide confidence intervals for the findings. However, the work indicates that such a trial could be run on a larger scale.

During the 1990s, Olsen published the results of a meta-analysis of observational home birth studies.[55] After the application of statistical testing for homogeneity (similarity of study profiles) and heterogeneity (differences in study profiles), results indicated that perinatal mortality was not significantly different between hospital and home birth groups. Lower frequency of low Apgars (1 and 5 minutes) and fewer severe perineal lacerations in the home birth group were the principal differences. This group also had fewer medical interventions (induction and augmentation of labour, episiotomies, assisted vaginal births and caesarean sections).

Although some of these differences may have been affected by bias, Olsen notes that RCTs have demonstrated clear benefit in a number of these areas for elements of the home birth 'package of care'. These include continuity of care during labour and birth and midwife-led care, both of which are probably universal aspects of home birth provision. The most convincing evidence is the large prospective comparative study undertaken in the USA by Johnson and Davis in 2000. This involved 5418 women, and concluded that there were no additional risks to low risk women booking home birth with midwives, when compared with similar US births over the same period.[56]

Though official UK government policy during most of the 1990s was to offer women a choice about place of birth, the national home birth rate is still only about 2% compared with 25% in the early 1960s.[57] Despite the rhetoric of choice, there are plenty of anecdotal stories of women being discouraged from choosing the home birth option. A recent National Childbirth Trust survey showed over 50% of GPs were reluctant to recommend home birth.[58] Unfortunately, in some countries which have opted for modernization in the American model, the option for home birth is being taken away from women entirely. In Egypt, home birth under the care of the daya was outlawed after a brief experiment in the late 1980s in Upper Egypt, where dayas were given additional training to provide care for poor rural women.[59] The women cited in El-Nemer's study either experienced childbirth at home while dayas were still allowed to practise, or they defied current convention because of their strong desire to maintain childbirth as a private, family-centred event.[60]

Birth centres

There are no randomized controlled trials and generally a paucity of good quality research in this area. Walsh & Downe's structured review found these environments lowered childbirth interventions but methodological weaknesses in all studies made conclusions tentative at best.[61] Stewart et al's commissioned review reached similar conclusions.[62] Interestingly, individual studies in both the USA[63] and the UK[64] have singularly influenced policy makers in both countries, but Walsh & Downe found both studies methodologically flawed.[61] This underlines the need for robust, prospective, multi-method studies which separate out modes of care from types of birthing centre.

Regarding integrated birth centres or alongside midwifery-led units, evaluations have shown no statistical difference in perinatal mortality and encouraging results regarding the reduction in some labour interventions.[41,65] Debate has continued to rage over the noted non-significant trend in some of the studies of higher perinatal mortality for first-time mothers. This is unlikely to be resolved until contextual studies exploring the interface at transfer, or clinical governance arrangements, or the impact of contrasting philosophies are examined in depth.

Qualitative literature on home birth and free-standing birth centres highlight two other aspects of care in these settings. These are to do with how temporality is enacted and how smallness of scale impacts on the ethos and ambience of care. The regulatory effect of clock time is much less in evidence both at home and in birth centres. Labour rhythms rather than labour progress tend to be emphasized by staff and there is usually greater flexibility with the application of partograms. Part of the reason for this lies in the absence of an organizational imperative to 'get women through the system'.[66] Small numbers of women birthing means less stress on organizational processes and a more relaxed ambience in the setting. This appears to suit women and staff well. It also appears to be attuned to labour physiology, which inherently manifests biological rhythms based on hormonal pulses of activity, rather than regular clock time rhythms.[67]

Beliefs about labour and birth

There is a burgeoning corpus of research that is helping us unpack the impact that beliefs, values and expectations have on the childbirth event. Green et al's seminal work revealed with some clarity how expectations shape outcome.[23] In other words, if women approached birth with an optimism and positive outlook, they tended to have more fulfilling, less interventionist birth experiences. In repeating this work more recently, Green & Baston have demonstrated that women's expectations have changed between the two studies, with a greater acceptance of interventions over time.[68] The recent data also suggested that greater acceptance of intervention resulted in more operative births. The use of epidural analgesia, in particular, mediated that link.

In the late 1990s, Esposito found that encountering an active birth philosophy in a birth centre changed many women's negative expectations of birth, and that a number of women in her study then went on to have empowering birth experiences.[69] Her work suggested that it was possible during pregnancy to gently challenge negative expectations of birth with a more positive take on normal, physiological birth.

Research in Australia demonstrated that women accessing birth centres expected to find a congruent philosophy in their midwife carers[70] and highlighted the importance of exploring practitioners' philosophy when appointing midwives to birth centre posts. Though it could be expected that a midwife who wants to work in a midwifery-led setting will have a philosophy of care that resonates with that setting, anecdotal experience reveals that some take a 'hospital mindset' into the birth centre. A fascinating paper by Regan & Liaschenko, from interviews with midwives in the USA, elaborates on how cognitive frames of references may predispose to a lower or higher caesarean section rate.[71] They deduced that three frames of reference were influencing the decision making of midwives working with normal birth: 'birth as natural process' (BNP), 'birth as lurking risk' (BLR) and 'birth as risky process' (BRP). These frames were reflected in propensity to use labour interventions like continuous fetal monitoring and early recourse to epidural anaesthesia.

Elsewhere, Bewley[72] revealed how personal circumstances (in her case, a study of childless midwives) subtly influence dialogue between midwives and women. Levy, in her illuminating study of Hong Kong midwives, coined the phrase 'gently steering' to capture the subtleties of how midwives presented information to women around labour choices.[73] These studies confirm that personal beliefs, experiences and values shape practice profoundly.

Evidence and labour care

Approaches to the latent phase of labour

The need to constrain labour to a specific normalizing time frame has created a situation where some women's accounts of their early labour cannot be counted as 'true'. When a woman comes into hospital describing labour pains for seven days, it is hard for staff to validate this, as 'normal' labour is not supposed to exceed 24 hours in most hospital settings. Euphemisms have been invented to overcome this dissonance for the staff: 'spurious labour', 'false labour' or, simply and starkly, 'you're not in labour'. Unfortunately, these euphemisms increase a sense of dissonance and uncertainty in the woman, who knows what she is feeling, but who finds the reality of her sensations dismissed by those in authority (midwives and doctors). Gross and colleagues[74,75] have illuminated our understanding of the phenomenon of early labour by revealing how eclectically it presents in different women and how women vary in their self-diagnosis. Less than 60% of woman experienced contractions as the starting point of their labours. The remainder described fluid loss (28%), constant pain (24%), blood-stained loss (16%), gastrointestinal symptoms (6%), emotional upheaval (6%) and sleep alterations (4%) as heralding the start of labour, none of which fit the classic textbook definition. Gross suggests we change the direction of our questioning from eliciting the pattern of contractions to simply enquiring 'how did you recognize the start of labour?'.

Burvill[76] and Cheyne et al[77] point out that the midwifery diagnosis of labour in hospital is not simply a unilateral clinical judgement, but a complex blend of balancing the totality of the woman's situation with institutional constraints like workloads, guidelines, continuity concerns, justifying decisions to senior staff and risk management. It appears that the more relaxed organizational and clinical parameters for home birth or free-standing birth centres allow more freedom for more flexible diagnoses,[78] but caregivers may still need to be aware of the need to justify their decision making in the event of a transfer to secondary care.

In 1987, Flint counselled that early labour was best experienced at home with access to a midwife,[79] and this remains the ideal for women who are labouring normally, and who are relaxed in the home setting. This approach to early labour has become increasingly acceptable, based on evidence that hospitalizing women too early results in higher rates of labour interventions.[80,81] Indeed, busy labour wards find it hard to cope with so-called 'nigglers'[82] who are labouring very slowly, and taking rooms from those who are in active labour. Recent studies have showed the value of triage facilities or early labour assessment centres if home assessment in early labour is not an option. Women who attend them have less labour interventions.[83] This finding of reduced intervention for women in early physiological labour has also been attributed to free-standing

birth centre care[84] and to caregiving by a midwife as compared to by a doctor.[85] Individualizing care, and ongoing informational and relational continuity, all appear to be important elements of best practice for the latent phase of labour.

The strong evidence base of these forms of care suggests a firm basis for practical application. Logistically, triage or assessment centres are not complex to set up, though providing home assessment in early labour might be. The Mother and Infant Research Unit at the University of York in England is currently running two trials (ELSA[86] and OPAL[87]) to investigate a range of outcomes (including cost-effectiveness) associated with home visiting, and to assess the impact of telephone contact with women in early labour.

Pushing/bearing down techniques

In 1979, Caldeyro-Barcia et al's seminal studies showed that prolonged breath holding in the second stage of labour decreased placental perfusion resulting in fetal hypoxia.[88] More recently, Aldrich et al have demonstrated that instructed pushing involving prolonged breath holding decreased fetal cerebral oxygenation.[89] These observational studies were added to by two RCTs in the 1990s. Thomson[90] showed that if coached pushing in the second stage lasted longer than an hour, then babies had a lower pH at birth. There were no differences between the two groups regarding type of birth and perineal outcome, though the spontaneous pushing group had longer second stages. Parnell and colleagues' RCT concluded that instructed pushing resulted in a longer second stage than spontaneous pushing with no differences in type of birth, fetal outcome and perineal outcome.[91] On the basis of these two studies, there is no evidence to support the practice of coached pushing. Despite this, the practice continues. For example, in 1999, an internal audit at a large UK maternity unit of midwives' practice with low-risk women indicated that only 8% encouraged spontaneous pushing.[92]

There have been a number of other concerns voiced about instructed pushing from a variety of observational studies over the past 20 years. These include:

- maternal exhaustion[93]
- more assisted vaginal births[94,95]

- more episiotomies and perineal tears[96]
- deleterious impact on the pelvic floor,[97] in particular urinary stress incontinence.[98]

In 2006, Bloom et al published the results of an RCT that concluded that instructed pushing had no benefit over spontaneous pushing except in shortening the second stage by 14 minutes; an interval deemed not clinically important.[99]

In an observational study, Sampselle and colleagues have classified behaviours that constitute instructed or spontaneous pushing, or bearing down.[100] These are helpful in delineating the differences between the two, as there can be a fine line between instruction and encouragement:

Spontaneous pushing

- Breathing pattern during contraction and pushing is self-directed.
- Time of initiating push is irregular (woman initiates push independently, and pushing often begins once contraction is well established).
- Pushing may be characterized by grunting with pushing, short and more frequent bearing down efforts with each contraction, or both.
- Open glottis pushing (i.e. grunting noise while pushing).
- Woman follows cues from her own body.
- No verbal instruction as to how to push is given.
- No non-verbal instruction is given (e.g. provider does not take a deep breath to provide a cue).
- Caregivers offer encouragement and praise only, not instruction.

Directed pushing

The woman follows verbal direction, demonstration or instruction from caregivers regarding:

- time of pushing (when to start/stop)
- length of pushing (how long to push)
- position for pushing
- breathing during pushing
- strength of push
- specific direction on how to push
- instruction to make no noise with pushing efforts.

Directed pushing also involves:

- actively positioning the woman in a certain way for pushing or verbally directing her to position herself in a certain way
- vaginal examination with concurrent direction such as 'push my finger out'
- vaginal examination actively stimulating Ferguson's reflex or manipulating or stretching the cervix or perineum
- following any non-verbal instruction regarding how to push.

Sampselle's study found that spontaneous pushing did not lengthen the second stage.

In a timely systematic review of types of pushing, Bosomworth & Bettany-Saltikov concluded from the examination of ten studies of Valsalva's manoeuvre (pushing while breath-holding) that the practice should be discontinued because of its negative effects on the fetal heart and on the perineum.[101] In this, they are supported by Enkin et al in the seminal *A Guide to Effective Care in Pregnancy and Childbirth*,[52] who state that forms of care unlikely to be beneficial include routine directed pushing, pushing by sustained bearing down and breath holding.

Apart from the overwhelming evidence over 30 years of the significance of continuous support in labour, there is no other area of normal birth where the research evidence is so unequivocal. In conclusion, the practice of instructed pushing is probably putting women and babies at unnecessary risk, and should be discontinued where women are labouring without an epidural and with no contraindications.

Systematic reviews of other beneficial/harmful routine interventions in normal labour

As well as the specific interventions outlined above, *A Guide to Effective Care in Pregnancy and Childbirth* has summarized areas of routine practice around normal birth where evidence is strong, areas where there is likely to be benefit and forms of care likely to be ineffectual or harmful (Box 10.2).[52] Although the latest version of the guide was

Box 10.2

Evidence relating to normal birth

1) Strong evidence
- External cephalic version at term to avoid breech birth
- Not offering induction of labour until after 41 completed weeks of gestation
- Providing continuous physical, emotional and psychological support for women during labour and childbirth

2) Likely to be beneficial
- Midwifery care for women with no serious risk factors
- Giving women a choice of companions
- Respecting women's choice of birth place
- Companion on admission
- Giving women as much information as they want
- Freedom of movement and choice for position of labour and birth
- Change of position for fetal distress
- Guarding perineum
- Position changes, distraction, counter pressure, heat to relieve labour pain

3) Forms of care likely to be ineffective or harmful
- Electronic fetal monitoring (EFM) without access to fetal scalp sampling during labour (or any continuous EFM where mother and baby are well)
- Requiring a supine, flat-on-back position in the second stage of labour
- Routine or liberal episiotomy for birth
- Routine restriction of mother–infant contact

Box 10.3

WHO ten principles of perinatal care
- Care for normal pregnancy and birth should be de-medicalized
- Care should be based on the use of appropriate technology
- Care should be evidence based
- Care should be regionalized
- Care should be multidisciplinary
- Care should be holistic
- Care should be family centred
- Care should be culturally appropriate
- Care should involve women in decision making
- Care should respect the dignity, privacy and confidentiality of women

WHO ten principles of perinatal care

The aim has been to provide an essential antenatal, perinatal and postpartum care course that includes a teaching pack and clinical practice evaluation package. It has been used in a range of countries. In an attempt to monitor and evaluate changes in practice in maternity services, key indicators, summarized under the title of the Bologna score (Box 10.4), were developed for the evaluation of effective care in normal labour. The Bologna score aims to measure how normal labour is managed within a given population in developed and developing countries.[103] The objective is to quantify the extent to which labours have been managed as if they were normal as opposed to complicated, both in the context of individual women and in a wider population.

The instrument has elicited criticisms, in that it assumes that normal birth is to be managed. It has also been argued that it omits some key aspects that women and midwives may value highly.[104]

published in 2000, many of the beneficial practices are still not universal, and some of the harmful practices are still widespread in some countries: specifically the liberal use of routine episiotomy, and mother–infant separation.

Examining systems of maternity care

There have been a number of international and national initiatives to underpin maternity care systems across the world on evidence. First, the World Health Organization (WHO) has developed ten principles of perinatal care (Box 10.3).[102] These are linked with an implementation strategy.

The CIMS Mother-Friendly Childbirth Initiative

The Coalition for Improving Maternity Services (CIMS) is a USA-based alliance of professional and consumer organizations and individuals, with a concern for the care and well-being of mothers, babies and families and for improving maternity services.[105] Their mission is to promote a wellness

Box 10.4

Assessing effective care of normal labour: the Bologna score

- Presence of a companion at birth
- Use of a partogram
- Absence of augmentation
- Use of non-supine position for birth
- Skin-to-skin contact of mother and baby for at least 30 minutes within the first hour after birth

model of maternity care that will improve birth outcomes and substantially reduce costs. The Coalition for Improving Maternity Services has proposed a model for evaluation of the efficacy of maternity care services in maximizing physiological birth. The model is promoted via the Mother-Friendly Childbirth Initiative. This is a self- and externally assessed exercise for maternity units, based on the ten steps strategy for mother-friendly hospitals, birth centres and home birth services proposed by CIMS. The initiative has some parallels with the Baby-Friendly Initiative which has been so successful in promoting breastfeeding worldwide.

The evidence base for the CIMS strategy has recently been published.[106]

Royal College of Midwives' campaign for normal birth

The Royal College of Midwives (RCM) in the UK has recognized that, while evidence-based care is essential, normal birth cannot be achieved if midwives don't believe in it, or if they do not have the skills to promote it. As a consequence, the college has established a Web-based campaign that uses both evidence and narrative to support midwives in the promotion and dissemination of capacity in this area.[107] The Web site provides summaries of evidence that underpin stories of unusual normal birth told by midwives and by childbearing women. This approach to knowledge generation and attitudinal change has generated interest in other European countries. However, as yet, there are no formal studies of the impact of the site on practice, attitudes or beliefs. The Web pages

and further details are available via the RCM Web site (http://www.rcm.org.uk/).

Other systematic approaches

There is worldwide interest in changing systems of maternity care to generate the potential for optimal, humane, physiological birth. Movements such as the Network for the Humanization of Childbirth (ReHuNa),[108] based in Latin America, are gaining momentum. These movements engage a range of formally trained and trained-by-experience practitioners, midwives, obstetricians, paediatricians and childbearing women. The kinds of evidence generated by these coalitions, and by initiatives such as the mother-friendly process and the narrative-based approach adopted by the RCM, hold out a fascinating promise of a more subtle approach to evidence in the area of normal childbirth in the future.

Conclusion

Continuity of carer initiatives, especially continuous support in labour by experienced women, make a difference to the caesarean section rate, operative delivery rate and vaginal birth rate. There is strong evidence of beneficial effects on other childbirth interventions, including some psychosocial outcomes. In addition, women like this model of care.

There is evidence from observational studies that midwife-led birth centres and the availability of a home birth service also contribute to normal birth outcomes. Large evaluations of these complex models of care would be helpful along with qualitative studies of how philosophies of care and beliefs about birth may contribute.

Although there is a good evidence base in maternity care about what specific clinical interventions may promote normality in childbirth, for example in the latent and second stage of labour, large variations in practice remain. Several attempts have been developed to change practitioner behaviour, but we don't yet have enough evidence to say whether they are working. Finally, Davis-Floyd[25] has pointed out in her work, on women who opted for either technocratic or 'natural births', that both were seeking empowerment, but using differing means to achieve it. This analysis directs attention away from the sterile debate of trying to define and reify 'normality', which attempts to classify an 'ideal' type of birth that focuses on what 'is done to' women, and towards seeing women as individuals with agency, and with a subjective sense of choice, power and control regarding childbirth. Further research is needed on the different strategies that women use in a proactive way to empower themselves, or not, and the relationship of labour support and expertise to the complex notion of 'control'.

References

1. Downe S, McCormick C, Beech B 2001 Labour interventions associated with normal birth. Br J Midwif 9:602–606

2. Mead M 2004 Midwives' perspectives in 11 UK maternity units. In S Downe (ed.) Normal childbirth: evidence and debate. Churchill Livingstone, London

3. Declerq E, Sakala C, Corry M et al 2002 Listening to mothers: report of the first national US survey of women's childbearing experiences. Maternity Center Association, New York

4. Roberts C, Algert C, Peat B et al 2002 Trends in labour and birth interventions among low-risk women in an Australian population. Aust N Z J Obstet Gynaecol 42:176–181

5. Ilich I 1976 The limits to medicine. Macmillan, London

6. McKeown T 1976 The role of medicine: dream, mirage or nemesis? Nuffield Provincial Hospitals Trust, London

7. Cochrane A 1971 Effectiveness and efficiency. Nuffield Provincial Hospitals Trust, London

8. Tew M 1990 Safer childbirth? Chapman & Hall, London

9. Chalmers I, Richards M 1977 Intervention and causal inference in obstetric practice. In: Chard T, Richards M (eds) Benefits and hazards of the new obstetrics. Spastics International Medical Publications, London

10. Wagner M 1994 Pursuing the birth machine: the search for appropriate birth technology. Ace Graphics, Sydney

11. Chalmers I 1989 Implications for the current debate on obstetric practice. In: Chalmers I, Enkin M, Keirse M J N C (eds) Effective care in pregnancy and childbirth. Oxford University Press, Oxford

12. World Health Organization 1985 Appropriate technology for birth. Lancet, August 24:436–437

13. World Health Organization 1996 Care in normal birth: a practical guide: report of a technical working group. WHO, Geneva

14. Reid M, McIlwaine G 1980 Consumer opinion of a hospital antenatal clinic. Soc Sci Med 14A:363–368

15. Cartwright A 1979 The dignity of labour? A study of childbearing and induction. Institute for Social Studies in Medical Care, London

16. Oakley A 1984 The captured womb. Basil Blackwell, Oxford

17. Chalmers I, Enkin M, Keirse M J N C 1989 Effective care in pregnancy and childbirth. Oxford University Press, Oxford

18. Department of Health 2007 Maternity matters: choice, access, continuity of care in a safe service. DoH, London

19. Department of Health and Human Services, Office of Disease Prevention and Promotion 2002 Healthy people 2010. US Government Printing Office, Pittsburgh, PA

20. Simkin P 1992 Just another day in a woman's life? Part II: nature and consistency of women's long-term memories of their first birth experiences. Birth 19:64–81

21. Gottvall K, Waldenstrom U 2002 Does a traumatic birth experience have an impact on future reproduction? BJOG 109:254–260

22. Soderquist J, Wijma K, Wijma B 2002 Traumatic stress after childbirth: the role of obstetric variables. J Psychosom Obstet Gynecol 23:31

23. Green J M, Coupland V, Kitzinger J V 1998 Great expectations. A prospective study of women's expectations and experiences of childbirth. Books for Midwives, Cheshire

24. Jacoby A 1987 Women's preferences for and satisfaction with current procedures in childbirth: findings from a national study. Midwifery 3:117–124

25. Davis-Floyd R 2001 The technocratic, humanistic and holistic paradigms of childbirth. Int J Gynecol Obstet 75:S5–S23

26. Davis-Floyd R 1992 Birth as an American rite of passage. University of California Press, London

27. Walsh D 2007 A birth centre's encounters with discourses of childbirth: how resistance led to innovation. Sociology of Health & Illness 29(2):216–232

28. Sackett D 1996 Evidence based medicine: what it is and what it is not. Br Med J 312:71–72

29. Walsh D 2007 Evidence-based care for normal labour and birth: a guide for midwives. Routledge, London

30. Hodnett E D, Gates S, Hofmeyr G J et al 2003 Continuous support for women during childbirth. Cochrane Database Syst Rev, Issue 3. Art. No.: CD003766. DOI: 10.1002/14651858.CD003766.pub2

31. Hodnett E, Lowe N, Hannah M et al 2002 Effectiveness of nurses as providers of birth labour support in north American hospitals. JAMA 288:1373–1381

32. Rosen P 2004 Supporting women in labour: analysis of different types of caregivers. J Midwifery Womens Health 49:24–31

33. Gagnon A, Meier K, Waghorn K 2007 Continuity of nursing care and its link to caesarean birth rate. Birth 34:26–31

34. Page L, McCourt C, Beake S et al 1999 Clinical interventions and outcomes of one-to-one midwifery practice. J Pub Health Med 21:243–248

35. North Staffordshire Changing Childbirth Research Team 2000 A randomised study of midwifery caseload care and traditional 'shared-care'. Midwifery 16:295–302

36. Benjamin Y, Taub N, Walsh D 2001 An evaluation of an alternative organisation of midwifery care: partnership caseload holding within a midwifery group practice. Midwifery 17:234–240

37. Sandall J, Davies J, Warwick C 2001 Evaluation of the Albany Midwifery Practice: final report. Nightingale School of Nursing and Midwifery, King's College London, London

38. Walsh D 1999 An ethnographic study of women's experience of partnership caseload midwifery practice: the professional as friend. Midwifery 15:165–176

39. Sandall J 1997 Midwives' burnout and continuity of care. Br J Midwif 5:106–111

40. Hodnett E D 2000 Continuity of caregivers for care during pregnancy and childbirth. Cochrane Database Syst Rev, Issue 1. Art. No.: CD000062. DOI: 10.1002/14651858. CD000062

41. Hodnett E D, Downe S, Edwards N et al 2005 Home-like versus conventional institutional settings for birth. Cochrane Database Syst Rev, Issue 1. Art. No.: CD000012. DOI: 10.1002/14651858.CD000012.pub2

42. Hatem M, Hodnett E D, Devane D et al 2004 Midwifery-led versus other models of care delivery for childbearing women. Cochrane Database Syst Rev, Issue 1. Art. No.: CD004667. DOI: 10.1002/14651858.CD004667

43. Biro M, Waldenstrom U, Pannifex J 2000 Team midwifery care in a tertiary level obstetric service. Birth 27:168–173

44. Hicks C, Spurgeon P, Barwell F 2003 Changing childbirth: a pilot project. J Adv Nurs 42:617–628

45. Homer C, Davis G, Brodie P et al 2001 Collaboration in maternity care: a randomised trial comparing community-based continuity of care with standard hospital care. Br J Obstet Gynaecol 108:16–22

46. Waldenstrom U, Brown S, McLachlan H et al 2000 Does team midwife care increase satisfaction with antenatal, intrapartum and postpartum care? A randomised controlled trial. Birth 27:156–167

47. Harvey S, Jarrell J, Brant R et al 1996 A randomised controlled trial of nurse/midwifery care. Birth 23:128–135

48. Bradley B, Tashevska M, Selby J 1990 Women's first experience of childbirth: two hospital settings compared. Br J Med Psychol 63:227–237

49. Tracy S, Tracy M 2003 Costing the cascade: estimating the cost of increased obstetric intervention in childbirth using population data. BJOG 110:717–724

50. Kitzinger S 2000 Rediscovering birth. Little Brown, London

51. Rosenberg K, Trevathan W 2003 Birth, obstetrics and human evolution. Br J Obstet Gynaecol 109:1199–1206

52. Enkin M, Kierse M, Neilson J et al 2000 A guide to effective care in pregnancy and childbirth. Oxford University Press, Oxford

53. Tew M 1998 Safer childbirth? a critical history of maternity care. Free Association, London

54. Dowswell T, Thornton J, Hewison J et al 1996 Should there be a trial of home versus hospital delivery in the United Kingdom? Br Med J 312:753–757

55. Olsen O 1997 Meta-analysis of the safety of home birth. Birth 24:4–13

56. Johnson KC, Davis BA 2003 Outcomes of planned home births in Washington State: 1989–1996. Obstet Gynecol 101:198–200

57. Department of Health 2002 NHS maternity statistics England 1998–99 to 2000–1. DoH, London

58. National Childbirth Trust 1999 Fifty per cent of doctors oppose home birth – results of survey of NCT branches. Press Release, 23 August, London

59. El-Nemer A, Downe S, Small N 2006 'She would help me from the heart': an ethnography of Egyptian women in labour. Soc Sci Med 62:81–92

60. Rashad R, Phipps F 2001 Different strokes for different folks: birth stories: varied perspectives. Third International Conference on Advances in the Delivery of Care. City University, London

61. Walsh D, Downe S 2004 Outcomes of free-standing, midwifery-led birth centres: a structured review. Birth 31:222–229

62. Stewart M, McCandlish R, Henderson J et al 2004 (revised 2005) Report of a structured review of birth centre outcomes. National Perinatal Epidemiology Unit. Online. Available: http://www.npeu.ox.ac.uk/birthcentrereview/ (accessed 23 August 2007)

63. Rooks J P, Weatherby N L, Ernst E K et al 1989 Outcomes of care in birth centres. The National Birth Centre Study. N Engl J Med 321:1804–1811

64. Saunders D, Boulton M, Chapple J et al 2000. Evaluation of the Edgware Birth Centre. North Thames Perinatal Public Health, Middlesex

65. Walsh D 2004 Birth centres not safe for primigravidae. Br J Midwif 12:206

66. Walsh D 2006 Subverting assembly-line birth: childbirth in a free-standing birth centre. Soc Sc Med 62:1330–1340

67. Adam B 1995 Timewatch: the social analysis of time. Polity, Cambridge

68. Green J, Baston H 2007 Have women become more willing to accept obstetric interventions and does this relate to mode of birth? Data from a prospective study. Birth 34:6–13

69. Esposito N W 1999 Marginalised women's comparisons of their hospital and free-standing birth centre experience: a contract of inner city birthing centres. Health Care Women Int 20:111–126

70. Coyle K, Hauck Y, Percival P et al 2001 Ongoing relationships with a personal focus: mother's perceptions of birth centre versus hospital care. Midwifery 17:182–193

71. Regan M, Liaschenko J 2007 In the mind of the beholder: hypothesized effects of intrapartum nurses' cognitive frames of childbirth caesarean section rates. Qual Health Res 17:612–624

72. Bewley C 2000 Midwives personal experience of their relationships with women: midwives without children. In: Kirkham M (ed.) The midwife–mother relationship. Routledge, London

73. Levy V 2004 How midwives used protective steering to facilitate informed choice in pregnancy. In: Kirkham M (ed.) Informed choice in maternity care. Palgrave Macmillan, London

74. Gross M, Haunschild T, Stoexen T et al 2003 Women's recognition of the spontaneous onset of labour. Birth 30:267–271

75. Gross M, Hecker H, Matterne A et al 2006 Does the way that women experience the onset of labour influence the duration of labour? Br J Obstet Gynaecol 113:289–294

76. Burvill S 2002 Midwifery diagnosis of labour onset. Br J Midwif 10:600–605

77. Cheyne H, Dowding D, Hundley V 2006 Making the diagnosis of labour: midwives' diagnostic judgement and management decisions. J Adv Nurs 53:625–635

78. Walsh D 2006 'Nesting' and 'matrescence': distinctive features of a free-standing birth centre. Midwifery 22:228–239

79. Flint C 1986 Sensitive midwifery. Butterworth-Heinemann, London

80. Hemminki E, Simukka R 1986 The timing of hospital admission and progress of labour. Eur J Obstet Gynecol Reprod Biol 22:85–94

81. Rahnama P, Ziaei S, Faghihzadeh S 2006 Impact of early admission in labour on method of delivery. Int J Gynecol Obstet 92:217–220

82. Hunt S, Symonds A 1995 The social meaning of midwifery. Macmillan, Basingstoke

83. Lauzon L, Hodnett E 2001 Labour assessment programs to delay admission to labour wards. Cochrane Database Syst Rev, Issue 3. Art. No.: CD000936. DOI: 10.1002/14651858.CD000936

84. Jackson D, Lang J, Ecker J et al 2003 Impact of collaborative management and early labour admission in labour on method of delivery. J Obstet Gynaecol Neonatal Nurs 32:147–157

85. Turnbull D, Holmes S, Cheyne H et al 1996 Randomised controlled trial of efficacy of midwifery-managed care. Lancet 348:213–218

86. Mother and Infant Research Unit (MIRU) Early Labour Support Assessment (ELSA) Trial. Online. Available: http://www.nrr.nhs.uk/2006AnnualReports/ProgrammeSameIDRecords.asp?Code=RR8&Title=Maternal+and+Infant+Research (accessed 31 August 2007)

87. MIRU Options for Assessment in Early Labour (OPAL) Study. Online. Available: http://www.york.ac.uk/healthsciences/miru/primresearch.htm (accessed 31 August 2007)

88. Caldeyro-Barcia R, Giussi G, Storch E 1979 The influence of maternal bearing down efforts and their effects on fetal heart rate, oxygenation and acid base balance. J Perinatal Med 9:63–67

89. Aldrich C, D'Antona D, Spencer J 1995 The effects of maternal pushing on fetal cerebral oxygenation and blood volume during the second stage of labour. Br J Obstet Gynaecol 102:448–453

90. Thomson A 1993 Pushing techniques in the second stage of labour. J Adv Nurs 18:171–177

91. Parnell C, Langhoff-Roos J, Iverson R 1993 Pushing method in the expulsive phase of labour. A randomised trial. Acta Obstet Gynecol Scand 72:31–35

92. Walsh D, Harris M, Shuttlewood S 1999 Changing midwifery birthing practice through audit. Br J Midwif 7:432–435

93. Knauth D, Haloburdo E 1986 Effects of pushing techniques in birthing chair on length of second stage of labour. Nurs Res 35:49–51

94. Fraser W, Marcoux S, Krauss I 2000 Multi-centre, randomised controlled trial of delayed pushing for nulliparous women in the second stage of labour with continuous epidural analgesia. Am J Obstet Gynecol 182:1165–1172

95. Hansen S, Clark S, Foster J 2002 Active pushing versus passive fetal descent in the second stage of labour: a randomised controlled trial. Obstet Gynecol 99:29–34

96. Sampselle C, Hines S 1999 Spontaneous pushing during labour: relationship to perineal outcomes. J Nurse Midwifery 44:36–39

97. Schaffer J, Bloom S, Casey B 2005 A randomised trial of the effect of coached vs uncoached maternal pushing during the second stage of labour on postpartum pelvic floor structure and function. Am J Obstet Gynecol 192:1692–1696

98. Handa V, Harris T, Ostergard D 1996 Protecting the pelvic floor: obstetric management to prevent incontinence and pelvic organ collapse. Obstet Gynaecol 88:470–478

99. Bloom S, Casey B, Schaffer J 2006 A randomised trial of coached versus uncoached maternal pushing during the second stage of labour. Am J Obstet Gynecol 194:10–13

100. Sampselle M, Miller J, Luecha Y 2005 Provider support of spontaneous pushing during the second stage of labour. J Obstet Gynecol Neonatal Nurs 34:695–702

101. Bosomworth A, Bettany-Saltikov J 2006 Just take a deep breath. MIDIRS Midwifery Digest 16:157–165

102. Chalmers B, Mangiaterra V, Porter R 2001 WHO principles of perinatal care: the essential antenatal, perinatal, and postpartum care course. Birth 28:202–207

103. Chalmers B, Porter R 2001 Assessing effective care in normal labour: the Bologna score. Birth 28:79–83

104. Downe S 2001 Review of Chalmers B, Porter R 2001 Assessing effective care in normal labour: the Bologna score. Birth 28:79–83 In: MIDIRS Review 2001

105. Coalition for Improving Maternity Services. Ten steps of the Mother-Friendly Childbirth Initiative. Online. Available: http://www.motherfriendly.org (accessed 31 August 2007)

106. Multiple papers/authors 2007 Evidence basis for the ten steps of mother-friendly care. J Perinat Educ 16(suppl 1):1–96

107. Royal College of Midwives Campaign for Normal Birth. Online. Available: http://www.rcmnormalbirth.org.uk/ (accessed 31 August 2007)

108. Editorial 2002 Humanising childbirth. Women's Health Journal (July). Online. Available: http://findarticles.com/p/articles/mi_hb343/is_200207/ai_hibm1G199289969 (accessed 31 August 2007)

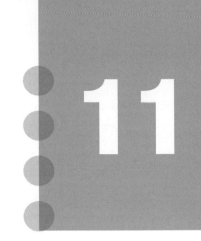

Aspects of a controversy: summary and debate

Soo Downe

I have stated on numerous occasions that there is no more need to interfere with the course of normally progressing labor than there is to tamper with good digestion, normal respiration, and adequate circulation.

Thaddeus Montgomery[1]

Different social and professional groups bring varying interpretations to the concept of normality. These sometimes seem to be based in widely varying philosophical and socioeconomic paradigms. In the context of childbirth, this results in a spectrum of belief about optimal maternity care, rather than a set of agreed definitions. The consequent lack of agreement can lead to a failure of communication and comprehension between those whose views lie at the extremes of this spectrum. Given these problems, it is not surprising that normality in birth is contentious. This book has evolved into an exposition of competing discourses in maternity care, embodied largely in the thoughts, lives and work of midwives and illustrated by stories of women and babies. It is intended both to provide evidence and debate and to critique the very structures on which these evidences and debates are based. In the process, a number of taken-for-granted assumptions within midwifery, and maternity care, are explored. This includes assumptions about medicalization and intervention, and about the inevitable women-centredness of birth centres. It includes how midwives practise in the context of normality. It raises the possibility that

there is not simply a 'medical model' or 'midwifery model', but a multitude of models of practice.

While the so-called medical model has been seen to hold authority over taken-for-granted concepts of midwifery, it is of interest to note that Bridget Jordan was clear that authoritative knowledge is not necessarily the knowledge of the elite but, specifically, the knowledge operating in a particular social context: 'By authoritative knowledge I mean … the knowledge that participants agree counts in a particular setting, that they see as consequential, on the basis of which they make decisions and provide justification for courses of action' (p 58).[2] The question becomes then, not what profession do I belong to but what do I believe and value, and how can I make it count?

Over the past 15 years or so, along with many others, I have been thinking about the issue of normality in childbirth, and the paradox between the claim of midwifery to be the guardian of normality while apparently actively participating in the reinforcement of technical ways of doing birth. Why do the caesarean section rates remain persistently high? Current popular explanations, such as women's desire for control, obstetricians' belief in technology and the rising rates of litigation or maternal choice, are not ultimately satisfying. Interventions designed to tackle separate elements of the issue, such as social support in labour, or audits to decrease rates of induction of labour do not seem to work as anticipated from meta-analysis.

Along with many others, some presenting their interpretations in this book, I have been trying to understand why the problems seem to be so clear but the solutions are so difficult to find. I have come to the conclusion that this is because the debate is founded in a discourse that is alien to the conversation we have been trying to have. The purpose of this book has been to begin to reframe the context for the debate and to provide some specific examples of areas we need to explore in trying to reach some conclusions about normal childbirth. The discussion of ways of seeing, which I undertook with Christine McCourt in Chapter 1, provides a first attempt at rethinking this area. In the deliberations we offer, we reach a position which suggests that individual interventions cannot work while they are superimposed on a system that still frames childbirth (and 'normality' within childbirth) on the basis of simplicity, certainty and pathology. This new framing tends towards the concept of unique normality, raised first, as far as we are aware, by Robbie Davis-Floyd[3] and Elizabeth Davis. In this process, we tentatively reach a conclusion that a system which responds to women's unique normality is one which is most likely to engage with complexity and uncertainty, and to maximize holistic well-being, while ensuring appropriate responses to pathology when it arises. We accept that this is our particular way of seeing. It is an approach that takes the debate beyond birth itself and into the areas of social capital and community well-being. While the other authors writing in this book were not aware of the conclusions to our chapter when they were writing their contributions, many of them have coincidentally illustrated elements of this way of seeing in their chapters. I see this as evidence of a change in the childbirth zeitgeist amid thinkers and practitioners in this field.

Birth, in this sense, is catalytic in women's lives and, beyond that, in the lives of their families and the wider society. The public health and social capacity potential of birth is in contrast to the usual media discourse, where 'bad' births and the destruction they cause are the meat and drink of newspaper stories and litigation. The issues discussed by many of the authors also raise an interesting point: what is the risk of losing the benefit of positive physiological birthing where pathology-based risk systems are dominant?

Many questions are raised by the discussions in the book, and most of them are open to research. We hope that some in the field will be inspired to undertake this research, and that future books in the area of normality will encompass findings based on different ways of seeing health and birth. As one of the respondents to Sue Crabtree's research stated:

> It [natural birth] needs to be reframed, so that people understand what natural is … It's not a rigidly determined thing. It's something that involves judgment, it involves process. It's processing with women and that is a really vague thing to transmit to people. (Sue, p 17)

I hope that this book has begun to find ways of capturing the nature of the elusive concept of unique normality so that it can be enacted in the practice of maternity-care providers and supporters, and in the lives of women and their babies, families and communities. However, there is much more to do. To repeat Thaddeus Montgomery's words at the beginning of Chapter 8:[1]

> … it is amazing how little of fact is known about the simplest phases of reproduction. The field for research here is widely open.

References

1. Montgomery T L 1958 Physiologic considerations in labor and the puerperium. Am J Obstet Gynecol 76:706–715

2. Jordan B 1993 Birth in four cultures, 4th edn. Waveland Press, Prospect Heights, IL

3. Davis-Floyd R, Arvidson P S 1997 Intuition: the inside story. Routledge, New York

Index